The Tropical World *of*
Samuel Taylor Darling

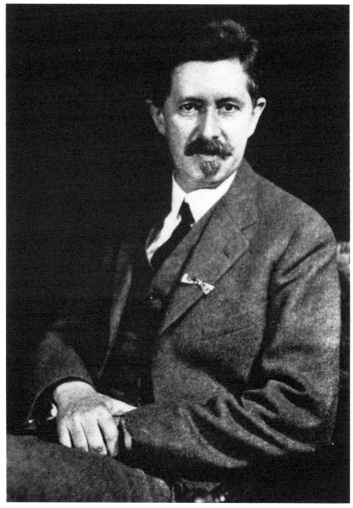

Samuel T. Darling, 1923, at age 51, portrait by Underwood & Underwood. Reproduced with permission, courtesy of Rockefeller Archive Center, Sleepy Hollow, New York.

Oh it is so good to be alive and to see all the wonders in this tropical world.

Samuel Taylor Darling

The Tropical World *of*
Samuel Taylor Darling
Parasites, Pathology and Philanthropy

E. Chaves-Carballo

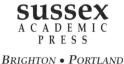

sussex
ACADEMIC
PRESS

BRIGHTON • PORTLAND

2 4 6 8 10 9 7 5 3 1

First published 2007 in Great Britain by
SUSSEX ACADEMIC PRESS
PO Box 139
Eastbourne BN24 9BP

and in the United States of America by
SUSSEX ACADEMIC PRESS
920 NE 58th Ave   Suite 300
Portland, Oregon 97213-3786

British Library Cataloguing in Publication Data
A CIP catalogue record for this book is available from the British Library.

Library of Congress Cataloging-in-Publication Data

Chaves-Carballo, E.
The tropical world of Samuel Taylor Darling : parasites, pathology, and philanthropy / by E. Chaves-Carballo.
   p. cm.
Includes bibliographical references and index.
ISBN-13: 978-1-84519-183-2 (h/b : alk. paper)
ISBN-10: 1-84519-183-8 (h/b : alk. paper)
   1. Darling, Samuel Taylor, 1872–1925. 2. Tropical
   medicine—Biography. I. Title. [DNLM: 1. Darling,
   Samuel Taylor, 1872–1925. 2. Tropical Medicine—
   history—Biography. 3. History, 20th Century—
   Biography. 4. Parasitology—history—Biography.
   5. Pathology—history—Biography. WZ 100 D219C 2007]

RC961.5.D37C53—2007
616.9'8830092—dc22
                                                         [B]
                                              2006038375

Typeset & Designed by SAP, Brighton & Eastbourne
Printed by The Cromwell Press, Trowbridge, Wilts.
This book is printed on acid-free paper.

Contents

Contents

Illustrations and Tables

Illustrations

Tables

Foreword by
Gerald L. Baum

In 1950, I first met Dr. Jan Schwarz, director of the Mycology Laboratory at Cincinnati General Hospital and associate director of the Jewish Hospital clinical laboratories in Cincinnati, and soon went to work with him in the field of medical mycology, especially the deep fungous diseases. This work became full time in 1956, and the major topic was histoplasmosis. I became fascinated with the life of the man who discovered this disease, Samuel Taylor Darling, and began to seek out information from a variety of sources. This led to putting together a monograph which was published in 1958 but then my life took me in other directions, leaving Dr. Darling behind, so to speak.

In the year 2004, two events occurred, almost simultaneously, that rekindled my curiosity about Samuel Taylor Darling; I was approached by Dr. Darling's granddaughter for information about her grandfather and I received a request for information about Dr. Darling from Dr. Enrique Chaves-Carballo who was in the midst of writing this current biography of the man. I could not get over the coincidence and was delighted to become involved with both information seekers. The granddaughter contact resulted in a delightful weekend meeting of our families and the author contact resulted in my becoming involved once again with the remarkable person that was Samuel Taylor Darling.

My personal point of departure was the fungal disease he discovered but as I have followed the progress of the development of this book I began to learn in even more detail what an excellent and industrious scientist Dr. Darling was and how much he was involved in his major interest, human parasitic diseases. This compelling curiosity led to his traveling all over the world and making significant contributions to the health systems of many countries and to the improved health status of the citizens of those areas. In addition his immersion in the subject and his lack of arrogance gave him the tools to be a fine teacher.

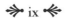

Often the complaint is leveled at a biography of a great scientist and achiever such as Dr. Darling that he emerges from the pages as a two-dimensional character without a unique personality. A measure of the quality of this biography by Dr. Chaves-Carballo is that Dr. Darling comes across as a very striking personality indeed, possessed of both humanity and an intense desire to learn.

Part of the importance of this book is that it explores a topic that has faded from medical headlines in the early twenty-first century due to the great advances in technology, genetics and subcellular approaches to human health and disease among other achievements. We all tend to lose sight of the fact that morbidity from diseases related to poverty, poor hygiene, crowding and lack of intensive public health measures affect a very large part of the world's population and thus information relative to these problems is of great significance to hundreds of millions of people. Human parasitic diseases are still extremely widespread and, along with tuberculosis, account for major morbidity and mortality in the world despite the fact that treatment exists and the means for cure are available. The failure to achieve better control of these problems is closely related not only to personal poverty but poverty of governments that cannot afford to establish effective public health systems. In addition the lack of means in a large part of the world results in the crowding and poor hygiene that foster the spread and persistence of these diseases.

Thus this biography emphasizes not only the remarkable person that was Samuel Taylor Darling but also redirects our attention to the terrible world of parasite infestation of humans. The shock comes from realizing that what Dr. Darling had to deal with almost one hundred years ago is still a major problem in a great part of the world.

GERALD L. BAUM, M.D.
Professor Emeritus of Medicine
Sackler School of Medicine, Tel Aviv University

Preface

After completing studies at the University of Oklahoma College of Medicine, I returned with my family to Panama to begin duties as an intern at Gorgas Hospital on July 1, 1963. The selection of Gorgas Hospital for a year of internship was not based on its reputation as a good teaching hospital or its prominence in the history of tropical medicine, but because of its geographical location. My wife and I had come to the United States from this tropical region (she from Panama and I from Costa Rica) and now, after a prolonged absence, we were both anxious to return home.

Despite an intern's busy schedule, sufficient time was available to visit the hospital's medical library in the evenings and on week-ends. The medical librarian, Virginia Ewing Stich, diligently helped interns and residents to find informative references about difficult clinical cases and exotic tropical diseases. Mrs. Stich (as she was respectfully known) was also eager to reminisce about the great accomplishments of Gorgas (Ancon) Hospital during the construction of the Panama Canal between 1904 and 1914.[1]

Protagonists such as William Gorgas, Henry Carter, Joseph Le Prince, Louis La Garde, and other notable members of the hospital staff and sanitation team, came out of the past and reenacted the gallant battle that defeated yellow fever and malaria in Panama. Among these charismatic figures, one person stood out in my mind above all the others. Samuel Darling toiled in relative obscurity in his laboratories in Ancon and found solutions to important problems that threatened to upset the delicate balance between health and disease on the isthmus. I was pleased to know that, almost six decades earlier, Darling had also been an "interne" at Ancon Hospital when he arrived in Panama in 1905.[2]

I began to share Mrs. Stich's admiration for this remarkable scientist and avidly read the reprints available in her files about his discovery of histoplasmosis, studies on malaria, research on amebiasis, and numerous reports on other tropical diseases. For a man who worked in isolation

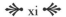

from peer scientists, Darling's scholarly output was impressive. More than a hundred clinical and scientific papers recorded the results of his innovative and meticulous observations in Panama. He also helped to organize the Canal Zone Medical Association and to establish the *Proceedings of the Canal Zone Medical Association*, a respected periodical which first published many of his original contributions. Before long, the world began to notice this outstanding pathologist, malariologist, parasitologist, bacteriologist, and epidemiologist. Darling was soon recognized worldwide as an authority on tropical diseases.

Mrs. Stich and I organized a library exhibit of Darling's memorabilia, including photographs, reprints, and original pages from his records of histoplasmosis cases. The inclement environmental conditions of heat and humidity inherent in Panama and Darling's bold, left-handed strokes made with black India ink, conspired to destroy some of these fragile documents. The three folios from Darling's first case of histoplasmosis suffered the most from the ravages of time and climate. Fortunately, someone came to the rescue. Charlotte Campbell, from the School of Public Health at Harvard University, had worked on histoplasmosis at the Middle America Research Unit (MARU) adjacent to Gorgas Hospital in Ancon.[3] Campbell made the necessary arrangements to have the fragile documents sent back to the United States, where they were restored by experts who applied techniques similar to those used to preserve the Dead Sea Scrolls. After several months, the rejuvenated autopsy records were returned to Gorgas Hospital and, once again, these were proudly displayed in the reading room of the medical library (commemorated years later as the *Samuel Taylor Darling Memorial Library*).[4]

After completing an internship in Panama and a pediatric residency in the United States, I returned to Gorgas Hospital in 1967 as a staff pediatrician and resumed my long conversations with Mrs. Stich about our favorite subject: Darling's life and work. My voluminous files on Darling continued to expand accordingly. Although I left Panama in 1972 to pursue a neurology residency at Mayo Clinic, Mrs. Stich and I continued our correspondence about Darling. We agreed that someone needed to write a full-length biography of this remarkable man. Gerald Baum's admirable account of Darling's life, a thirty-five page repository of tantalizing glimpses and illustrations published in Cincinnati as a limited and private edition, had long been out-of-print and was difficult to access.[5] A more exhaustive biography written by Michael Takos, a former pathologist at Gorgas Hospital, unfortunately, did not find a receptive publisher and the whereabouts of his manuscript were unknown.[6]

Mrs. Stich retired in 1972, after serving for more than thirty years as medical librarian at Gorgas Hospital, and went to live in New Orleans. I visited her whenever possible and continued to enjoy our ongoing discussions about Darling. During one of these visits, Mrs. Stich asked me if I would be willing to write Darling's biography. As an enticement, she entrusted me with many of the papers she had collected about Darling throughout the years. I hesitated initially, not confident in my abilities to fulfill our common dream. The real challenge, however, was to find sufficient primary sources and the time necessary to write a more complete biography. As a busy academician, all I could muster in the ensuing years was a handful of articles about Darling and Ancon Hospital published in diverse English and Spanish periodicals.[7–11] Only after my retirement as a teacher and researcher, was I able to dedicate myself full-time to this endeavor.

Forty years after my introduction to Darling in Panama, efforts to write Darling's biography have now come to fruition. I hope Mrs. Stich will be pleased (if only belatedly) as much as I am to share with others our admiration for this remarkable scientist, widely regarded during his lifetime as America's outstanding tropical parasitologist and pathologist.[12]

ENRIQUE CHAVES-CARBALLO
Department of History and Philosophy of Medicine
Kansas University Medical Center

Acknowledgments

I wish to thank the following persons and institutions for their willingness and generosity in helping me to find information, correspondence, and photographs about Samuel Taylor Darling.

First and foremost, I must acknowledge the inspiration and reverence with which Virginia Ewing Stich kept Darling's publications, records, and a complete set of the *Proceedings of the Isthmian Canal Zone Association*, while she was medical librarian at Gorgas Hospital in the Canal Zone. She was also responsible for preserving Darling's autopsy records of cases of histoplasmosis, at a time when the ravages of time and a tropical climate threatened to destroy those precious documents. Through her perseverance, the Gorgas Hospital medical library was dedicated in 1972 as the *Samuel Taylor Darling Memorial Library*, and she kept copies of nearly every article published about the medical history of the isthmus of Panama. Although Mrs. Stich died in 1989, I hope that she will be pleased with this effort and forgive me for taking so long to complete Darling's biography.

More recently, I am indebted to Gerald Baum, Professor Emeritus of Medicine at Sackler School of Medicine, Tel Aviv University, and author of *Samuel Taylor Darling*, the only extant biography of Darling. This thirty-five page monograph was published privately in Cincinnati in 1958 and has long ago been out-of-print. Nevertheless, nearly fifty years later, Dr. Baum has been most generous, not only in his willingness to share and allow me to quote freely from his work, but in accepting to critically review what I have written and encouraging me to complete this work. His magnanimity and industriousness have also been a source of inspiration for me. I am grateful and honored that he consented to write the foreword for this book.

To Darwin H. Stapleton and Kenneth W. Rose, of the Rockefeller Archive Center (RAC) in North Tarrytown and now Sleepy Hollow, New York, I am indebted for giving me unqualified access to Darling's papers, including Darling's personnel files. I also wish to thank the RAC for

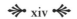

honoring me with a grant-in-aid that allowed me to make trips to North Tarrytown and spend several weeks there to review the correspondence between Darling and the International Health Board. Thanks to the commitment of the RAC staff to preserve historical documents and to make these accessible to researchers, it was possible to reconstruct in detail Darling's decade of work for the Rockefeller Foundation's International Board of Health.

Many others have assisted generously and willingly in different aspects of this biographical work and I wish to acknowledge with gratitude their contributions. Marjorie Ciarlante and Fred Romanski at the Textual References Branch, National Archives in College Park, Maryland, located most of the pertinent records of the Isthmian Canal Commission; the staff at the History of Medicine Division of the National Library of Medicine in Bethesda, retrieved documents about William Gorgas, malaria, and yellow fever; Michael Rhode, head archivist at the National Museum of Health and Medicine in Washington, D.C., and custodian of unique records and photographs pertaining to malaria and yellow fever, as well as of the priceless volumes of autopsy records made by Darling and his colleagues at Ancon Hospital, allowed me to view and photograph most of these extensive holdings; the staff at Linda Hall Library of Science, Engineering, and Technology in Kansas City, Missouri, a repository for the fragile pages of the *Bulletin du Canal Interocéanique*, textbooks about the Panama Railroad Company, and valuable transcripts of oral history by former employees of the Panama Canal Company, was always helpful and informative; the photographic staff at the Herbert Hoover Presidential Library in West Branch, Iowa, painstakingly restored by hand each of the photographs of Darling's autopsy records on cases of histoplasmosis; the staff of the Library of Congress retrieved contemporary issues of newspapers such as The *Star and Herald, Panama-American, La Estrella de Panamá, The New York Times* and The *Baltimore Sun*, in response to my attempts to reconstruct the weather, baseball events, and national politics from 1905, and allowed me to review the microfilm reels containing thousands of photographs taken during the construction of the Panama Canal; the staff of the Photographic Division of the National Library of Medicine supplied photographs of Ancon Hospital, William Gorgas and Samuel Taylor Darling; Microfilm Documents of Lawrence, Kansas, copied more than two thousand documents pertaining to the early history of Ancon Hospital; the staff of the Technical Resources Center in Balboa, Panama, helped me to review their valuable collection of texts and monographs about health and sanitation in the Canal Zone, especially documents about Ancon Hospital; Itza Pinilla of the Panama Canal Company provided a complete list of William Gorgas' publications; Robert Karrer of the Panama Canal Museum in Seminole, Florida, shared photographs from his extensive Panama postcard and book collection; Virgilio and Pauline Peralta from Panama City, Panama, listed trees and flowers seen along the Panama Railroad route; J. P. Dubey, U.S. Department of Agriculture Animal Parasitic Diseases Laboratory in Beltsville, Maryland, provided information on *Besnoitia darlingi*; William E. Collins, Division of Parasitic Diseases, Centers for Disease Control and Prevention, in Atlanta, offered references on *Anopheles darlingi*; Richard J. Behles, Historical Librarian/Preservation Officer, University of Maryland Health Sciences and Human Services Library in Baltimore, allowed me to review textbooks about the Baltimore medical schools and their faculties at the time of Darling's enrollment and, to my delight, found the actual log of class records and grades given to medical students (including Darling) at the College of Physicians and Surgeons; Noel R. Rose of the Johns Hopkins School of Hygiene and Public Health, kindly determined that the Samuel Taylor Darling Library (once containing about two hundred books and several thousand pamphlets donated by Mrs. Darling) dissipated through the years; Christopher Crenner, chairman of the Department of History and Philosophy of Medicine, Kansas University Medical Center, accepted me into his fold and cheerfully agreed to the onerous task of reviewing the manuscript; and Dawn McInnis, Rare Book Librarian at the Kansas University Medical Center Clendening History of Medicine Library, enthusiastically obtained elusive reference material on the history of malaria and yellow fever.

This book would not have been possible without the interest and support of Anthony Grahame, editorial director at Sussex Academic Press, and his helpful professional staff.

I am especially indebted to Darling's family, who generously shared with me memories, letters, documents, and photographs of their illustrious relative. Ruth Darling Mannhardt of Cromwell, Connecticut, at age 97, evoked a particularly fond and emotive account of her brother; Virginia Darling of Charlottesville, Virginia, freely shared letters, certificates, and photographs of her notable father-in-law; and Ed and Nina Curran of Williamsburg, Virginia, provided a copy of the Darling family crest. More recently, I had the pleasure of contacting Mary Darling Lloyd, Darling's granddaughter, of Charlottesville, Virginia, and Darling's grandson, Samuel Darling, of British Columbia, who followed in his grandfather's footsteps by developing an effective and economical mosquito repellent for use in malaria endemic regions and established the Puerta del Cielo Foundation to benefit underprivileged natives in Guatemala. I hope to repay all of them for their kindness by utilizing most of what they so willingly shared with me.

Finally, I am most grateful to my wife, Vilma, and our children, Rick, Maria, Andy, Karen, and Eunice, for generously and patiently allowing me the time required to collect all the information that somehow, some day, would come to light. In this sense, Darling frequently was a welcome visitor at our dinner table and an honored guest in our home.

Chronology of Samuel Taylor Darling

April 6, 1872	Born in Harrison, New Jersey.
April 30, 1903	Graduates first in his class (Gold Medal) from College of Physicians & Surgeons of Baltimore.
	Appointed instructor in histology and pathology at his alma mater.
	Appointed resident pathologist at Baltimore City Hospital.
	Appointed instructor in bacteriology at Women's Medical College in Baltimore.
February 12, 1905	Accepts position under Col. William Gorgas as "Interne" at Ancon Hospital, Panama Canal Zone.
February 18, 1905	Marries Nannyrle Llewellyn, a student nurse from Virginia.
February 20, 1905	Departs from New York City to Panama on Panama Railroad Company steamship.
February 28, 1905	Arrives in Panama to start work as interne in Ancon Hospital.
June 1, 1905	Appointed "Physician" at a salary of $125 per month.
July 1, 1905	Appointed "Pathologist" at a salary of $200 per month.
August 16, 1905	Performs his first autopsy in Panama.
December 7, 1905	Performs autopsy #252 on a 27-yr-old carpenter from Martinique and discovers a new disease, histoplasmosis.
January 30, 1906	Performs autopsy #306 on a 21-yr-old Martiniquan (second case of histoplasmosis).
February 23, 1906	Given temporary position as "Pathologist in

	charge of the Board of Health Laboratory," Canal Zone.
August 6, 1906	Performs autopsy #572 on a 55-yr-old Chinese (third case of histoplasmosis).
October 5, 1906	Promoted to "Chief of the Board of Health Laboratory" at a salary of $333.33 per month.
October 16, 1913	Accompanies Col. William Gorgas to South Africa to investigate high mortality from pneumonia among Rand Mine workers (until April 8, 1914).
January 2, 1915	Accepts appointment to head a commission to investigate the effect of hookworm disease on the working efficiency of the people of Malaya, Java and Fiji, offered by the International Health Board of the Rockefeller Foundation.
May 23, 1915	Resigns Panama post.
April 6, 1915	Sails from New York to London.
May 29, 1915	Arrives in Singapore.
June 2, 1915	Arrives in Kuala Lumpur.
August 4, 1916	Departs Sumatra to Java.
April 6, 1917	Departs Singapore.
May 18, 1917	Arrives in Fiji.
August 13, 1917	Departs Fiji.
August 28, 1917	Arrives in Victoria, Canada.
September 4, 1917	Arrives in New York.
September 17, 1917	Accepts appointment to establish a Department of Hygiene at the Facultade de Medicina e Cirugia in São Paulo, where he serves as professor of hygiene and director of the Laboratory of Hygiene until 1920.
December 16, 1917	Departs New York for Rio de Janeiro.
January 6, 1918	Arrives in Rio de Janeiro.
April-Nov 1920	Develops weakness of his left arm and leg.
April 27, 1920	Departs Rio de Janeiro for health reasons.
May 16, 1920	Arrives in New York from Brazil.
June 1920	Seen by Drs. Barber and Dandy at Johns Hopkins.
September 16, 1920	On sick leave at Johns Hopkins Hospital and Esmont, Virginia.
November 15, 1920	Admitted for treatment of a brain tumor to Johns Hopkins Hospital.
November 18, 1920	Dr. Walter Dandy removes a glio-sarcoma.
January 27, 1921	Discharged from Johns Hopkins Hospital to convalesce in Esmont, Virginia.

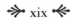

August 23, 1921	Moves with family into new home in Baltimore.
September 15, 1921	End of sick leave and appointed as fellow by courtesy at Johns Hopkins School of Hygiene.
January 27, 1923	Leaves Baltimore for a tour of the Southern states (North Carolina, Georgia, South Carolina, Alabama, Mississippi, and Louisiana) to survey malaria conditions and to select site for a malaria field station.
February 28, 1923	Returns to Baltimore.
March 27, 1923	Arrives in Leesburg, Georgia, to establish a Station for Field Studies in Malaria under the auspices of the Rockefeller Foundation (where he remains for two years).
March 21, 1925	Leaves Baltimore to join the Malaria Commission of the League of Nations for the Third Tour to Palestine, Lebanon, and Syria.
May 21, 1925	After completing work in Palestine and while returning to Beirut, Darling, at age 53, is fatally injured in a motorcar accident.

This book is dedicated to
Virginia E. Stich, medical librarian
at Gorgas (Ancon) Hospital, Canal Zone,
who kept the memory of Samuel Taylor Darling alive.

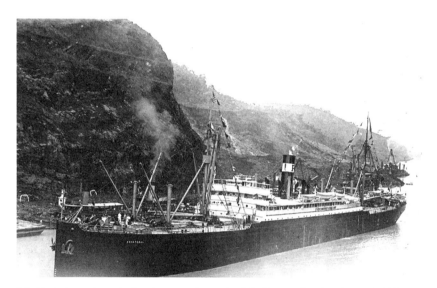

S.S. Cristobal completes the first interoceanic transit of the Panama Canal on August 3, 1914 (twelve days before the official inaugural canal crossing by the S.S. Ancon). About two hundred guests were on board invited by chief engineer Col. George Goethals, undated postcard.

Prologue
Aboard the *Cristobal*, 1914

On August 3, 1914, the S.S. *Cristobal* began the first complete passage across the Panama Canal.[1,2] The test voyage from Cristobal on the Atlantic to Balboa on the Pacific was scheduled by chief engineer George Goethals in anticipation of the official opening of the canal to world commerce twelve days later. The *Cristobal* traversed the fifty-mile channel and reached Balboa almost twelve hours later without any "operation incident."[1,2] The elusive strait that Columbus sought in vain four centuries earlier finally had become a reality. The Panama Canal was hailed as a triumph of engineering and sanitation.

Among the nearly two hundred passengers invited by Goethals to accompany the *Cristobal* on her inaugural canal crossing was Samuel Taylor Darling, chief of the Board of Health Laboratories at Ancon Hospital.[1] Other notable guests aboard included Philippe Buneau-Varilla, fiery French engineer who was instrumental in convincing the Americans to discard the Nicaragua canal plans for the Panama route; Joseph Bucklin Bishop, scholarly secretary of the Isthmian Canal Commission and subsequent author of several authoritative books on the canal enterprise; J. J. Moran, heroic participant in the yellow fever human experiments conducted by Walter Reed in Cuba that proved the mosquito-vector hypothesis; and Henri Pittier, indefatigable Swiss naturalist who spent years studying the flora and fauna of the isthmus.[1] The group of older employees and honored guests had taken a special train from the Pacific side at 5 o'clock that Monday morning for the two-hour trip by rail across the isthmus. From the terminal station in Colon on the Atlantic side of the isthmus, the passengers were transferred to the *Cristobal* in time for the historic maiden canal crossing.[1]

The progress made by the *Cristobal* along the canal route was recorded in characteristic detail by the weekly official publication, the *Canal Record*.[2] The 9,606-ton Panama Railroad Steamship Line vessel, constructed by the Maryland Steel Company and at one time engaged in trade between Puget Sound and the Orient, left the port of Cristobal shortly after 7 a.m.; stopped before the lower gates of Gatun locks at 8:15 a.m.; arrived in Gatun Lake shortly after 11 a.m.; entered Culebra Cut at 1 p.m.; reached Pedro Miguel at 2:30 p.m.; entered Miraflores Locks at 3:40 p.m.; reached the Pacific channel about 5:45 p.m.; and arrived opposite Balboa on the Pacific side at about 6:30 p.m.[2,3] Except for minor difficulties with the mules (towing locomotives) at Gatun and Pedro Miguel locks, the test voyage was a success.

The audacious crossing of the interoceanic canal by the *Cristobal* rivaled Jules Verne's fantastic voyages to the moon, center of the earth, or twenty-thousand leagues under the sea. Culmination of Columbus' dream to establish a shorter route to the fabled Indies, however, came at a staggering cost. Expenditures for the combined French and American efforts were estimated at $670 million ($13.1 billion in today's dollars) and the loss of at least 28,819 lives.[4,5] Construction of the Panama Canal could be given a price tag of $14 million and 576 lives for each one of the fifty miles spanning the interoceanic waterway.[6] Although the cost in dollars spent, cubic yards excavated, and thousands of workers hired could be roughly anticipated, the sacrifice in human lives far exceeded all expectations. Malaria, yellow fever and other tropical diseases exacted a heavy toll "as a divine punishment," according to a Jesuit priest, upon those who "dared to alter the form which the Creator, with supreme wisdom and forethought, designed for the structure of this universe."[7]

Control of yellow fever and malaria played a decisive role in the excavation of the Panama Canal. French records disclosed how yellow fever decimated the engineering corps and claimed the lives of many administrators, nurses, and laborers. Despite an excellent hospital system and competent medical staff, the French were handicapped by a lack of knowledge that both yellow fever and malaria were transmitted by mosquitoes.[8] Carlos Finlay, a Cuban physician educated in Philadelphia, had incriminated the mosquito as vector of yellow fever as early as 1881, but his ideas were met with incredulity and ridicule.[9] It was not until twenty years later, when Walter Reed proved beyond any doubt the important role of the mosquito in the transmission of yellow fever, that these diseases were effectively controlled — too late for the French enterprise which had curtailed much of its activities on the isthmus by 1889.[10] After an estimated loss of $287 million and 22,000 lives, the French abandoned the interoceanic project and transferred their properties to the Americans on May 4, 1904, for a lump-sum payment of $40 million, defeated by poor administration, debauchery, and tropical diseases.[11–13]

Darling was keenly aware about the deadly consequences of tropical diseases among the workers of the Panama Canal. As chief pathologist, he had supervised more than four-thousand autopsies among employees who died during the American period of construction of the isthmian canal between 1904 and 1914.[14,15] His vast experience with the pathology of malaria, yellow fever, tuberculosis, amebiasis, hookworm, and other local scourges, gave him a valuable perspective on tropical diseases. Darling's laboratories became the uncontested center for the investigation of relevant human and animal diseases in Panama. The results of his imaginative research provided the scientific basis for converting the isthmus from a nidus of pestilence to a healthy place in which to live and work.[16]

Although Gorgas was rightfully credited for the successful sanitation of Panama, it was Darling who investigated and offered solutions for many of the health problems that threatened to derail the engineering effort in Panama. Gorgas was dismayed to see that the sanitation measures that he had applied so successfully in Havana were ineffective against malaria in Panama. The rate of malaria among canal workers increased until it surpassed the worst figures experienced during the years of French excavation, reaching 821 per thousand workers in 1906.[13] Darling studied in his laboratories the different species of mosquitoes found in Panama and elucidated their feeding and breeding habits, as well as their propensity to carry malaria. He identified *Anopheles albimanus* as the only important vector and suggested species-specific anti-mosquito measures to render the sanitation efforts more effective and less expensive in the fight against malaria.[17] The different habitats and breeding characteristics between *Aedes egypti*, the yellow fever vector, and *Anopheles albimanus* accounted for the initial lack of success of the anti-malaria campaign in Panama.

Darling was 32 years old when he joined Gorgas' sanitation team in Panama. He departed from the United States scarcely two days after his wedding to Nannyrle Llewellyn, a student nurse from Virginia he had met in Baltimore, and arrived on the isthmus on April 28, 1905. She would join him eight months later when living quarters became available for married employees.

Darling had graduated from the College of Physicians and Surgeons of Baltimore in 1903 and received a gold medal for leading his class in the final examination.[18] He was qualified for a higher position than was available in Panama because of his post-graduate training in pathology, bacteriology, and laboratory sciences. Nevertheless, at the recommendation of William Welch, dean of Johns Hopkins School of Medicine, Darling accepted an offer for employment as an "interne" in Ancon Hospital, at a monthly salary of $50, including board, lodging, and laundry.[19] Working on the premise that he would be promoted according to his demonstrated skills, his superiors soon recognized his exceptional qualities as a physician, pathologist, and scientist. His titular rise among the ranks was swift: from interne he was ascended to physician in charge of one of the wards, then to pathologist at Colon Hospital and, within twenty months after his arrival in Panama, to the important post of chief of the Board of Health Laboratories.[16] His superior skills as a pathologist led him to the discovery of a new disease he named histoplasmosis.[20,21] Darling remained as head of the laboratories for eight years until his departure from Panama in January 1915. During this time, he recorded the results of his clinical and scientific investigations in more than a hundred original publications. His laboratories became a mecca for malariologists, parasitologists, helminthologists, pathologists, and other interested scientists who came to Ancon, Panama, to learn from this remarkable scientist.[16]

Almost two weeks after the first canal crossing by the *Cristobal*, the official opening of the Panama Canal to world traffic took place on August 15, 1914.[3] The S.S. *Ancon* ("nearly" twin-sister ship to the *Cristobal*) left its berth and began the scheduled canal trip at 7:30 a.m.[3] Secretary of War Lindley M. Garrison invited a couple hundred officials and dignitaries to participate in the inaugural voyage.[3] The distinguished entourage included Panama's president Belisario Porras and his cabinet, government officials, members of the diplomatic corps and resident consuls-general, and officers of the Tenth Infantry and Coast Artillery Corps.[3] A gift of champagne from the Swiss–Italian Colony winery in San Francisco ensured that this would be a jovial event. Nine hours and forty minutes later, the *Ancon* reached the end of a dredged channel five miles out in the Bay of Panama and returned to anchor in Balboa, as thousands gathered to witness the historic event.[3]

Secretary Garrison extended official recognition to all those involved in the successful completion of the canal:

> On behalf of the Government of the people of the United States, I express to you and through you to all concerned in the achievement, the intense gratification and pride experienced today. By the successful passage of vessels through the Canal the dream of centuries has become a reality. Its stupendous undertaking has finally been accomplished and a perpetual memorial to the genius and enterprise of our people has been created. The fully earned and deserved congratulations of a grateful people go out to you and your cola-borers [*sic*].[22]

President Woodrow Wilson had created a committee composed of six members of the Isthmian Canal Commission under the direction of the governor of the Canal Zone to "arrange and provide suitable ceremonies for the official and formal opening of the Panama Canal."[23] As part of the planned events, an international fleet of more than a hundred warships was scheduled to depart Hampton Roads, Virginia, cross the Panama Canal, and arrive in San Francisco in time for the opening of the Panama-Pacific International Exposition on February 20, 1915.[24] The inauguration of the Panama Canal, however, lacked the expected show of world pride, pomp, and circumstance. Most of the scheduled official ceremonies were canceled because of the recent outbreak of war in Europe.

True to his reputation as a "benevolent despot," Colonel Goethals also managed to deflate some of the celebratory mood experienced by his invited employees aboard the *Cristobal* on her first canal crossing with a terse memorandum:

> There appears to be some misconception regarding the time taken off by employes [sic] invited by me to make one of the trips through the Canal. There is no authority to carry this as gratuity time, and the day required for the trip will, therefore, be charged against the employe in every instance. Report of absence should be sent in on Form P. C. 484 for each employe absent."[25]

Most of the employees who participated in the building of the Panama Canal knew that the time had come to make important decisions about their future. Some were happy to return home and join their families in the Caribbean, Europe, and Asia. Others preferred to cast their lots with the fledgling but promising new country of Panama. By now, Darling was decidedly enamored of the tropics and eagerly awaited for new challenges and opportunities "to see all the wonders in this tropical world."[26]

PART I

Formative Years
1872–1905

1

Scottish Ancestry

Samuel Taylor Darling was born of good New England stock on April 6, 1872, in Harrison, New Jersey.[1] His parents were Edmund Adams Darling, born on January 18, 1849, and Sarah Ann Patterson, born on March 23, 1852. Edmund and Sarah were married at St. Paul's Church, Newark, New Jersey, on June 7, 1871, when he was twenty-two and she was eighteen.[2] Samuel was the eldest of seven siblings, two of whom did not reach adulthood (Herbert Emerson and Sarah Emily). The surviving five siblings (Samuel Taylor, Chester Morton, Annie Taylor, Ruth and Florence) spanned a child-bearing period of twenty-three years. Samuel's mother was 43-years old when she gave birth to her youngest daughter, Florence.[2]

Samuel represented the fifth generation to carry the surname Darling[1] since Dennis Darling arrived from Scotland in 1661 and settled in Braintree, Massachusetts, a coastal farmland community twelve miles south of Boston.[2,3] Seventy-five years later, Braintree consisted of white clapboard farmhouses surrounded by wooden fences or low walls made from the "ubiquitous rock and stone."[4] Its inhabitants experienced an "austere struggle" due to "reluctant crops of corn and wheat," and "every able inhabitant worshipped twice on Sunday and once in midweek."[4] In 1792, the northern part of Braintree become Quincy, the birthplace of John Quincy Adams, the sixth president of the United States. Quincy's father was John Adams, one of the founders of the new nation and its second president. John Adams was born, raised, and died in Braintree, Massachusetts.[5,6]

Dennis Darling married Hannah Francis and died at an undetermined age on January 24, 1717, in Mendon, Massachusetts.[2] The Darling side could trace back their ancestors to Abigail Adams, wife of president John Adams, whose home was also in Braintree, Massachusetts.[1,3] On the maternal side, Sarah Ann Patterson traced back her lineage to John Taylor and Anne Perkins, who were married at St. Saviour's Parish in Southward, County of Surrey, England.[2] Following the death of her husband, Anne Perkins Taylor came to America with her four daughters and made a living as a dressmaker. One of her daughters, Sarah Harding Taylor, married David Patterson on October 28, 1847, and they had four children, including Sarah Ann Patterson, Samuel's mother.[2] After the death of her husband, Sarah Harding Taylor, Samuel's maternal grandmother, was married on October 5, 1875, to Robert H. Orr, a minister at the Holy Trinity Church in Brooklyn, New York.[2] No children were recorded from her second marriage.[2] Samuel's maternal grandmother, Sarah Harding Taylor, and the founding father, Dennis Darling, stand out among his ancestors as imbued with the hardy and independent New England spirit which would later guide Samuel's own life trajectory.

Edmund Adams Darling (Samuel's father) died when Samuel was at an early age.[1] His mother moved with the remaining family to Pawtucket, Rhode Island, where he attended public schools.[1] Samuel's religious upbringing was rigid, as among his ancestors were several Episcopalian ministers and, in Pawtuckett, he and his mother lived with a cousin who was an Episcopalian minister.[1,7] When Samuel was about fourteen, plans were made against his wishes for him to attend a college preparatory school in Andover. In an act of rebellion, he ran away to New York, where he lived in Brooklyn with his maternal grandmother, Saran Ann Patterson, and Robert H. Orr.[1,2,7]

This was a time of doubts and wandering, during which Samuel was unable to define his future goals. He worked as a "druggist" or apothecary for Parke-Davis, in New York City, and later completed a three-year chemistry curriculum (1895–1898) at the Cooper Union Institute, but did not receive a diploma.[1,2,7] He took and passed "with honors" the New York State Regents' examination in 1897 but he had no immediate plans to attend college.[1,7] He remained undecided until two years later, when he reached a momentous decision to pursue a career in medicine. At age 27 and older than most applicants, Samuel sought admission and was accepted at the College of Physicians and Surgeons of Baltimore, for the first year course starting on October 1, 1899, at the advent of the new century.[7,8]

Darling's earlier wanderings and indecision had come to an end at the same time the 1800s concluded and the arrival of the 1900s was greeted with great expectations. The spirit of the new century may have emboldened Darling's aspirations for the future — a future he now faced more confidently.

2

New Century

The turn of the century was a propitious time for America, when optimism appeared to be boundless. Scientific and technological advances fueled an unprecedented confidence in the future. The promise for a better life brought waves of immigrants who were now poised to reap the benefits of their earlier struggles. Other countries in Europe and Asia looked with awe at this young nation as it rose from the devastation of a civil war to a position of prominence and leadership in the world.

Many new inventions for work or pleasure appeared at this time. These included the telephone, the phonograph, the typewriter, and the sewing machine. Housewives found stores well-stocked and prices affordable: eggs were one cent apiece, sirloin steak twenty-four cents a pound, and a turkey dinner was twenty cents.[1] *The 1902 Sears, Roebuck Catalogue*, distributed to 600,000 customers, reflected a cornucopia of abundance by listing in its pages more than 100,000 items.[2] Sears abolished C.O.D. (cash on delivery) orders to reduce clerical expenses and raised the minimum order to fifty cents. A set of fifteen slides of president McKinley's assassination was available for $7.50, with "realistic views of the assassination, of the assassin himself, taken within ten minutes of his capture by the police, and beautiful illustrations of the funeral cortege, in fact, a complete illustrated history of the most terrible tragedy of the present century."[3] This was a magnificent example of early American entrepreneurial spirit at its best!

Among the musical instruments, Sears, Roebuck and Company advertised a twelve-pound roller organ for $3.25, and a dozen popular song and dance rollers for $2.16, from a selection list of such favorites as *Old Folks at Home, Home Sweet Home, Yankee Doodle, Oh My Darling Clementine, My Old Kentucky Home, and Red, White and Blue*.[4] A ladies' 1902 Model Edgemere bicycle with pneumatic tires cost only $8.95.[5] For baseball fans, a Victor League baseball "guaranteed to hold its shape for nine innings" cost ninety cents, a professional model bat made of the best quality "second growth wide grain ash" was fifty-five cents, and a men's glove made of "Napa tanned horsehide" was listed for $1.[6] A leather-quarter top buggy sold for $34.95, a Smith & Wesson revolver for $11.25, and a wide selection of family bibles ranged in prices from $1.10 to $6.65 — the most expensive version offered a marriage certificate, a family record, and a family temperance pledge — all "beautifully bound in genuine Turkey morocco leather."[7-9]

A popular and controversial item in the catalogue was *Dr. Hood's Plain Talks and Common Sense Medical Adviser* about "nature, sexual physiology, natural relations of the sexes, civilization, love and marriage," plus a thirty-two-page pamphlet with twenty-nine special plates illustrating the female "productive" organs.[10] A twenty-eight page Drug Department described "almost every known patent medicine."[11] Among these, *Sure Cure* for the tobacco habit was said to "rejuvenate the weak and unstrung nerves caused by over indulgence in this poisonous weed." *Somone*, a vegetable preparation, quieted "the nervous excitement and muscular trembling caused by the excessive use of liquor." Dr. Rose's *Obesity Powders* reduced "corpulency in a safe and agreeable manner." And Sears' popular *Little Liver Pills* cured constipation — mankind's main affliction:

> [A]s we say that nine-tenths of human sickness is due to this one thing. When the bowels do not move regularly the natural drainage tract in the human system is dammed up, decomposition ensues and poisonous gases and liquids are carried all through the system. The result is jaundice, torpid liver, biliousness, sallow skin, indigestion, foul breath, coated tongue, loss of appetite, pimples, belching foul gases, blotches, boils, dizziness, headaches, cramps, colic, etc.[12]

Such extravagant claims seldom, if ever, were substantiated by any sort of reasonable — much less scientific — analysis. Patent medicines, as their name implied, were composed of ingredients purportedly granted exclusivity by the Patent Office. Most of the remedies, however, contained only vegetable extracts diluted with alcohol and laced with morphine, opium, or cocaine. Little wonder, then, that a soft drink patented in Atlanta in 1886 and containing small amounts of cocaine, was accordingly named Coca-Cola, and gained unprecedented popularity. Finally, propelled by widespread indignation after Upton Sinclair's description of the unsanitary conditions at meat packing plants in Chicago in *The Jungle*, as well as persistent efforts by professional and temperance groups, Congress passed the Pure Food and Drug Act on June 30, 1906, under the Theodore Roosevelt administration.[13]

The first self-propelled flight by the Wright brothers and the advent of the automobile prophesied faster travel to distant places. On a cold and windy December 17, 1903, Orville and Wilbur Wright, bicycle mechanics from Dayton, Ohio, after four years of experimentation with kites and gliders, maneuvered the first manned flying motor machine for twelve seconds and a hundred and twenty feet at Kitty Hawk, North Carolina.[14] Three more flights that day extended the time and distance in the air to fifty-nine seconds and eight hundred and fifty-two feet. Except for the innovators themselves, few took notice or cared about this milestone at the time. Only the editor of the Norfolk, Virginia, newspaper, *Virginian-Pilot*, considered the event sufficient news to place it in the front page. A year later, upon receiving the news that Theodore Roosevelt had won the presidential election, the Wright brothers celebrated the victory by taking their flying machine on a three-mile flight that lasted over five minutes, the longest to date. No one at the time could envision what the future held for this airborne contraption in terms of passenger travel, mail delivery, or military strategy.[14]

Transportation for people and goods was the domain of the railroads and in 1900 the nation was connected by almost 200,000 miles of track overrun by speeding "iron horses," as the steam locomotives were known. Yet American individualism toyed with the motorcar (also known by different names such as locomobile, motocycle and petrocar) and by 1900 Americans owned eight-thousand horseless carriages.[15] In 1903, Henry Ford organized in Detroit the Ford Motor Company with twelve partners and a capital of $28,000. Despite early competition by established automakers such as Buick, Cadillac, Packard, Oldsmobile and Studebaker, Henry Ford's idea of building a motorcar for the great multitudes became a reality. By the end of the decade, the Model T (affectionately known as the Tin Lizzie) became affordable, starting at a little less than $1,000 in 1909 and dropping to $295 in the ensuing years.[16] In the summer of 1903, America's early fascination with the motorcar peaked when E. T. Fetch and M. C. Krarup made the first coast-to-coast trip on a Packard Pacific from San Francisco to New York in fifty-two days and captured the nation's attention.[17] Americans became enamored of speed, independence, travel, and adventure. Although promotion of an interoceanic canal was motivated mainly by national and political interests, the opportunity to travel faster and more economically from coast to coast through a narrow isthmus was also appealing to the average citizenry.

No one in politics embodied the vitality and cocksure spirit of the United States at the turn of the century better than did Theodore Roosevelt. Whether carrying a pistol to patrol the streets as New York City's police commissioner or hoisting a sword to lead a cavalry charge during the Spanish–American War, Teddy Roosevelt exuded energy and stood above any other man of his time in America. At age 42, he became the youngest president six months after being elected vice president when

William McKinley was assassinated in September 1901. Four years later, Roosevelt was elected president by the largest plural majority of any previous candidate.[18] His vision that an isthmian canal was necessary to place the United States as a dominant maritime power emboldened his aspiration to construct a canal under American control. In the end, the successful completion of the Panama Canal was his own triumph, commensurate with his grand persona and his famous credo, "Speak softly and carry a big stick." Yet he spoke with more of a "high-pitched, staccato bark" and only when provoked or animated he became "a human volcano, roaring as only a human volcano can roar! — leading the laughter and singing and shouting, like a boy out of school, pounding the table with both noisy fists."[18] Such was the exuberance of the man who led the country into the new century and who would build the Panama Canal. The president's enthusiasm was contagious and even Darling, a non-Republican, may have joined those who saw the advent of a bright and promising future under Roosevelt's leadership.

3

College of Physicians and Surgeons of Baltimore

Darling matriculated as a first-year student at the College of Physicians and Surgeons of Baltimore for the winter session starting October 1899.[1] At age twenty-seven, he was older than most of his classmates when he enrolled in medical school. His physical appearance at the time was fondly recalled by a classmate:

> He was . . . tall and slender, with a remarkably handsome head. His hair was light brown, and he wore a full blonde beard. His wonderful brown eyes were full of expression — the eyes of a poet. His complexion was ruddy and clear. . . . His voice was deep, melodious, and resonant. Altogether his personality was one of the most attractive that it has ever been my good fortune to encounter.[2]

In addition, his vast knowledge of the English literature "was manifested in a beautiful English style of expression."[3]

Students were instructed to register as soon as they arrived in the city to the dean's office, in the College Building at the northwest corner of Calvert and Saratoga Streets. Darling recorded his name in his own bold, left-handed strokes in the matriculation records of the College for 1882–1912 and listed his home address as 28 Brook St., Pawtucket, R[hode] I[sland].[4] Following registration, the new students were placed under the guidance of a janitor in charge of the baggage, finding a suitable boarding house, and furnishing all required information.[1]

Requisites for admission to the medical college consisted of an entrance examination in algebra, higher arithmetic, elements of physics, Latin prose, and an English composition of two hundred words.[1] Darling had passed the New York State Regents' examination and, therefore, was probably exempt from this requirement.[3]

✦ 15 ✦

Darling's decision to study medicine in Baltimore likely resulted from a measured analysis of available options for a future career. The sketchy records remaining from this early period of his life show that he enrolled in evening classes at the Cooper Union Institute in New York City in 1895 and completed there a three-year course in chemistry (but did not receive a degree).[3] He was employed at Parke-Davis pharmaceuticals and possibly acquired in that connection a reasonable working knowledge of *materia medica*.[5] While concocting prescriptions, he probably learned something about the diseases for which physicians dispensed those remedies. His preparation in chemistry would have given him additional insight on the beneficial and toxic properties of chemical compounds.

Physicians at the turn of the century were more likely to prescribe a combination of medicinal ingredients rather than to dispense patent or already prepared medications. The pharmacist not only had the onerous task of deciphering the handwritten list of ingredients along with their individual amounts written in Latin and in apothecary measures (ounces, drams, scruples, and grains), but also of preparing these as well using a graduated cylinder, mortar and pestle, and weighing scales, and presenting the final product in the form of a liquid (elixir, syrup, or tincture), powder (usually dispensed in paper packets), or gelatin capsules.[6] Patients often consulted pharmacists for advise on how to treat ailments and to directly obtain from them non-prescription (patent) medications readily available on the premises.[7] Pharmacists were not competing with doctors in this role but provided assistance to a clientele that eagerly sought their help. In fulfilling this role, a pharmacist was both a healer and a businessman who made a living by selling his products and obtained the satisfaction of helping friends and neighbors through his knowledge and expertise.

Although regarded as apocryphal, an anecdote told by Darling's wife years later may have had some basis on truth. Sir William Osler, the venerated physician and teacher at Johns Hopkins and author of the authoritative *The Principles and Practice of Medicine*, visited Cooper Union and saw Darling dissecting a bovine heart with such dexterity that he predicted Darling would some day become a prominent physician.[3] If so, this brush with greatness may have stimulated Darling to gaze far into his future and inspire him to reach for the stars.

Darling's choice of medical school could have been influenced by several factors, including location, cost, and curriculum. Baltimore as the city of choice to begin his medical studies was not as far-fetched as it may seem. Prior to Flexner's 1910 scathing report on the state of medical education in the United States criticizing the proliferation of mediocre medical schools and a lack of quality control in medical education, an abundance of these proprietary institutions concentrated in large cities such as New York, Philadelphia, and Boston.[8]

Baltimore had at least one advantage that was in ferment at the time Darling entered medical school. Visionary medical educators in that city were placing the foundations of what would become a model of excellence in medical education. William Halsted, William Welch, William Osler, and Howard Kelly came together to form the great team at Johns Hopkins School of Medicine and their careful planning and execution would revolutionize American medical education.[9] The proximity of the College of Physicians and Surgeons of Baltimore to Johns Hopkins may have exerted some beneficial influence and one can sense from the College's description of the curriculum that the emphasis on laboratory training in the different disciplines of chemistry, physiology, and histology, responded to a genuine desire for improvement, if not outright competition. Following the session of 1891–1892, a regular three-year graded course was required by the College of Physicians and Surgeons of Baltimore for obtaining the degree of Doctor of Medicine.[10]

Accessibility to Baltimore from Pawtucket, Rhode Island, was facilitated by an extensive railroad network that linked the country from the Atlantic to the Pacific. Travel from Darling's home to Baltimore required only a few hours and an affordable passenger ticket. By the second year of studies, Darling no longer listed his residence as Rhode Island and by the third gave his home address as the College of Physicians and Surgeons itself.[11] Baltimore was a city of 400,000 inhabitants by the year 1900. The College announcement of courses extolled the virtues of Baltimore as having "an advantageous location, salubrity of climate, cheapness of living, genial hospitality of its citizens, which combined to make it the great medical center of the country."[12] A convenient line of cable and electric cars simplified personal transportation from anywhere in the city to the College.[13]

A New England upbringing, a strict religious background, a home without a father at an early age, and a mother who moved to seek a better plight for her family — all point to hardship and frugality as underlying themes in Darling's formative years. His financial resources were very meager.[2] Cost of a medical education was, undoubtedly, also an important issue. College fees for the 1899–1900 winter session consisted of a $5 matriculation fee and a $100 charge for professors' fees for the winter session payable on entering; there were no fees for laboratory work and dissections.[1]

The cost of available medical textbooks for the 1899–1900 session was quite reasonable. Some of the textbooks recommended for the first year class and their listed prices were: Physiology (Kirke's $3.25), Chemistry (Simon's Manual $3.00), and Medical Dictionary (Dunglinson $5.60).[1] Other textbooks listed for future courses included Surgery (American Text-book of Surgery $7), Practice of Medicine (Strumpell $4.80), Obstetrics (American Text-book $4.00), Diseases of Children (Smith

$3.60), Nervous Diseases (Dana $2.60), Mental Diseases (Savage on Insanity $1.60), and Hygiene (Rohes Text-book on Hygiene $3.00).[1] Dr. Thomas Opie, dean of the college, stated: "We believe that in no other large city of the United States can the same educational facilities be furnished at so low a cost."[1] The College offered residence to twelve students at a rate of $12 weekly and satisfactory board could be had for $3 a week. Such a reasonable cost of living and the opportunity to work as a pharmacy or laboratory assistant may have been important considerations for Darling to select Baltimore over New York, Boston, and Philadelphia as the preferred site for his medical studies.

The year Darling entered medical school marked the twenty-ninth annual session of the College of Physicians and Surgeons of Baltimore. The college had been founded in 1872 after a disagreement among the faculty members of the Washington University of Medicine.[14] The dissatisfied faculty members, joined by recently arrived physicians and led by Dr. Edward Warren, organized and incorporated the new school under the general laws of the State of Maryland. Five years later, because of declining enrollment and prestige, Washington University of Medicine transferred all of its franchises and property to the college and the two schools were consolidated by an act of the legislature.[14] The new college continued to prosper and announced that "important accessions have been made to the corps of teachers" since the previous session, including new chairs of obstetrics and hygiene and clinical medicine, as well as additional instructors and demonstrators in anatomy, clinical medicine, microscopy, and pathology.[15] The list of the faculty roster was impressive, consisting of seventeen professors, fifteen associate professors, and eleven demonstrators and assistant demonstrators (see Appendix B: Faculty Listed at Commencement Exercises, 1903). Baltimore physicians were proud of their history: they had founded the fourth medical college (Maryland Medical University in 1807) and the third medical journal in the United States, as well as the first college of dentistry in the world in 1839.[16]

A new college building had been erected in 1891 at the northwest corner of Calvert and Saratoga Streets.[17] The dominant thought in the construction of the college building had been to adapt it to the needs of the modern medical student, bringing student and teacher in close and intimate contact and giving less emphasis to lecture-room work and more importance to clinics, laboratory work, quizzes, and bedside instruction.[15] The first floor was devoted to dispensary work. The second floor was arranged into two large classrooms, a clinical laboratory, and library. The third floor housed two amphitheaters, and clinical, pathology, physiology, and chemistry laboratories. The fourth floor was devoted to clinical work with a modern amphitheater seating four hundred students, surrounded by a large suite of accessory rooms for sterilization, anesthesia, dressings, and minor surgery, as well as a well-equipped bacteriology laboratory.[15]

Adjoining the College Building were the Baltimore City Hospital and a "Hospital for the Colored Race."[15] The Maryland Lying-in Asylum was an obstetrical facility located at 115 West Lombard Street, about a five-minute walk from the college. Members of the graduating class were required to register at the asylum and were "summoned to the clinic upon the occurrence of labor cases by prompt messenger service or telegraph."[15] Bay View Hospital, located in the eastern suburbs of Baltimore, contained about two-thousand beds for the insane. The Nursery and Children Hospital, located at the corner of Franklin and Schroeder Streets, accommodated one hundred and fifty beds devoted entirely to diseases of infancy and childhood. In addition, the dispensary on the first floor of the college building offered an abundance of clinical material. It was staffed daily from noon to 2 p.m. by one or two attending staff and by fourth-year medical students. The dispensary registered 20,350 patients and dispensed 19,000 prescriptions during the previous year.[15]

The curriculum for the first year consisted of anatomy, physiology, chemistry, materia medica, histology, osteology, and chemical, histological, and anatomical laboratories.[15] The course in anatomy included lectures, recitations, and demonstrations as well as dissections under supervision of the demonstrators in anatomy. Physiology was taught didactically by lectures and recitations three hours weekly, and by laboratory courses in practical physiology and physiological chemistry. Chemistry "embrace[d]" lectures on inorganic and organic chemistry and a practical course on qualitative and quantitative analyses. Materia medica, pharmacology, and therapeutics were imparted by the Department of Pharmacology in the form of didactic lectures, together with demonstration of drugs using "lower animals." Six hours a week were devoted to histology laboratory work and two hours to didactic instruction.[15]

The college announcement emphasized that the laboratory facilities had been greatly increased. Complete laboratory courses were given in anatomy, osteology, histology, chemistry, physiology, physiological chemistry, materia medica and pharmacology, pathology, bacteriology, hygiene, and clinical medicine.[15] These laboratories were furnished with the most modern equipment and "every effort was put forth to make this important branch of the curriculum as complete and thorough as possible."[15] If Darling was interested in laboratory work, this description of his future experience in the college would satisfy a growing hunger for knowledge in the laboratory sciences.

The class schedule for the first year students is shown in Appendix B (see Daily Order of Lectures — First Year, 1900–1901). Classes were usually held Monday to Saturday for one-hour periods from 9 a.m. to 3 p.m.[15]

Darling's academic performance for the first year was outstanding. He was at the top of his class of sixty-one students and the next highest average score was more than five points below his.[4] Darling's grades for the 1900–1901 session were recorded in the ledger as follows: Physiology 100; Inorganic Chemistry 100; Materia Medica 100; Histology 93; and Osteology 99, for an average of 98 (see Appendix B: Student Registration and Grades).[4]

The course in histology offered during the first year was Darling's introduction to the microscope, a tool that would become indispensable in his future work. During this course, he studied the elementary tissues and then followed "a careful study of the various organs."[15] The textbooks used for instruction in histology were those by George Piersol and E. Klein. His first encounter with the course of pathology came in the second year and it is likely that this experience cemented his attraction to the field, revealing through the microscope disease manifestations in full color and undeniable beauty.

Other courses during the second year were anatomy, chemistry, bacteriology, medical jurisprudence, pharmacy, and hygiene. His scores for these subjects were even higher than those he had obtained the year before: Anatomy 98; Physiology 100; Chemistry 100; Bacteriology 100; Pathology 100; Medical Jurisprudence 100; Pharmacy 100; and Hygiene 98, for an average score of 99.0 (See Appendix B: Class Registration and Grades).[4]

Darling's superior performance during the second year of medical studies evidenced his dedication to study and to learn, but more than that, intimated that he had now found his true calling in life. According to a classmate, Edgar Friedenwald:

> From the very beginning of his medical training he applied himself to his work with earnestness and enthusiasm. The laboratories afforded an outlet for his scientific interests, and wherever opportunity offered for laboratory investigation or study, he embraced it eagerly and intelligently, whether in pathology, bacteriology, or anatomy. . . . I remember during our early days in medical school we often met in a tiny, unpretentious students' laboratory. One day Dr. Darling remarked that he would be entirely satisfied if he could only have a place like that to work in all the rest of his life.[2]

Darling most likely found a teacher or mentor who nurtured his thirst for knowledge and directed him to acquire a solid foundation in the field of pathology. That influential figure was probably Nathaniel Garland

Keirle, a professor of pathology and medical jurisprudence at the College of Physicians and Surgeons of Baltimore.

Nathaniel Keirle served three important functions in the City of Baltimore. He was professor at the college, medical examiner for the City of Baltimore, and director of the laboratory at the Pasteur Institute.[18] Born and educated in Baltimore, Keirle was an indefatigable worker whose energy and enthusiasm could have easily inspired Darling to emulate him.

As professor of Pathology and Medical Jurisprudence at the College of Physicians and Surgeons of Baltimore, Keirle gave didactic lectures in pathology and legal medicine, demonstrations of gross pathological anatomy, and imparted instruction in microscopic examination and diagnosis of morbid growths, urinary deposits, and other pathological secretions and products.[1] His role as medical examiner allowed him to demonstrate cases of medico-legal interest before the class. He conducted post-mortem examinations in a "commodious and well-lighted amphitheatre" where students were allowed to inspect morbid lesions *in situ*.[1]

In 1897, Keirle became director of the Pasteur Institute. As part of the City Hospital, the institute was founded and directed by the college "for the preventive treatment of hydrophobia according to the Pasteur method."[19] Patients were instructed to come without any delay directly to the institute where they would be received by a resident physician and given suitable accommodation. Patients were quarantined for twenty-three days. Further instructions were given to persons bitten by animals suspected to be rabid to make every effort to keep the animal under observation or, if the animal was dead, to bring the animal packed in ice to prevent putrefaction.[19] Up to June 1902, 322 cases had been admitted to the Pasteur Institute under Keirle, and two-hundred nine (65 per cent) proved to be bitten by rabid animals. Only one death was reported, and this was ascribed to an "incomplete period of immunization."[18] All cases admitted were charged a uniform fee of $150, which included board and lodging at the institute.[19]

Keirle was highly regarded among his colleagues and by the citizens of Baltimore. His dedication to medical education, service as medical examiner, and stewardship of the Pasteur Institute, elevated him prominently as a man who dedicated his life to the service of the city.[20] Furthermore, Keirle was a local product: he was born, educated, and resided all his life in Baltimore. He was described as short in stature, with "closely-cut hair, mustache and beard, with a scholar's head," so that he was "a distinguished figure wherever he appeared."[20] Keirle continued to function as director of the Pasteur Institute for ten years and as city medical examiner for thirty years. He had been witness in almost every murder trial in the Baltimore courts and judges and lawyers alike esteemed him as a careful, exact witness, whose testimony always weighed heavily in determining a case.[20] As for his personal life, he had married at an advanced age in 1870 and had three children. Ten years later, two of his children died shortly after their mother had succumbed. He remained single but comforted by his only son, Nathaniel G. Keirle, Jr. (graduated from the college at the top of his class the year before Darling enrolled), who faithfully accompanied his father, so that the two were described as "inseparable."[20] Keirle experienced the irreparable death of his son in 1908 and became a lonely, single man until, at the age of 80, he married a woman thirty-two years his junior. His second wife remained devoted to him until his death six years later.[20]

Darling worked as a laboratory assistant to Keirle at the Pasteur Department, where he aided in the preparation of viruses, inoculation of animals, and many other such chores, all of which were within his field of special interest and helped to prepare him for his ultimate place in the medical world.[3] Darling often assisted Keirle in autopsy examinations. The two men became life-long friends as a result of this association.[3]

The curriculum for the third year students at the College of Physicians and Surgeons of Baltimore listed Medicine, Surgery, Obstetrics, Therapeutics, Gynecology, Clinical Medicine, Diseases of the Eye and Ear, Diseases of the Nervous System, Genito Urinary Diseases, Applied Anatomy, Diseases of the Stomach, Dermatology, Physical Diagnosis and Clinical Laboratory.[19] The initial class of sixty-one students had now increased to eighty-two and Darling continued to lead the group with an average score of 93.9 (see Appendix B: Student Registration and Grades).[4] He achieved perfect scores (100) in Eye and Ear, Therapeutics, and Clinical Laboratory. His lowest scores for that year were in Obstetrics (88) and Surgery (94).[4] For the fourth and last year of instruction, the curriculum listed Medicine, Surgery, Obstetrics, Therapeutics, Gynecology, Clinical Medicine, Operative Surgery, Daily Ward Classes and Dispensary Work in Medicine, Surgery, Obstetrics, Gynecology, Nervous Diseases, Diseases of Eye and Ear, Diseases of Stomach, Pediatrics, Laryngology, Medical Electricity, Genito Urinary Diseases, Dermatology, and Mental Diseases.[19] Darling's average score was 93.83, which led the class once again. His grades for the four years averaged 96.27 (his closest classmate was T. J. Cummings of New Jersey, with an average score of 95.70).[4]

The College recognized Darling's stellar performance by awarding him the Gold Medal for achieving first place in the final examination among a class of seventy-six graduating students at the thirty-first annual commencement of the College of Physicians and Surgeons held on April

30, 1903.[21] Additional gold medals were given for second, third, and fourth place standings in the graduating class, and the respective recipients were T. J. Cummings, F. W. A. Mayer (both from New Jersey), and William S. Evans (from Utah).[21]

Darling was the academic and social leader of his class or, as he later called it, the class of "naughty-three."[3] He also participated in extracurricular activities and was responsible for establishing in Baltimore the Zeta chapter of Phi Beta Pi, one of several medical fraternities in the country formed mainly to offer room and board at a more affordable rate to medical students.[3] He was described as "extremely popular" and "he entered into all the activities and frivolities of his classmates, and was the gayest and most jovial among them."[2] At times he would be absent for two-to-three day periods associated with excessive alcohol consumption, but such interludes were reportedly infrequent.[3]

Following graduation, Darling became an active alumnus and in the list of officers for 1903–1904 appeared as first vice president of the Alumni Association of the College of Physicians and Surgeons.[22] By now he had decidedly cast his lot in the field of pathology, attracted by both the anatomical and the laboratory aspects of this branch of medicine. He was appointed instructor in histology and pathology at his alma mater, resident pathologist at Baltimore City Hospital (later known as Mercy Hospital), visiting pathologist at Bay View Hospital, and instructor in bacteriology at the Women's Medical College of Baltimore.[3,15,23,24] He gained much valuable experience in these various posts under the tutelage of Keirle and other influential faculty members.

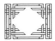

Another towering figure who may have influenced Darling directly or indirectly during his early training in pathology and bacteriology in Baltimore was William Welch at the Johns Hopkins University School of Medicine. Although the two medical schools were physically and ideologically separate, Johns Hopkins already was forging a successful experiment in medical education as a graduate school rather than a private or propietary enterprise. It is plausible that some difficult pathology cases may have required the expertise of Welch, who had been trained among the finest pathologists in Europe.[9,25,26]

Welch would become a pivotal figure in the change of American medical education from mediocrity to excellence, from private and proprietary schools to centers of learning based on scientific and technological advances.[27] He was a pathologist, a bacteriologist, a laboratory man. He was also a leader of men and an organizer who could inspire those around him to perform at or beyond their capabilities.

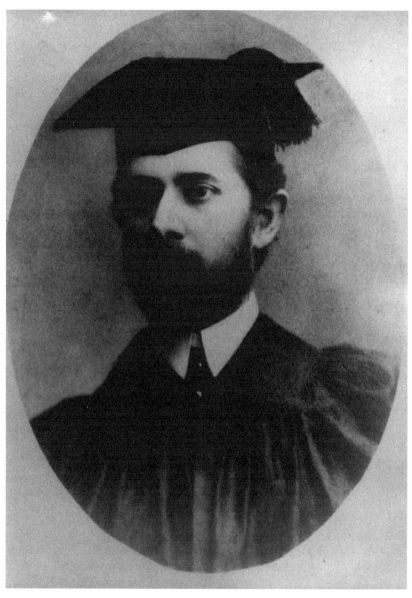

3.1 Darling at graduation from College of Physicians and Surgeons of Baltimore in 1903, at age 31. Reproduced with permission, courtesy of Gerald L. Baum.

Welch, like Darling, was an admirer of the classics. As an undergraduate at Yale University, Welch's aspiration was to become a tutor in Greek.[28] However, his attention turned to medicine at his father's insistence and he became receptive to the exciting advances in bacteriology coming from the laboratories of Koch and Pasteur in Europe. As a medical student at the College of Physicians and Surgeons in New York, he excelled as a prosector in anatomy and, as an intern at Bellevue, came under the favor of Francis Delafield, a pathologist, who entrusted him to make entries in the pathology book and to act as summer curator of the pathological specimens at Bellevue.[29] By now Welch was excited at the prospect of becoming part of the Johns Hopkins' medical revolution as a pathologist, and prepared himself accordingly by traveling to Europe to learn from Ludwig, von Recklinghausen, Hoppe-Seyler, Waldeyer, Weigert in Strassbourg, Leipzig, and Breslau.[30] After spending nearly two years learning in the laboratories of these giants, Welch returned to America in 1878.[31] Unable to obtain sufficient space for setting up a laboratory at his alma mater, Welch opted for a modest beginning at Bellevue. He was given three rooms and some kitchen tables without any equipment (he estimated the administration spent "fully twenty-five dollars" on his behalf) to set up the first teaching pathology laboratory in America.[32] Belatedly, the College of Physicians and Surgeons of New York realized the missed opportunity and now found what they thought would be sufficient space and money to lure the prize back. However, Welch's dream to become a professor of pathology at Johns Hopkins prevailed and he declined the offer. In 1884, at the age of thirty-four, Welch was offered and he accepted an appointment as the first professor at the Johns Hopkins School of Medicine.[33]

The lure of Johns Hopkins for men such as Welch was the promise that the Baltimore institution would revolutionize medical education in this country.[26] By emphasizing laboratory-based teaching to medical students and employing a full-time faculty, without the distractions of private practice or fees-for-classes, the new medical school would set a better standard for quality medical education. This lofty ideal was supported by a generous gift of $7 million in 1867 from Johns Hopkins, an unlikely benefactor, who stipulated that a university and hospital were to be created with the goal of encouraging research and of advancing individual scholars who, by their excellence, would advance the sciences they pursued and the society where they dwelled.

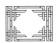

By the time Darling graduated from the College of Physicians and Surgeons of Baltimore in 1903, he had already expressed a desire to spend

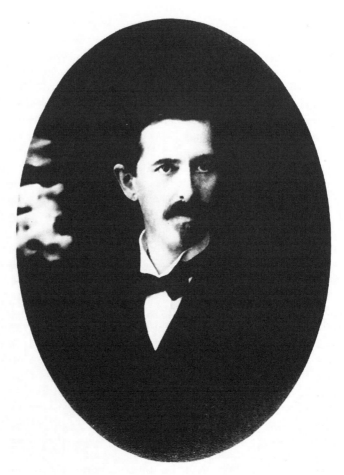

3.2 Darling as a young man, possibly in 1905, at age 33, at the time of his wedding. Reproduced with permission, courtesy of Gerald L. Baum.

the rest of his life working in a laboratory — not dissimilar to the goals a young William Welch had espoused early in his medical career. Having benefited from a medical curriculum which now required laboratory-based basic sciences in the first two years of training, Darling had essentially become the type of medical graduate that Johns Hopkins strived to nurture. In addition, by emphasizing the value of research among its faculty and recruiting prominent role models of the stature of Welch, Kelly, Halsted, and Osler, the success of Johns Hopkins may have strengthened Darling's resolve to strive for a career in laboratory medicine. The lure of pathology for both Welch and Darling was based on the ground-breaking hypothesis proposed by Rudolf Virchow that all diseases could be explained at the cellular level.[34] The examination of tissues would reveal in most instances a pattern of injury peculiar to a specific disease and, therefore, post-mortem examinations became an essential requisite for confirmation of a clinical diagnosis and for a better understanding of the mechanisms of disease.

Darling had readily adopted Baltimore as his new residence. He was content with his life, medical education, and pathology training. Baseball, his only distraction, was available when the Baltimore Orioles played at home and, when they went to New York, he could catch a game there if time and duties permitted. As he settled into the familiarity of his daily routine, a major disaster was waiting in the wings — the Great Fire of Baltimore.

On Sunday February 7, 1904, a fire alarm at 10:48 a.m. summoned firefighters to the John E. Hurst & Company building located between Hopkins Place and Liberty Street in the business section of Baltimore.[35] The fire spread quickly, aided by a southwest wind and, despite intervention by all of twenty-four Baltimore engines and additional aid summoned from Washington, D.C., Philadelphia, Wilmington, Atlantic City, and New York City, more than 1,500 buildings were destroyed over an area of one hundred and forty acres. Thirty-one hours later, the fire was contained on Monday at 5 p.m. A total of 1,231 firefighters and fifty-seven fire engines participated in the conflagration. Despite the loss in millions, only one death was reported — that of a firefighter.[35]

The proximity of the College Building and Baltimore City Hospital to the fire as it started to spread eastward resulted in preparations for evacuation of patients and specimens. This was done with the help of workers and volunteers, including medical students, some of whom distinguished themselves "nobly."

Fortunately, the fire changed course and stopped a few blocks from Calvert and Saratoga Streets, and the college and hospital buildings were spared.[35,36]

Darling's busy schedule as demonstrator, instructor, and resident in pathology in Baltimore must have been demanding. Yet it was while on duty that he met his future wife. Suspected cases of typhoid fever in Baltimore were further investigated using a recently introduced serological agglutination Widal test. Darling was sent to obtain a blood sample for this purpose from a student nurse at her home. On first encounter, she thought "he looked like Jesus himself" and that "he behaved as an ill-bred bore."[3] These initial impressions were only transient and in further meetings a more lasting relationship developed, perhaps fueled by a first kiss in a bundle room at the city hospital.[3]

Nannyrle Llewellyn came from a traditional family in Virginia and had been educated in private schools. Charles Marshall Llewellyn, her father, owned a thirteen-hundred acre plantation near Danville, close to the southern border between Virginia and North Carolina.[3] According to his daughter, Charles would supervise his land from the verandah "with a mint julep in his hand" and would sell a bit of his plantation each year to pay taxes.[3] Not surprisingly, Nannyrle's family opposed her wishes to become a nurse but she enrolled anyway in the nursing school in Baltimore. Superficially, it would seem that this couple had little in common, other than both being hard-headed and Episcopalians.[3] The romance took unexpected urgency when Darling began to consider taking a position in Panama. And so, on February 18, 1905, they were married and two days later Darling left for an uncertain future, leaving his newly acquired spouse behind until she could join him in Panama eight months later.[3]

The advantages of a tropical climate may have been romanticized in Darling's mind by the fact that the winter of 1905 in Baltimore was one of the most severe. The *Baltimore Sun* reported that it had snowed twenty-two times already by February 13, for a total of 39.1 inches — a remarkable record.[37] By contrast, Panama's weather in February was predictably balmy and had averaged 80.9 degrees Fahrenheit over a four-year period.[38] As a bonus, no rainy days were recorded in January or February 1905, on the Pacific side (La Boca).[39] If Darling had any remaining doubts about the soundness of his decision to seek his fortune in Panama, a comparison of the contrasting climates between Baltimore and Panama may have been persuasive.

But more important was the prospect of participating in the culmination of one of man's most ambitious dreams: the construction of an interoceanic canal on the isthmus of Panama. On the eve of Darling's wedding, The *Baltimore Sun* carried the news that on Thursday late afternoon, February 16, 1905, Congress had passed the "Panama bill," authorizing President Roosevelt to have complete control over the construction of the Panama Canal.[40] Everything seemed to be coming together quite well for the realization of Roosevelt's dream of constructing an isthmian canal. Darling surely must have been aware of the important role sanitation would play in the successful completion of this engineering feat. Roosevelt had already entrusted William Gorgas to do what the French had failed to accomplish in Panama: conquer yellow fever and malaria. And now Darling had chosen to become part of the American effort to control tropical diseases. One can only imagine the anticipation and excitement Darling must have sensed as he envisioned his new life in a tropical world.

PART II

Panama Years
1905–1915

4

Isthmian Explorations

The discovery of the New World by Columbus in 1492 posed an unexpected obstacle to his obsession to find a shorter route to *Cipango* (Japan) and *Cathay* (India). The cities of these far-away and exotic lands, according to Marco Polo, were so wealthy that their palaces were lined with gold and precious jewels.[1] Reaching the coveted riches and spices would have to wait until a passageway to Asia was found. Columbus firmly believed that such a path leading to the Indian Ocean existed west of the Indies.[2] A diligent search for the "elusive strait" would be the main objective of the Admiral's last voyage to the New World.

Columbus obtained permission and ten thousand golden pesos from the Spanish crown to prepare for his fourth and final voyage of exploration.[3] The Admiral, now aged fifty-one, sailed from Cadiz on May 9, 1502, and after two days' delay from a *vendaval* (strong wind), sailed west equipped with four ships and accompanied by one-hundred and forty men, including a brother, Bartholomew, and a son, Ferdinand.[3] After further delays from stops in Morocco and in the Canary Islands, Columbus started the ocean crossing on May 25. Twenty-one days later, on June 15, the fleet reached Martinique, making this the fastest voyage he had experienced to the Indies.[3]

On August 14, 1502, the Admiral and his fleet alighted in proximity to Central America (Honduras) and from there systematically explored the coastline for a passage to the East.[4] The poor condition of the vessels, raging storms, and dissension from the crew forced the explorers to remain near the isthmus of what is now Panama. The incessant storms battered the ships and despaired the crew, including Columbus, for twenty-eight days.[4]

Columbus had experienced hurricanes at least twice during previous voyages and, according to Samuel Eliot Morison, the Admiral's biographer, had learned to recognize the signs of an impending storm:

Oily swell rolling in from the southeastward, abnormal tide, an oppressive feeling in the air, low-pressure twinges in his rheumatic joints, veiled cirrus clouds tearing along in the upper air while light gusty winds flew on the surface of the water, gorgeous crimson sunset lighting up the whole sky. . . . [3]

The crippled fleet sailed along the coast and went by *Porto Bello* (Beautiful Port), *Nombre de Dios* (Name of God), *Bastimentos* (Provisions), and *Retrete* (Retreat) Bay — names found to this day in Panama maps. Although Columbus was reluctant to accept the reality of a new continent (he still felt he was on the eastern shore of Asia), by 1498, during his third voyage, he realized that the great expanses of land and major rivers were part of a continent and not an island, and named them *Tierra Firme* (Firm Land).[2]

Throughout all his explorations, Columbus held steadfast to his quest for a new route to the Orient. Had he known how close he was to the narrowest part of the isthmus (about ten leagues or thirty-five miles wide), he may have seen this as a divine sign guiding him in the right direction. However, his scouts and interpreters received no indications from the natives that another ocean lay only a few more days on foot across the land. Finally, having failed to find a passageway, Columbus left the Coast of *Contrastes* (Contrarieties), as he called it, and sailed toward Jamaica. Two of the ships had been abandoned due to damaged wood from *broma* (mollusks) and those remaining were in no condition to carry him back to Spain. After twelve months marooned in Jamaica, reluctant help came from his enemy, Nicolás de Ovando, who had been unwittingly appointed governor and supreme justice of the Indies by the Spanish sovereigns as an affront to the Admiral.[5] Columbus returned to Spain on November 4, 1504, after twelve years of hardship, in disgrace and in poor health, unable to find a passageway to the fabled Orient.[6]

Among those who came to the New World with Rodrigo de Bastidas in 1500 was a young, tall man who later hid as a stowaway to escape from his debtors in Hispaniola.[2] Not lacking in leadership skills, Vasco Núñez de Balboa promptly showed his bravery and fairness as a leader to this group of adventurers and rose in ranks to become *alcalde* (mayor) of the village of Santa Maria Antigua in Darien.[2,7] This time favorable reports were received about a large body of water that lay only a few days' journey across the isthmus. On September 1, 1513, Balboa set out with one hundred and ninety armed Spaniards (among these was Francisco Pizarro, who would conquer Peru and the Incas six years later), several hundred natives, and a pack of fierce dogs, including Balboa's own *Leoncico* (Little Lion).[8] The expedition encountered a litany of tribulations as they crossed the jungles of Darien: hostile natives, oppressive heat and humidity, implacable insects, horrible mountains, and many great rivers, desolate places and craggy rocks, wild beasts, and deadly diseases.[8] On September 25, 1513, Balboa reached a promontory (exact location is unknown) in Darien from where he could see a vast expanse of water, the South Sea. Four days later, in full armor and carrying a banner, he claimed the main, sea, and all adjacent lands to the dominion and empire of Castille.[8] Balboa's discovery of the South Sea gave tantalizing evidence that a narrow isthmus existed and that the elusive passage to the Orient was no longer doubtful but feasible. Search for a natural waterway continued, but only in Nicaragua was a possible route found through the San Juan River and Lake Nicaragua.

Charles V, grandson of King Ferdinand and heir to the Spanish throne in 1516, had a constant and keen interest in a waterway between the two oceans and in 1534 decreed a survey be made between the Chagres River and the South Sea.[9] Charles V sent a Portuguese navigator and naturalized Spaniard to look for the hidden strait. Ferdinand Magellan found one in 1520 at the tip of the continent and transited it in thirty-eight days.[10] However, the new strait was not only distant (about four thousand miles) but dangerous as well, due to storms and treacherous waters. Magellan gave the South Sea its present designation of Pacific Ocean, as he entered a welcoming calm sea following his ordeal in the strait that now bears his name. Even though Magellan's discovery was of little practical importance to those seeking a shorter route to India, it did confirm that America was a continent and not an island, and that the world was, indeed, round. (Although Magellan was killed in 1521 in the Philippines, one of his ships, the *Victoria*, manned by Juan Sebastián Elcano, returned to Spain to complete the first circumnavigation of the globe.)

In 1534, Charles V instructed the governor of the Panama region to make the Chagres River navigable and authorized him to spend up to a thousand golden pesos for that purpose.[9] A second, more specific order authorized and commanded exploration of the region, and enabled a commission of experts to report on whatever was necessary to excavate a waterway between the Chagres River and the South Sea. Furthermore, it requested information on problems caused by tides, elevations of the land, cost in money of the project, number of men needed, and time required for completion.[11] The response to the King was far from encouraging and admonished that "all the gold in the world would not suffice for its execution . . . " Charles V, nevertheless, remained interested but unable to further pursue these pretensions due to European wars during the last few years of his reign, which he abdicated in 1556. His son, Phillip II, succeeded him as King of Spain but not as an enthusiastic follower of his father's interest in building an isthmian waterway. Perhaps fueled by Gomara's flattery that "for a King of Castille, few things are impossible . . . " he tolerated a few proposals but nothing tangible in this regard resulted during his forty-two year reign.[11] A Jesuit priest who proclaimed such an enterprise to be impossible, may have dampened whatever enthusiasm the king, a devout Catholic, may have had for the project:

> I believe that no human power is capable of tearing down the strong and impenetrable mountain that God placed between the two seas, with hills and rocky crags able to withstand the fury of the seas on either side. And even if it were possible for men to do it I believe it would be very reasonable to expect punishment from Heaven for wishing to improve the works that the Maker, with sublime prudence and forethought, ordered in the fabric of this world.[12]

Although several enterprising minds obtained concessions for the study or building of an interoceanic canal, little if anything was accomplished despite the pressing need for a more efficient route between the two oceans. The conquest of Peru required the transfer of vast cargoes of gold and silver bullion across the isthmus for shipment to Spain.[13] For this purpose the first trans-isthmian route was established from Panama on the Pacific coast to Nombre de Dios on the Atlantic coast. This pathway, known as the *Camino Real* (Royal Road), was marked by a line of posts extending for about ninety miles.[9] By 1519, the road was paved with stones to facilitate the transport of precious goods and merchandise by mules and porters for safe storage at the customs house in Porto Bello until the Spanish treasure fleet arrived. This semestral event was an open invitation for the Caribbean corsairs to plunder the coveted loot. Among these, Francis Drake, Henry Morgan, and John Hawkins were repeatedly successful despite increasingly daunting fortresses constructed to guard the Spanish Main.[14]

Gold was discovered in California in 1848 and, once again, a more practical transit route across the isthmus became a necessity. This revived interest in the canal project but a more immediate and practical means of transportation meant the financing and construction of an isthmian railroad. William Aspinwall, Henry Chauncey, and John Stephens (of earlier fame as explorer of Maya ruins in Yucatan) obtained permission from the government of New Granada (Colombia) to build a railway and work was begun in August 1850.[15] Although it was said that construction of the railroad exacted a human life for each railroad tie laid across the forty-seven mile stretch across the isthmus, this was most likely an exaggeration. Laborers were difficult to obtain and the work faltered for almost a year. The Irish workers were unable to endure the effects of the climate and their numbers were decimated by sickness and death. Amassing a force of seven thousand men from Ireland, India, China, England, France,

Germany, and Austria, the company renewed the construction efforts.[15] However, of a thousand Chinese brought to the isthmus by the company along with their rice, tea, and sufficient quantities of opium to last for several months, scarcely a month after their arrival, the entire body became affected by a melancholic, suicidal tendency and scores of them ended their unhappy existence by their own hands.[15] The advent of the rainy season brought sickness, caused by exposure to the incessant rains, working waist-deep in the water, and an atmosphere saturated with "malarious poison."[15] Those who were not hospitalized deserted, frightened by the fevers or attracted by the higher wages in California. On the 27th of January, 1855, at midnight, in darkness and battered by rain, the last rail was laid, and on the following day a locomotive passed from ocean to ocean.[15] The total cost of the construction of the Panama Railroad was $8 million and the loss of lives remains speculative.

As the United States emerged as an economic and military power at the dawn of the twentieth century, the importance of building a transcontinental waterway became more obvious.

Panama was founded in 1519 and granted status as a city (*muy noble y leal ciudad*) by Charles V in 1581.[16] The name Panama, according to early reports, meant a place of fishermen or abounding with fish.[17,18] Other interpretations were a place of many butterflies, the name of a *cacique* (Indian chief), and of a large indigenous tree (*Sterculia apetala*).[19] Despite its obscure etymological origin, Panama was recognized as the first continental city to be founded by Europeans in the New World.[18]

Before news of Balboa's momentous discovery reached Spain, King Ferdinand had christened Panama (including the region extending from Honduras to Darien) *Castilla del Oro* (Golden Castille) and appointed an elderly aristocrat by the name of Pedro Arias de Ávila (Pedrarias) as governor.[20,21] The cruel and ambitious Pedrarias mounted a personal vendetta against Balboa, which eventually resulted in unfounded charges of treason and the execution of the *conquistador* in Acla, Panama, on an ignominious day in January 1517.[22]

Pedrarias had recruited about two thousand *hidalgos* and "distinguished men" to settle Panama.[23] The *hidalgos*, mostly soldiers of fortune attracted by prospects of a leisurely life of wealth and splendor on rich plantations manned by readily available slaves, were unprepared for the health conditions awaiting them when they arrived on the isthmus in 1514. "Being in a very wet country of swamps and overflowed land from which dense and sickly vapors rise, the men began to die and there died two thirds of them."[24] Another casualty was Francis Drake, the famous

English privateer who repeatedly sacked the Spanish Main and claimed vessels, riches, and slaves for the English crown. Drake met his fate on January 28, 1596, in the form of a fever and dysentery, and was buried in a lead casket off the coast of Porto Bello in Panama.[25] An occasional and daring traveler alighting on the isthmus would mostly corroborate the dire health conditions on the isthmus and Panama became synonymous with pestilence and death.[26] The lesson learned from history was that, notwithstanding valor and ambition, tropical diseases were the deadly enemy and the few who dared to challenge them would pay the ultimate price.

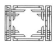

The success of the French in opening a waterway between the Mediterranean and the Red Sea in 1865 gave impetus to the idea of achieving a similar triumph in the American continent. Ferdinand de Lesseps surmounted the political and financial obstacles that obstructed the Suez enterprise and, as a result, *le grand français* became the toast of the world. Although already in his seventies, de Lesseps never lacked the enthusiasm or confidence necessary to tackle another seemingly impossible job.[27] Neither did he, at age sixty-four, lack the manly vigor to marry a much younger woman, Louise-Hélène Autard de Bragard (then only twenty), who bore him twelve additional children. The youngest child would be born in 1885 when de Lesseps was eighty. This charismatic figure became convinced that his next role was to give France the glory of uniting the Atlantic and Pacific Oceans. In 1879 he convened in Paris many of the world's engineering experts at the International Congress for the Studies of the Interoceanic Canal and ably led the discussions.[28] As expected, the delegates agreed with de Lesseps that the best route for the proposed waterway was in Panama. He believed that a sea-level canal could be built more expeditiously than one with multiple locks. Although enthusiasm was lacking among investors for funding the new venture, de Lesseps convinced the cautious and the incredulous that building a canal in Panama would be an easier task than it had been at Suez.

De Lesseps arrived on the isthmus on December 30, 1879, and charmed everyone with his enthusiasm and energy.[29] Ferdinande, his daughter, gave the first *coup de pioche* (strike of the pick-axe) and formally initiated the digging of the Panama Canal.[30] The world watched in anticipation for another engineering triumph by de Lesseps. Death and failure, however, awaited the French on the isthmus. Of thirty French engineers who arrived in Panama in October 1886, thirteen died within a month.[31] More poignant was the tragedy suffered by the general director of works of the French company, Jules Dingler, who buried his wife, a son, a daughter, and her fiancé in Panama from the malignant fevers.[32] After ten years of what would be described as the French debacle, the French abandoned the enterprise and transferred the equipment and buildings to the Americans on May 4, 1904, for a lump sum of $40 million.[33] Although the subsequent scandal uncovered the poor administration and debauchery of the French enterprise, there was little to criticize about their engineering and health planning efforts. De Lesseps and his engineers came to realize that to surmount the highest point of the intercontinental divide in the planned route (Culebra cut) a lock system would be necessary, and they discarded the sea-level canal plans. However, the French capitulated after an investment of $287 million and an estimated loss of 22,000 lives.[34,35] The real enemy was not poor judgment or corruption, but disease in the form of two deadly maladies: malaria and yellow fever.

5

Lure of Panama

Arthur Richards arrived in Panama in May 1904 and spent the next five years working as an engineer for the Isthmian Canal Commission. Sixty years later, he recalled the place (the Canal Zone) where he "went to work, live and suffer":[1]

> The most unattractive spot of land in the western hemisphere. It was a stretch of snake-infested, insect-ridden jungle between the Atlantic and Pacific about fifty miles long and ten miles wide, landscaped with bottomless swamps and mud flats, crossed by the lowest mountains between the Americas; a land of torrential rains which made floods forty feet deep in many gullies, and a wet season extending from about the 4th of July to Christmas, each and every year.
>
> Mosquitoes swarmed down upon both man and beast, omnivorous ants of many kinds could strip a garden, a tree, or even you, in a very short time. Ticks, redbugs and sand flys [sic] gnawing under the skin were a pestilence. Tarantulas, scorpions and poisonous snakes were everywhere, especially in the rainy season.
>
> And alligators, iguan[a]s, lizards unlimited, bees of many stings, tapirs, and yellow fever. Also flying cockroaches, bugs and insects of very many descriptions, with the sultry, hot, humid, wet and moldy atmosphere within your domicile.[1]

Despite such negative experiences and an established reputation as a nidus of pestilence, Panama nevertheless remained an attractive destination for many who sought better wages, a different way of life, or participation in one of the world's greatest engineering feats. Much as de Lesseps had attracted the funding and manpower necessary to launch the failed French transoceanic canal enterprise two decades earlier, so did Theodore Roosevelt capitalize on the American dream and inspire the young, strong, and visionary to help him "dig the big ditch."

The United States Civil Service Commission announced opportunities for employment in Panama in the latter part of 1904.[2] Nearly five thousand applications were received in Washington, D.C., in response to the announcement. Applicants included 1,198 office clerks, 1,061 skilled laborers, 1,044 engineers, and 266 book keepers.[3] In addition to the basic requirements of "being physically sound and in good health," candidates for employment were required to take an examination to be held on January 18, 1905, at any one of the 184 cities throughout the country "at which civil-services examinations [were] regularly held."[2]

The *Journal of the American Medical Association* announced on December 17, 1905, opportunities for employment in Panama for the positions of surgeons, physicians, pharmacists, hospital internes, and trained nurses.[2] As a result, applications were received from 285 doctors, 85 pharmacists, and 68 trained nurses.[3]

The required examination for physician applicants consisted of letter writing, anatomy, therapeutics, bacteriology and hygiene, obstetrics and gynecology (five per cent each); physical diagnosis, including questions relating to tropical diseases (twenty-five per cent); general pathology and practice, including questions relating to tropical diseases (twenty-five per cent); and practical experience (twenty-five per cent).[2] Special credit was given to applicants who had experience in the treatment of tropical diseases.

Salaries offered for physicians were $150, $200, and $250 per month, depending upon qualifications and experience. Other benefits included free transportation from New York, New Orleans, or San Francisco (and return transportation on completion of satisfactory service); free housing; and free "medical attendance, medicines, and care at hospitals when sick." Each employee was allowed six weeks' leave of absence annually on full pay, and transportation for him and members of his family at special rates of $25 between New York or New Orleans and Panama or $75 between San Francisco and Panama.[2]

A "final rigid" physical examination by one of the commission's doctors was an indispensable requirement for all appointees.[4] Grounds for rejection or dismissal from the service included diseases such as rupture, weak lungs or heart, venereal diseases, varicocele, varicose veins, piles, epilepsy, chronic alcoholism, deformed limbs, loss of fingers, defective eyesight and hearing, and other "serious" bodily defects.[4]

If Darling was interested in applying for a position in Panama at the time the announcement was made, no records are available to indicate this. It is more likely that, if interested, he would have preferred to wait until after completion of his residency in pathology. Furthermore, he was at a disadvantage, since he had no experience with tropical diseases. All this would have made sense, except for the fact that Gorgas needed three physicians to work under his supervision at Ancon Hospital in Panama.

Gorgas turned to William Welch, his trusted and influential friend in Baltimore, for help.

On January 27, 1905, D. I. Murphy, Secretary of the Isthmian Canal Commission, addressed a brief letter to Welch, Dean of Johns Hopkins University Medical School, asking him to recommend three physicians for the posts of "internes" on the medical service of the isthmus.[5] Five days later, Welch replied:

> In accordance with your letter of January 27th I have endeavored to find three physicians whom I could recommend for Internes on the medical service of the Isthmus. I have found only one whom I can recommend at present. At this time of the year it is difficult to secure young men for the most part for such service, as our graduates for the most part are occupying positions which they cannot relinquish before the summer or early autumn, and members of our graduating class who might be available will not be able to leave before June. If at that time there are such positions to fill, I could doubtless find suitable candidates to recommend. The candidate whom I can now recommend is Dr. S. T. Darling, at present pathological interne at the City Hospital in Baltimore. He is a graduate of the College of Physicians and Surgeons of this city, and has had a good experience in laboratory methods and work. I have had an interview with him. He is, I think, fitted for a higher position in the service than that of interne, and would be reluctant to take this position unless there was a fair prospect of promotion, provided his work and qualifications proved satisfactory. . . . My judgment would be to give such a man a trial, as in this way it may be possible to fill the higher positions with those already known to Dr. Gorgas and others in charge of the hospital and laboratory work.[6]

A week later, on February 8, 1905, Darling was offered a position as interne at Ancon Hospital and a corresponding salary of $50 per month, including board, lodging, and laundry, "providing you can get away at an early date."[7] Assurance for promotion was also given: "It is the intention of this Commission after a service of not less than one year to promote all Internes to the rank of Physician at $1500 per annum, providing their services have been satisfactory."[7] Four days later, Darling replied:

> I accept the offer of the position of Interne upon the Isthmus of Panama. I shall be able to leave Feb. 21. Do you require any special form of certification of physical fitness? Can you favor me with any information regarding clothing etc. required at the Isthmus as to the character and quantity and whether it must be purchased before leaving or can be obtained there?[8]

In this brief correspondence, Darling made no mention of his plans to marry before departing for Panama. His reticence may have been due, at least in part, by the Isthmian Canal Commission's requirement that new employees should work for eight months before bringing their spouses and family to Panama. Family living quarters were not readily available during the first few years of canal construction.[9] The commission also thought it wise to allow time for new employees to acclimatize and make certain they intended to remain for extended periods before bringing their families to Panama. Another possible reason for Darling's failure to report his status was the abruptness of his decision to marry.

On February 20, 1905, two days after his wedding to Nannyrle Llewellyn, Darling departed from New York aboard one of the Panama Railroad Line steamships which regularly carried freight and passengers weekly between ports in the United States and Colon, Panama. These ships were the *Alliança*, *Uranga*, *Advance*, *Yucatan*, and *Finance*, one of which left New York on Tuesdays at one p.m. from Pier Fifty-seven at the end of Thirty-seventh and West North River Street.[10] Advertisements in the local Panama newspapers described the vessels as "equipped with electric lights and all modern conveniences, offering the passengers everything required for their safety and comfort."[10] Each ship had on board a physician, a steward, interpreters for French and Spanish travelers, and first class cuisine."[10] The regular tariff for travel from Colon to New York was $85 to $100 for cabin and $90 for deck accommodations. Darling traveled as a guest of his new employer, the Isthmian Canal Commission.[10]

Henry Carter, Chief Quarantine Officer for the Isthmian Canal Commission, accompanied Darling during the trip from New York to Panama. Carter was also responsible for the organization, management, and personnel of the Canal Zone hospital system.[11] Carter, who was directed by Gorgas to interview Darling in Baltimore, was reportedly "charmed to find so interesting and promising a young man to add to the medical staff of the isthmus."[11,12] Although Darling was qualified for a better position than that of intern, Carter promised that he would be promoted quickly and according to his demonstrated abilities, once he assumed his post in Panama. Carter kept his part of the bargain and Darling recompensed his employer manifold by becoming the foremost scientific contributor to the sanitation effort in Panama.[13]

Carter's efforts to entice Darling to come to Panama were facilitated by his reputation as an expert in yellow fever. His epidemiological studies helped to convince Walter Reed of the possible role of the mosquito as vector for yellow fever in Cuba. Carter had described in a seminal paper a two-week period of "extrinsic" incubation between the appearance of the initial case of yellow fever and subsequent victims in the same household, suggesting the presence of an intermediate host, such as the mosquito which Finlay had proposed almost twenty years earlier.[14,15]

Reed and members of the U.S. Fourth Yellow Fever Board carried out human inoculations which proved the mosquito-vector hypothesis and allowed William Gorgas to eradicate yellow fever from Havana for the first time in one hundred and fifty years.[16] Following the unprecedented success of Gorgas' sanitation program in Cuba, Theodore Roosevelt realized that building an American isthmian canal would require a similar program and protection of the workers from yellow fever and malaria. His appointment of Gorgas to head the sanitation effort in Panama was a logical choice. Carter, along with Joseph Le Prince, Chief Sanitary Inspector of the Isthmian Canal Commission, completed the triumvirate of experts in charge of making the Canal Zone a salubrious place to live and work.

William Gorgas, Henry Carter, and Joseph Le Prince were experts in the public health aspects of yellow fever and malaria control.[14,17,18] Each one had made important contributions to assure the control of these diseases in endemic regions such as the South and Cuba. But none of them were true scientists in the strict definition of the word. Rather than "thinkers," they were "doers" and they had to have the scientific information on hand before they could proceed effectively. Gorgas, for example, refused to accept the important role of the mosquito in the transmission of yellow fever, even after Finlay had discussed this with him for several years.[17] Gorgas believed that sanitation meant the elimination of filth. Despite his efforts to clean Havana by removing trash, cleaning the streets, providing potable water, and reducing sewage, the toll from yellow fever worsened. At this point he was dismayed by the lack of success from his sanitation campaign in Havana. Only after Reed and his colleagues were able to demonstrate by careful human experiments that *Culex* (renamed *Stegomyia* and later *Aedes*) mosquitoes transmitted yellow fever did Gorgas add mosquito-control measures to his sanitation program.[17] Carter was an epidemiologist who made careful observations of the appearance and course of public health ailments such as yellow fever and malaria. His epidemiological studies in Orwood and Taylor, Mississippi, supported Finlay's hypothesis and raised the possibility that mosquitoes and not miasmas were responsible for these tropical scourges.[14] Le Prince was the warrior who, given the identity and location of the mosquito enemy, was able to mount an all-out attack with an army of inspectors and laborers using sulphur and pyrethrum to fumigate houses and spreading oil to kill mosquito larvae breeding in stagnant water.[18] What was Darling's role in this important war, a war lost by the French and now facing the American effort in Panama?

Carter's conversations with his new recruit during the trip to Panama must have given him evidence for the missing piece of the puzzle. What was needed to complement the sanitation team was a "laboratory man" who not only had the knowledge required to run effectively a hospital laboratory, perform autopsies, and examine surgical specimens to aid in the diagnosis of diseases, but also a scientist who would investigate unforeseen problems as these would arise during the construction of the canal and apply the scientific methods necessary to solve them. Carter undoubtedly recognized in Darling a scientific mind who would join in the impending fray to conquer tropical diseases in Panama. Carter's delight in finding such a promising young man would be more than justified in the ensuing decade as Darling assumed within two years the important post of chief of the Board of Health Laboratories.[11]

At this juncture in his life, Darling was thirty-two years old, mature, and confident in his abilities. Yet, in a period of less than one week, he had chosen a companion for the rest of his life and cast his lot with a team of visionaries. As Darling sailed aboard a company steamship for Panama, he must have reflected on recent events and wondered if he had made the right choices. After a long journey of uncertainty and preparation, he was now well on his way across the Caribbean to meet his destiny in Panama. Was it the lure of the tropics and the challenge of exotic and deadly diseases, or was it the prospect of participating in one of the world's greatest engineering works by contributing to the sanitation effort as part of the American confidence and know-how to achieve what the French had been unable to do, or was it personal ambition to join Gorgas, the hero of Havana, and share the future accolades given to the man responsible for defeating yellow fever and malaria that attracted him to Panama? We have no answers to any these intriguing questions.

Eight days after sailing from New York City on a Panama Railroad Steamship Line vessel, Darling and Carter arrived in Colon on February 28, 1905, at the Atlantic terminus of the isthmus of Panama. Escorted by Carter, the transfer of baggage and personal belongings by porters to the railroad station a few blocks away, was expected to be prompt and efficient. The train scheduled four trips daily from Colon to Ancon on the Pacific side, leaving at 6:45 a.m., 8 a.m., 12:45 p.m. and 4 p.m. The first class passenger trains ran every day at 8 a.m. and 4 p.m. The train journey from Colon to Panama City spanned forty-seven miles, took two hours and twenty minutes, and passed by twenty-seven stations — some with exotic names such as *Ahorca Lagarto* (Hang Alligator), *Bailamonos* (Dances with Monkeys), *Bohio* (Native Hut), *Culebra* (Snake), *Empire*, *Gatun, Lion Hill, Mamei* (a tropical fruit), and *Matachin*.[19]

The luxurious vegetation and exiguous living conditions of the natives in a tropical environment were soon apparent as the passenger train traversed the isthmus of Panama. Darling may have felt rejuvenated as he recalled the severe winter conditions he had just left behind in Baltimore.[20] The distinction between winter and summer was much less stark in Panama, where the average daily temperature did not fluctuate much throughout the year. The only palpable change in the weather was the presence or absence of abundant rain. The months of December, January, February, and March represented the dry season or "summer," while the rest of the year was the wet season or "winter." To someone arriving in February to Panama for the first time from northern latitudes, the climate was a most welcome change. The heat and the humidity could be regarded as better than freezing weather. However, in a few months the rainy season would start and the skies would open with torrential downpours that persisted for several days. It was preferable to arrive in Panama before the rains began and allow some time to better acclimatize to the tropics. The rainfall records for February 1905 showed no measurable rain on the Pacific side (La Boca) and only 1.13 inches of rain on the Atlantic side (Cristobal).[21] By May 1905, the amount of rainfall would rise to 22.96 inches on the Atlantic and 3.16 inches on the Pacific terminals. The total yearly amount of rain recorded for the previous year was 126.9 inches in Cristobal and 62.42 inches in La Boca.[21]

The city of Colon (previously known as Aspinwall, in honor of William Aspinwall, one of the builders of the Panama Railroad) was the main port terminus on the Atlantic side of the isthmus of Panama. It had little of interest to offer the newcomer and already had a bad reputation as unclean and unhealthy.[22] Passengers from the steamships arriving in Colon were usually whisked away quickly to the railroad depot for the trip to Panama City on the Pacific side.

Once aboard the train, the passengers usually waited with eager anticipation the whistle from the steam locomotive engineer signaling the start of the trip. Excitement increased as the train left Colon and the landscape changed. A third of a mile later brought into view the swamps commonly blamed for the poisonous vapors or *miasmas* that caused disease among the inhabitants of Colon. The swamps were lined with dense mangrove bushes whose branches and roots interlaced into an impassable network of dense vegetation.[22] About a mile further appeared Mount Hope, site of the general cemetery of Colon and final resting place for many of the victims from malaria and yellow fever. Near Mindi, the traveler encountered many varieties of palm trees as well as some cultivation of land with bananas, plantains, corn, and sugar cane. About five miles south of Gatun was the infamous Black Swamp (at places 185 feet deep) responsible for numerous sinkings and displacements of the railroad.[23] After seven miles of swamp land, the train arrived at Gatun Station located on the eastern bank of the Chagres River. Although only about fifty yards wide in the summer, this mighty waterway was to later become a major challenge to the engineers in charge of the construction of the Panama Canal. How to diverge its waters during the rainy season would occupy a good deal of their time and effort. A few hundred yards later, the train crossed over the Gatun River on an iron bridge about one hundred feet in span. Ahorca Lagarto was the next station and now the swamps were replaced by forests with large trees, some of which were a hundred feet tall and used by the natives to make canoes for transportation of people and goods over the rivers.[22]

The train followed the course of the Chagres for a while and then arrived at the Frijoles station. A display of colorful flowers here greeted the passengers, particularly the scarlet passion flower, and many varieties of birds including *oropendolas* (basket-weavers), parrots, toucans, and hummingbirds. Among the many varieties of indigenous animals the passengers might see were monkeys, opossums, ant-eaters, peccaries, sloths, and deer; but the most unusual was the *iguana*. This lizard, from three to six feet in length, was considered a local delicacy and sought avidly for its delicate-tasting meat and eggs — a thought that usually made newcomers cringe in disgust.

After Frijoles, the mighty Chagres was once again encountered and crossed this time at Barbacoas on a 625-foot iron bridge. Half a mile from the bridge came San Pablo Station, followed by Mamei, Gorgona, and Matachin. Here the stately royal palms (*Oredoxa regia*) dominated the landscape. Brought from Cuba in the 1850s, these beautiful palms often reached a height of sixty feet and Darling would encounter them again later that day as he entered the garden-like landscaped grounds of Ancon Hospital. Large *ceiba* trees lined the shores of the Obispo River, the largest tributary of the Chagres. Now followed a luxurious woodland cultivated with delicious native fruit trees: *mango, zapote, nispero,* and *guava.* From there the train ascended for about three miles until it reached Empire Station and Summit, the highest elevation on the railway. Nearby, a small settlement named Culebra (Snake) marked where the railroad ended in 1854 and passengers had to be carried on mules the remaining twelve miles before reaching Panama City. The last stretch offered the most profuse and gorgeous vegetation, with thick and tall tress named *ceiba, cedro,* and *malvicino.* The incessant chatting of hordes of green parakeets, clouds of gigantic blue (*Morpho*) moths, and the colorful plumage of songbirds, added to the exuberant growth of flowers and trees. Finally, after passing by some cocoa tree groves, a view of Ancon hill emerged, announcing the end of the transcontinental trip.[22]

Ancon hill stood at 660 feet as a green sentinel overlooking the Bay of Panama. Its name was derived from the Spanish term *ancón* which means cove or inlet (from the Latin *anconeus* or elbow); other interpretations are roadstead or anchorage.[24] The French had selected this site to build their main hospital on the Pacific side of the isthmus, as it was favored by refreshing ocean breezes which not only helped to make the tropical heat more bearable but, more importantly, ventilated the buildings with "healthy air" to counteract the dreaded miasmas blamed for causing malaria and yellow fever. Darling may have given Ancon hill a long and pensive look, as this was now his designated home and place of work.

As the train came to a stop at the Pacific terminus of Panama, Darling and Carter transferred their luggage to a horse-driven car sent by the hospital to greet them. Shortly afterwards, the two men crossed the entrance of the hospital grounds, at the foot of Ancon hill, and advanced along the winding La Boca Road, flanked at each side by wooden buildings set on stone pillars — a total of some thirty buildings constructed originally by the French during their futile attempt to dig a sea-level canal in Panama. Rows of royal palms also lined the road and thousands of flowering shrubs adorned the hospital grounds. Near the top of the hill, Carter showed Darling his new living quarters. Even though Darling had been used to frugal living conditions in Baltimore, he may have been surprised by what greeted him at the end of the long journey. Although accommodations may have been improved in the interim, an employee from Oelwein, Iowa, arriving in 1907, recalled:

> The first quarters assigned to me after my arrival on the Isthmus, July 1, 1904, were in an empty ward at Ancon Hospital, which lies just outside Panama city. There were as near as I can recollect about thirty single iron beds of French make, ranged hospital style, a row on each side of the room. Our conveniences there were far from deluxe. One single straight-backed chair was made to do duty for the entire bunch, and this useful article was generally found in the morning alongside the bed of the one who was last in at night. We had but one lamp, and this was usually empty. There were no mirrors, and the fortunate possessor of an individual looking glass was to be envied. Some combed their hair and shaved with the aid of the swinging glass windows backed up against the wall. There were but two washstands for all of us, but thanks to the French, there were a couple of pretty decent shower baths.[25]

At a starting salary of $50 a month, Darling was to be assigned (according to regulations) only a square foot of living quarters per dollar of monthly salary.[26] But thanks to his hospital contract and Carter's administrative influence, Darling was probably spared such sparse domiciliary constraints.

The view from Ancon hill more than compensated for any temporary discomforts the recently arrived traveler may have experienced. Marie Gorgas, Colonel Gorgas' wife, recalled this magical experience:

> There is an alluring something about a night in the tropics . . . It was a beautiful and starry evening. Beyond stretched the great Pacific, the dotted islands in the distance dimly seen in the misty moonlight, every place teeming with the history of the departed glory and vast enterprise . . . The road was bordered by a row of stately royal palms,

planted by the French some fifteen years before. Beyond a stretch of green valley the hills and mountains were seen emerging from the heavy mist which often envelops them by night. The sun rising from the Pacific, a strange phenomenon, and the rays gave a jeweled appearance to the dew-soaked plants and the leaves of the trees.[27]

Gorgas himself also described in detail the building (previously known as the St. Charles yellow fever ward and reputedly the site where more people had died from yellow fever than any other building then standing in the world) where he and Carter lived with their families during the first few years in Panama:[28]

> This building was about the center of the hospital grounds, and occu-
> pied a most attractive site. It was situated about two hundred feet up
> the side of the mountain looking to the northeast. A macadam road
> skirted the building on the down side, and the masonry retaining-wall
> supported this road on the lower side. Between the border of the road
> and the retaining wall was a superb row of stately royal palms. Behind
> the building rose the mountain for four hundred feet, covered by a
> perfectly impenetrable tropical forest, giving to the picture the
> deepest possible dark green background. The view to the north and
> east extended for miles and miles. To the east, over the bay of
> Panama, dotted with its forest-clad islands, I have many times
> watched from the gallery of this building that anomaly, so generally
> remarked in Panama, the sun rising from the Pacific. To the north
> and east were in view the various ranges of the Andean mountains
> which make up the backbone of the Isthmus. From this point, four
> or five ranges of mountains could be seen, and in the evening, when
> the sun was setting behind the Ancon mountain at one's back, the
> play of colors was superb; light green upon the nearer ranges,
> changing into deep azure upon the further ranges, with the mountain
> tops and higher valleys covered here and there with a robe of white
> mist.[29]

Darling's first impressions of Panama, Ancon, or Ancon Hospital are not recorded in available documents. Panama's verdant jungle, colorful flowers, and brightly plumaged birds must have pleased him. Yet he knew that behind nature's beautiful façade lurched insects and parasites capable of decimating human populations. A combination of nervous anticipation and mature confidence in his abilities to face whatever challenges lay ahead may have ultimately prevailed as he gazed at Ancon Hospital and pondered about his future on the isthmus of Panama.

6

Ancon Hospital

Theodore Roosevelt recognized the important role that sanitation would play in the successful completion of an isthmian canal.[1] "I desire that every possible effort be made to protect our officers and workmen from the dangers of tropical and other diseases, which in the past have been so prevalent and destructive in Panama," he wrote to Secretary of War, William H. Taft, on May 9, 1904.[2] Roosevelt sought advice from prominent individuals and groups to help him designate the best qualified person to rid Panama of the tropical scourges responsible for the French debacle. The unanimous choice was William Gorgas of the U.S. Army.[3]

Gorgas, a man of impeccable credentials, had been recently promoted from major to colonel in recognition for his outstanding sanitation work in Havana. Although initially not an adherent to the yellow fever mosquito-vector hypothesis, he nevertheless implemented in February 1901 the recommendations promulgated by Walter Reed and the Fourth U.S. Army Yellow Fever Board.[4] Eight months after the introduction of mosquito-control measures, Gorgas eliminated yellow fever in Havana for the first time in one hundred and fifty years. This unprecedented achievement in public health elevated Reed and Gorgas to the status of medical heroes: Reed for carrying out the meticulous experiments that proved beyond doubt Finlay's mosquito-vector hypothesis, and Gorgas for the practical application of preventive measures that controlled the propagation of yellow fever in Havana.[5]

Gorgas made a preliminary visit to Panama in April 1904, to assess the magnitude of the sanitation problem that he would face and, among other things, to inspect the medical facilities abandoned by the French.[3] He was accompanied on this trip by John W. Ross, of the U.S. Navy, Louis A. La Garde, of the U.S. Army, and Cassius E. Gillette, of the Corps of Engineers.[6] Gorgas conducted a detailed inspection of the hospital facilities and concluded that, notwithstanding almost fifteen years of neglect and progressive deterioration from the relentless heat and humidity, most of the buildings were in fair condition and could be salvaged or repaired.[7]

The French first arrived in Panama to begin the construction of the sea-level canal in 1881, well aware of its reputation as one of the most insalubrious places on earth. Travelers to the isthmus had encountered the ravages of malaria and yellow fever and labeled both Colon and Panama City as pestholes.[8-10] Although Carlos J. Finlay, a Cuban physician educated in the United States, had proposed at about the same time (1881) the hypothesis that yellow fever was transmitted by a mosquito, few paid any attention to the insistence of this "mosquito man."[11] The common belief was that the locally prevalent fevers, including Panama fever, Chagres fever, and swamp fever, were caused by miasmas that resulted from putrefaction of vegetable and animal matter in nearby swamps and humid tropical soils.[12] In the evenings, gentle breezes would transport these "bad airs" to populated areas and render the inhabitants sick with malaria and other putrid fevers. As late as 1905, respected medical journals such as *Lancet* continued to expound on the poor salubrity due to the climate conditions and miasmas in Panama:

> Near the sea and along the greater part of the line of the projected canal, much of the land is low-lying swamp, the washings of the soil, full of vegetable remains, brought down by the rivers in their flood. For miles round the country reeks with exhalations from decomposing organic matter, and the deleterious effects of these emanations, considered not only as agencies of specific diseases but as unwholesome gases, are evident on all sides. All the physiological consequences of life in the tropics are found in exaggerated forms. The abnormal moisture of the atmosphere lessens evaporation from the skin and lungs, and this condition, in alliance with the continuous heat, readily induces languor, loss of appetite, depression of spirits and dullness of the entire nervous system, with consequent reduction of the pulse-rate, decrease in respiratory action, poverty of the blood, softness of the tissues, disorders of the kidney, stomach, and intestines, and a tendency towards congestion of the liver and spleen.[13]

The only effective remedies known at the time to combat miasmas were fresh air and cleanliness. Construction of homes and buildings was predicated on such preventive measures. Direct contact with the soil was avoided by placing stone or concrete pillars upon which the dwellings were erected and ventilation was enhanced by surrounding open windows and tall ceilings.

The French hospital system was designed to complement in every possible way the engineering effort needed to construct the isthmian canal. According to Gorgas, "The hospital built by them was well manned and equipped, and was a very much better institution than any hospital in America that I know of at the same period carried on by a firm or a corporation."[7]

The site selected for the construction of the main French hospital on the Pacific side was an eighty-acre tract of land known as *La Huerta de Galla*, located on the northeastern slopes of Ancon hill and favored by refreshing ocean breezes and spectacular views of the Panama bay.[14] A well-equipped, five-hundred bed hospital, *L'Hôpital Central du Panama*, completed after eighteen months of planning at a cost of $5,600,000 (although Gorgas gave a more conservative estimate of $400,000), was formally dedicated on September 17, 1882.[14] A smaller hospital was built on the Atlantic side in the city of Colon and a number of district and sub-district (rest camps) hospitals were distributed along the fifty-mile isthmus.[15]

The French hospital complex at Ancon consisted of one-story, wood-frame buildings of the pavilion type, surrounded by verandahs, and covered by roofs with Marseilles tiles, spaciously distributed over the terraced grounds and interconnected by walkways and loggias to facilitate traffic and protect visitors from the inclement weather.[12] In keeping with the current explanations for the causation of tropical diseases such as yellow fever and malaria as due to poisonous vapors that emanated from swamps and decomposing filth, the distribution and construction of the buildings favored spaciousness and good ventilation. Each patient ward measured 85×35 feet and accommodated only twenty-four patients, so that each bed was allocated a commendable twelve-hundred cubic feet of air space.[14]

The hospital entrance at the foot of Ancon hill led to a porter's lodge, a dispensary, and the bishop's residence.[14] A series of buildings then followed a winding road (known as La Boca Road) stretching for about a mile up to an elevation of one-hundred eighty feet above sea level. The buildings included, in addition to patient wards, servant halls, kitchens, a servant lodge, a chaplain lodge, a chapel, a school for orphaned children, and a residence for the Sisters of Charity.[14] Altogether, the complex consisted of some thirty buildings distributed in a "most beautiful and picturesque manner," among carefully prepared grounds adorned with all kinds of tropical shrubs and flowering plants.[7]

Gorgas returned to the United States to obtain $50,000 in essential medical supplies and personnel.[15] In June 1904, Gorgas again sailed for Panama on the S.S. *Alliança*, accompanied by the newly appointed members of the Medical Department: John W. Ross (U.S. Navy), Director of Hospitals; Henry R. Carter (U.S. Health and Marine Hospital Service), Chief Quarantine Officer; Major Louis A. La Garde (U.S. Army), Superintendent of Ancon Hospital; Captain Theodore Lyster, ophthalmologist; J. C. Perry, U.S. Public Health Service; C. C. Pierce, U.S. Public

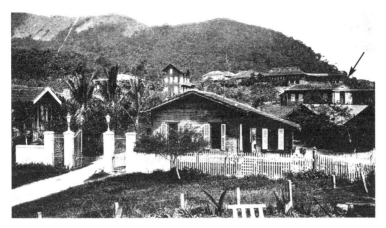

6.1 Ancon Hospital entrance, from a postcard by M. Espinoza dated 1905. Darling's laboratory (arrow) is located to the right and above the porter's lodge.

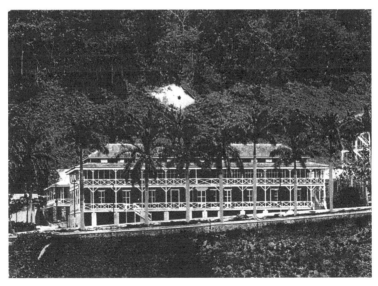

6.2 Ancon Hospital building. One of about thirty pavilion-type buildings erected on concrete pillars and surrounded by verandahs left by the French and repaired by the Americans in 1905, undated postcard.

Health Service; Joseph Le Prince, Chief Sanitary Inspector of the Canal Zone; Louis Balch, Health Officer of Panama; Major James Turtle; and Mary Eugenie Hibbard, director of nurses, and her two assistants, Mary C. Markham and A. McGowan, from Bellevue Hospital in New York.[15,16] They were joined a week later by A. B. Herrick, chief surgeon; Edward P. Beverly, assistant physician; A. I. Kendall, chief of laboratories; and Lloyd Nolan, assistant surgeon.

Gorgas' power of persuasion and influence were evident in the number and quality of these recruits, considering that most of them were already familiar with the tragic consequences suffered by those who had preceded them during the excavation period in Panama two decades before. Yellow fever had claimed the lives of most of the French corps of engineers brought by Ferdinand de Lesseps to the isthmus. Most heart-wrenching was the story of Jules Dingler, director-general of the French Canal Company, who refused to leave Panama despite the exodus that followed the path of destruction and death left by the tropical fevers. Within six months after his arrival, Dingler had lost his wife, a son, a daughter and her fiancé, to yellow fever.[17]

The Sisters of Charity of St. Vincent de Paul, wearing their traditional dark blue robes and white-winged bonnets, attended the sick at the French hospitals. Under the supervision of Mother Superior Marie Roleau, the sisters carried their duties with "compassion, cordiality, and devotion."[14] Although they were not trained nurses, the sisters took temperatures, made beds, changed linen, and attended wounds but were not allowed by their order to take pulses.[14] Among other duties was the beautification of the hospital grounds by planting many varieties of flowers and shrubs, some of which came from the French colonies in the South Pacific.[14]

Twenty-one of the initial group of twenty-four sisters who arrived in Panama to serve in the French hospitals died of tropical fevers — presumably yellow fever.[18] By 1887, only fourteen sisters remained to perform the hospital duties in Panama.[14] As the French company abandoned the canal project in 1889, the number of patients admitted to the hospitals decreased precipitously. The sisters tried to subsist with their meager income (they received five francs for each patient daily) but were forced to supplement revenues by selling flowers, fruits, and vegetables grown in the hospital grounds.[14]

Between 1889 and 1904, the sisters worked with Dr. Jean Pierre Lacroisade, the only French doctor to remain as an attendant at the hospital after the French departure, until doctors and nurses were recruited from the United States.[14] As better trained personnel began to arrive in Panama, the limited services of the sisters became dispensable. The remaining ailing and elderly sisters were asked by the Americans to vacate their living quarters to free needed space.[19] A letter was sent to the Governor complaining about this unfair treatment.[20] Despite apolo-

gies and promises for proper restitution, including payment of transportation costs to return the sisters to Colombia, El Salvador, and
France, the incident caused resentment among religious and political
leaders in Panama.[19,21] The prevalent sentiment in support of the sisters
was voiced by Gorgas, "they deserve[d] a great deal of credit for the
brave and successful struggle which they made in supplying the wants of
the sick entrusted to them."[22] A subsequent request for additional sisters
to be sent to Ancon Hospital as aids to the American nurses was respectfully declined by the head of the religious order community in
Maryland.[23]

The French surrendered their property and holdings, including the railroad and hospitals, to the Americans on May 4, 1904, and the first eighty
patients in the French registry were transferred to the care of Gorgas' team
of doctors and nurses.[24] The hospital buildings were repaired and
equipped with the first water and sewage systems, electricity, and laundry
facilities, at an initial cost of $50,000.[7]

On July 13, 1905, Governor George E. Davis officially changed the
name of *L'Hôpital Central du Panama* to *Ancon Hospital* and the first
patients were admitted two days later.[23] Before the end of the year, 1,174
patients were admitted to the Ancon facility and the wards were so
crowded that patients were refused admission every day.[23] A year later,
7,561 patients were admitted, treated, and discharged at Ancon
Hospital.[23] From July 15, 1905, to July 23, 1908, a total of 43,243
patients were treated at Ancon Hospital and it became the largest hospital
in the western hemisphere south of the United States capable of handling
any type of medical or surgical problem.[24,25]

Further repairs and renovations were necessary as the older facilities
deteriorated. Between 1904 and 1909, about half a million dollars was
spent on repairs and the hospital complex expanded to 96 buildings,
1,170 hospital beds, and a staff of 509.[23] A more detailed description of
Ancon Hospital was given by the Chief Sanitary Officer in 1908:

> In the reservation are 96 buildings, most of which are of frame
> construction and thoroughly screened. . . . Among them are 18 quar-
> ters for married employe[e]s, four quarters for nurses, one large
> building for bachelors, 47 wards in 32 buildings, and a chapel for
> Roman Catholics with a priest's house adjoining. . . .
>
> Of the 47 wards, 23 were for medical cases, 8 [for] surgical [cases],
> 3 [for] eye and ear [cases], one [for] isolation cases, one [for]
> tubercul[osis cases], and 11 [for the] insane. The wards are divided
> into sections of two wards each with a building between in which are

the kitchen, dining room, linen room and a room for personal effects of patients. The ward equipment includes white enamel iron beds (United States Army standard), with [horse] hair mattresses, hair and feather pillows; white enamel iron bedside tables with glass tops; medicine closets; linen closets; nurses' desk and chairs; and each ward is provided with lavatories, closets, shower and tub baths.

The tubercul[osis] ward is a two-story building . . . with a capacity of about twenty-five beds and four private rooms for special cases. The isolation building is a separate structure of six private rooms and two small wards, with baths, linen rooms and diet kitchens. In a small adjoining building is a morgue, with a special room for the sterilization of all infected clothing. . . .

The operating room . . . has a concrete floor and a floor space of 1400 square feet, and is well lighted from two sides and the roof. The equipment is thoroughly modern and complete, comprising operating tables, instrument cases, dressing and solution cases, and white enamel sinks. In the same building are a surgeon's office, dressing room, sterilizing room connected with a central steam plant, two dressing and instrument sterilizers with condensing water tanks, an anaesthetising [*sic*] room, and closets for surgical dressings and appliances. In order that emergency cases may be operated on at night the surgery is provided with special electric lighting facilities, which include a large stationary light, numerous stationary 16-[candle power] lights, and portable lights with reflectors. This building is easily accessible to the surgical wards, and patients are carried to and from it on hand litters. Surgical cases from private rooms in building further away are carried in the rubber tired ambulance.

Near the operating room is a building containing the library of reference books and many of the current medical magazines, consulting offices, waiting rooms, office of the resident chaplain, and the X-ray laboratory, where all sciagraphs [roentgenograms] are made and cases of injury or disease examined. . . .

The nurses' [quarters] consist of four buildings in which are dormitories, reading rooms, two large recreation rooms, and a library. The floor of each building was provided with modern lavatories and bathrooms. A ward of sick beds in a small building . . . is reserved for sick nurses. . . .

The main kitchen is provided with a large range, a sterilizer, in which all water used in the hospital was sterilized, and a steam cooking outfit which included coffee boilers, soup, and vegetable kettles. The ice box has a capacity of three thousand pounds of ice and a cold storage area of about fifty square feet, where a sufficient supply of fresh meat, butter and eggs was kept to provide for any emergency that may arise. Staple supplies are delivered three times a month . . . [while] cold storage supplies are delivered daily. . . .

A dairy of fifty-four cows provides about 130 gallons of milk daily at a net price of about thirty-two cents per gallon. . . . A poultry yard contains some two thousand hens.[24,26]

The excellent sanitation system, including the hospitals and dispensaries, initially devised by the French, was nevertheless insufficient to counteract the onslaught caused by tropical diseases, particularly from malaria and yellow fever. Lack of knowledge about the crucial role played by mosquitoes in the transmission of these diseases assured failure. According to available records, the French lost 22,189 personnel during the nine-year period from 1881 to 1889 of active excavation in Panama.[27] Of a total of 5,518 documented hospital deaths, 1,368 were from malaria and 1,026 from yellow fever.[22] Gorgas projected that an American working force subjected to similar morbidity and mortality rates during the construction of the isthmian canal, would have reached a staggering total of 78,000 deaths.[28]

The American personnel put their lives and trust in Gorgas, confident that he would be as successful in Panama against the yellow scourge as he had been in Cuba. However, none of them, including Gorgas, were prepared for the bureaucratic entanglements that awaited his efforts and threatened to defeat the sanitation plan.

The members of the Isthmian Canal Commission carried their mission from afar and had little knowledge of the prevailing health conditions in Panama.[29] Even worse, most of them did not believe the mosquito-vector hypothesis and soon began to respond accordingly to Gorgas' seemingly outlandish requests for materials and supplies. The chief engineer, Colonel George W. Goethals, objected to the mounting expenditures of the Department of Sanitation and once recriminated Gorgas that to exterminate each mosquito cost the government ten dollars. Gorgas replied, "But just think, one of those ten-dollar mosquitoes might bite you, and what a loss that would be to the country!"[30] The disbelief and intransigence that threatened to derail Gorgas' sanitation program was, however, beyond wry humor. Gorgas detailed his tribulations with Admiral Walker, chairman of the commission:

> Day after day I would go to . . . Admiral [Walker] with requisitions for various things needed and we would talk the matter over. He would always get on the subject (of economy). "Gorgas there is one thing certain: whether we build the canal or not we will leave things so fixed that those fellows up on the hill can't find anything in the shape of graft". After this he would take my requisition and stick it in a drawer where it would remain for an indefinite time.[31]

An initial requisition for eight tons of insect powder estimated by Gorgas to be needed for insect fumigation, resulted in "shock[ed] and surprise[d]" by the reviewing authorities, and was used to demonstrate the "wildness" of the estimates.[32] When the sanitary authorities urged more extensive preparations and larger expenditures, the commission thought of them as "visionary" and lost confidence in their sanitation plan. Yet, by the end of the first year of sanitation activities, one hundred and twenty tons of insect powder (100 tons of pyrethrum and 20 tons of sulphur), representing the whole supply of the United States for a year, had been used in Panama, or fifteen times the amount initially requested.[17,32]

Despite his patience and "imperturbability" during these frustrating encounters, Gorgas was unable to convince the members of the Isthmian Canal Commission of the soundness of his approach to the sanitation problem and the commission requested for his dismissal.[33] The American Medical Association was closely monitoring the situation and underscored the commission's disregard for the importance of sanitation by showing the disparity between the annual salaries of the chief engineer ($25,000), an administrative commissioner ($12,000), and the salary of the chief of sanitation officer ($7,500).[34] Secretary of State Taft entrusted Charles A. L. Reed, a surgeon from Cincinnati and former president of the American Medical Association, to confidentially investigate the precarious situation in Panama. Reed's report, which appeared (to Taft's consternation) in the widely-read *Journal of the American Medical Association* on March 11, 1905, vindicated Gorgas' methods and blamed the commission for the recent resurgence of yellow fever in Panama.[35] Although Gorgas remained in his post, he continued to be under the authority of the reorganized commission. Within eight months, in June 1905, the new commissioners once again requested that Gorgas, Carter, and those who believed with them in the mosquito theory, should be relieved and men with more practical views be appointed in their stead.[36] This time the request was endorsed by the Secretary of State Taft himself and forwarded to Roosevelt for executive action. Roosevelt consulted prominent medical leaders, including William Welch of Johns Hopkins, who assured him that Gorgas was the right man for the job. Alexander Lambert, the president's personal physician and a close friend, sternly admonished Roosevelt:

> You are facing one of the greatest decisions of your career. Upon what you decide depends whether or not you are going to get your canal. If you fall back on the old method of sanitation you will fail just as the French have failed. If you keep Gorgas and his ideas and let him make his campaign against the mosquito, then you get your canal.[37]

Roosevelt acquiesced and directed that every possible support and assistance be extended to the sanitary officials.[36] Gorgas was eventually promoted to equal membership in the commission and given full voting rights.[38]

Before the end of the year after his arrival, Gorgas turned to his colleagues as they surrounded an autopsy table and prophesied, "Take a good look at this man . . . for it's the last case of yellow fever you will ever see. There will never be any more deaths from this cause in Panama."[39] Except for an inconclusive case seen in Colon in May 1906, no further cases of yellow fever originating in Panama were documented thereafter.

Gorgas now turned his attention to other tropical diseases that threatened the well-being and stamina of the canal workers.[23] Particularly, malaria would prove to be an even more formidable health problem to the laborers than yellow fever. The sanitation measures that controlled yellow fever were relatively ineffectual against malaria.[40] In 1906, the number of hospital admissions for malaria reached 821 per thousand (21,795 cases among 26,500 laborers) and 233 employees died of malaria, for an annual death rate that exceeded even those recorded for French canal workers in any one of the years from 1888 to 1903.[41]

Quinine administration was predicated on a voluntary basis.[22] Known under the various designations of *Peruvian bark*, *Jesuit's bark*, *cascarilla*, and *cinchona bark*, quinine had demonstrated its efficacy against intermittent fevers for almost three hundred years.[42] Gorgas believed that if everybody took five grains of quinine daily, this would prevent the propagation of malaria in Panama.[22] Quinine "dispensers" were stationed along each district and laborers were allowed to chose among tablets, capsules, or quinine tonic (each ounce contained five grains of quinine). An educational campaign was waged and quinine tablets and tonic were placed on the tables of "eating-houses and messes" for voluntary consumption. The success of this campaign was measured by the maximum total number of doses given daily (forty thousand) and the average number of pounds of quinine given to employees yearly (2,600).[22,43] Gorgas noted that "a certain number of men" managed to throw their quinine tablets out of the dispensary window. An old turkey gobbler readily gobbled these up and "became so dissipated in this way that he finally developed quinin[e] amblyopia [blindness]."[22] Control of malaria required more than just prophylactic quinine administration and a detailed sanitation plan also was enforced.

The sanitation plan consisted of (1) segregation of patients in screened hospital wards and rooms; (2) fumigation to kill active mosquitoes; (3) drainage of all stagnant pools and waterholes by ditches; (4) spraying to kill mosquito larvae; and (5) rigid quarantine of ships arriving on the isthmus.[44] These measures had proved to be highly effective against the *Stegomyia* (now *Aedes egypti*) which transmitted yellow fever. But malaria was a recalcitrant enemy. The anopheles mosquito that carried malaria had different habitat and breeding practices, so that the sanitation plan was less effective against this hardy, vigorous, and highly-adaptable mosquito.[45] Gorgas was fortunate to have at his side able men such as Henry Carter, who had studied the epidemiology of yellow fever, and Joseph Le Prince, who knew more about mosquito control than anyone else in Panama.[46] However, it took a scientific approach to elucidate the morphological characteristics and susceptibility of different anopheline species to the malaria parasite and redirect the sanitation program based on a novel, more efficient, and economical concept of "species-control." This crucial information was provided by Darling and the Board of Health Laboratories.

7

Board of Health Laboratories

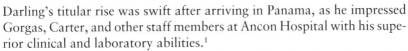

Darling's titular rise was swift after arriving in Panama, as he impressed Gorgas, Carter, and other staff members at Ancon Hospital with his superior clinical and laboratory abilities.[1]

Following his appointment as an "Interne" assigned to the medical wards at a salary of $50 per month on February 21, 1905, he was soon promoted to "Physician" on June 1, 1905, with a corresponding raise in salary to $125 per month. On July 1, 1905, he was appointed "Pathologist" at Colon Hospital (on the Atlantic side) at $200 per month, and to the temporary position of "Pathologist in charge of the Board of Health Laboratory" (in the absence of Arthur Kendall, first appointed director of the laboratory).[1,2] On October 5, 1906, Darling was named "Chief of the Board of Health Laboratory" at a monthly salary of $333.33 and remained in that capacity until his resignation on May 23, 1915.[1] His service records in Panama showed an additional salary increase on September 1, 1909, to $375 per month.[1] Thus, within a period of less than twenty months, Darling was promoted from interne to chief of the Board of Health Laboratory. Darling had proved his worth convincingly and Carter had kept his promise by increasing his salary accordingly.

The Board of Health had been created in agreement with the Panamanian authorities so that all matters pertaining to the health and sanitation of the Canal Zone, particularly relating to the terminal cities of Panama City on the Pacific and Colon on the Atlantic, would be under the responsibility of the Americans.[3] The Board consisted of four members: the Chief Sanitary Officer, the Director of the Hospitals, the Chief Quarantine Officer, and the Chief Sanitary Inspector of the Canal Zone.[3]

Bacteriological and chemical examinations of water and milk samples, as well as patient diagnostic tests, required support from a laboratory facility. On June 14, 1905, a resolution by the Executive Committee of the Isthmian Canal Commission established a laboratory under the Health Department, appropriately named the Board of Health Laboratories.[4] The following personnel and corresponding annual salaries were also authorized: chief of the laboratory, $4,000; pathologist, $3,000; bacteriologist, $3,000; and two attendants with quarters and laundry, $600 each.[4] Darling's initial staff included George V. Ridley, pathologist; Ralph W. Nauss, interne (chemistry); Paul M. Carpenter and Harry O'Connor, laboratory assistants (see Appendix D: Personnel and Staff, Board of Health Laboratories).[4] Although not listed among these, Alleyne became Darling's trusted autopsy assistant (Darling abhorred the term *deaner*) and over the following forty years the skilled Jamaican native would assist in more than 15,000 post-mortem examinations performed at Ancon (later Gorgas) Hospital.[5]

The Board of Health Laboratories were responsible for all the pathological, toxicological, and research work; the chemical and bacteriological analyses of water from streams, reservoirs, condensers, delivery carts, and faucets; the chemical analyses of food, soils, rock, silt, and such supplies for canal work as chemicals, oils, lubricants, and explosives.[6] Many of these analyses were related to the technical and engineering aspects of the canal operation. Other tests were part of the routine and specialized services necessary for patient care at hospitals.

Undaunted by what initially may have seemed an impossible task, Darling took his escalating duties with enthusiasm and rose to the challenge. The many functions of the laboratory soon required additional space and one of the old French buildings which housed the pharmacy was handed over to Darling.[7] The building was a one-story, wooden-frame structure, topped by a roof made of native red tile, with a series of rooms built around a paved central court-yard.[2,7] The structure stood at the foot of Ancon hill, immediately after the main entrance to the hospital grounds, on the right (east) side of La Boca road, and only a short walk from Darling's living quarters.[7] Darling used the front rooms for laboratory space and the rear housed the morgue and autopsy room.[7] A small detached building adjacent to the laboratory housed the mortuary and crematory services. Any American who died while employed in Panama was guaranteed that the body would be embalmed and shipped back to the United States at the expense of the Commission.[8]

The Board of Health Laboratories remained the locus of Darling's prodigious activities from 1906 to 1915. Several visitors had the opportunity to observe Darling in his laboratory:

> In a small, unpretentious building, Dr. Darling carries on his multifarious duties and researches . . . his laboratory . . . examines

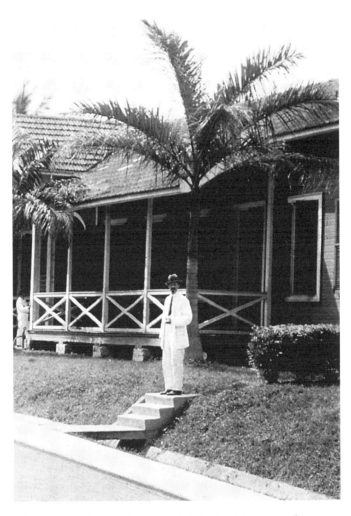

7.1 Darling standing outside the Board of Health Laboratories in Ancon, undated. Reproduced with permission, courtesy of Mrs. Virginia E. Stich.

everything from throat swabs for diphtheria to gear greases from engines. Fire clay and malignant tumors are equally seen for examination. Apart from all this work, which although routine, is of the highest value to the community, Dr. Darling has found time to carry on research work on a number of important subjects.[9]

Another visitor reported:

One of the most important sections of the Isthmian Canal Commission is the laboratory of the Board of Health, forming part of the department of sanitation, in charge of Samuel T. Darling, M.D., chief of the laboratory. Through the courtesy of Dr. Darling I was permitted to observe the methods of work carried on in the laboratory, which made my visit full of interest. The equipment of the laboratory is complete, the Government, through the Canal Commission, providing all that is necessary to conduct the important work of this department. The routine work in the laboratory includes examinations, pathological and bacteriological, for the hospitals, autopsies, surgical pathological studies, Wasserman reactions, blood cultures, vaccines, chemical analyses for the Commission and chemical examinations for the Ancon and other hospitals of milk and foods (toxicological), special examinations of urine, etc., chemical, bacteriological, and microscopic examination of all Zone water supplies, including five reservoirs. The research work involves various subjects, reports upon which have been published by Dr. Darling.[10]

A considerable amount of clinical material was sent to Darling's laboratories from the patient wards of the adjacent Ancon Hospital. In 1907, for example, 562 autopsies, 3,795 celloidin sections, 738 bacterial cultures, and 146 tissues and neoplasms were examined.[11] Darling's wish to spend the rest of his life working in a laboratory uttered when he was a medical student had been answered and he must have been more than happy to be immersed in this type of work.[12] This vocation, however, demanded long hours and painstaking work. To run a laboratory which provided important services not only to the medical community but to the engineering department must have taxed both his physical and mental powers. The bureaucratic tangles that resisted Gorgas' attempts to sanitate Panama and obstructed the effective control of disease would not have spared Darling's need for equipment and chemicals necessary to do the laboratory work in a timely and efficient manner. Again, his frugal upbringing, fierce independence, and dogged persistence related to his New England background, must have marked him early in Panama as a man not easy to contend with when priorities such as accurate and timely results were at stake.

One of Darling's first assistants, Herbert C. Clark, who joined him in 1909, recalled his experiences in the laboratory:

A brief acquaintance with him at that time would have left the true personality of Dr. Darling quite unknown to me. He gave me the impression at first, of a critical, merciless task-master, but after I came to know him through the stress of a long service and learned how completely he submerged everything for the benefit of his professional duty and ambition, I could not help but develop a very great admiration for the man and a loyal spirit of co-operation. . . . As I look back to his days in Panama, it seems impossible that one man could have done so much research work in connection with his routine duties. He was without the stimulus of associates in his own line, he had very limited access to library privileges and many times had to improvise very crude apparatus and methods with which to approach quickly an unexpected problem. He loved to work in complete isolation, and his devotion to his work and his ability to improvise and meet all problems never failed him.[13]

The routine performance of autopsies on all deaths occurring at Ancon Hospital and other Commission hospitals resulted in a large number of post-mortem examinations and pathological studies, most of which were performed by Darling himself. Even later, when he was able to delegate some of the routine work to his assistants, Darling continued to perform the autopsies and considered this aspect of his work to be a most important part of his duties.[14] Less than a year after his arrival in Panama, Darling's dedication to the study of tropical pathology led him to a momentous discovery.

Sir Ronald Ross, who had deciphered in 1897 the mode of malaria transmission by mosquitoes, visited Panama in 1904.[15] Ross was familiar with *kala-azar* (Hindi for "black sickness"; also known as Oriental sore or leishmaniasis), a systemic disorder prevalent in India, manifested by splenomegaly, emaciation, cachexia, irregular pyrexia, and the presence of intracellular protozoa denominated as Leishman–Donovan bodies (name which he had coined). Ross suggested that this parasite might also be found in tropical America but, despite looking throughout the wards at Ancon Hospital for a case of splenomegaly associated with the typical symptoms of kala-azar, none was found.[15] Darling continued to look for Leishman–Donovan bodies by examining microscopically smears obtained from spleen, liver, and "rib-marrow" in all deaths found to have splenomegaly.[15]

Scarcely four months after performing his first autopsy in Panama (dated August 16, 1905), Darling had the "good fortune" to discover a new disease which he named *histoplasmosis* (see Appendix E: Discovery and Pathology of Histoplasmosis). On December 7, 1905, he examined and recorded his findings at the autopsy of a 27-year-old carpenter from Martinique.[16] He found the lungs "studded with pale gray hyaline miliary

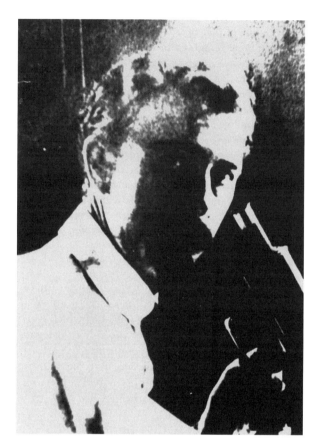

7.2 Darling at work in the laboratory behind his home in Ancon, circa 1912. Reproduced with permission, courtesy of Gerald L. Baum.

7.3 Last page of autopsy record No. 252, performed by Darling in Ancon Hospital on December 7, 1905, showing a pathological diagnosis of "Protozoan infection, Histoplasmosis, Histoplasma capsulatum." This was the first case of histoplasmosis discovered by Darling. Reproduced with permission, courtesy of Otis Historical Archives, National Museum of Health and Medicine, Armed Forces Institute of Pathology, Walter Reed Army Medical Center, Washington, D.C.

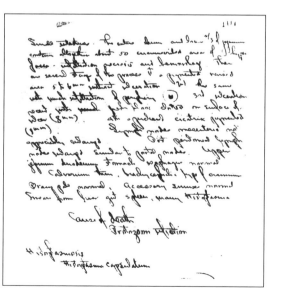

tubercles from 2 to 3 mm in diameter. . . . The tubercles were not as closely packed or as numerous as is often found in miliary tuberculosis . . . "[16] The gross anatomic diagnosis was acute miliary tuberculosis, pulmonary type. However, later in the day, he examined smears from a peculiarly white atypical tubercle in the lung and from the spleen, liver and bone marrow and, to his amazement, found "intense invasion of large endothelial-like cells by small round or oval micro-organisms."[16] He meticulously studied their morphology and realized that a new micro-organism capable of causing fatal disease in man had been discovered. Within one year, he encountered the same micro-organism twice more. In his own words: "On January 31, 1906, I duplicated that experience in another native Martiniquan. Again, on August 6, 1906, from a Chinese who had lived on the isthmus fifteen years, I had the pleasure of renewing my acquaintance with this peculiar little protozoon which had caused the deaths of the Martiniquans."[17]

Although Darling had described accurately a new micro-organism, he reached the wrong conclusion in calling it a protozoon. His observations of some flagellated forms (probably an artifact) in a section from the lung from one of the cases and relying heavily on the respected opinion of Ross, who had reviewed Darling's material and agreed that it resembled the protozoon described by Leishman, Donovan, and Wright in 1903 as causing kala-azar, affirmed Darling's erroneous conclusion.[17] His attempts to cultivate the new micro-organism in vitro and in laboratory animals were unsuccessful, otherwise he would have seen the budding yeast characteristic of a fungal organism. He selected the name *Histoplasma capsulatum* to emphasize that it invaded the cytoplasm of histiocyte-like cells and that each was enveloped by a capsule, and signed out the autopsy reports of his three unusual cases as due to *histoplasmosis*.[16] Many years later, while working in the same laboratory, Grocott would apply silver stains to facilitate demonstration of the capsule of *Histoplasma capsulatum* and aid in the classification of the micro-organism as a fungus.[18] With proper scientific objectivity, Darling wrote: "Cultural experiments and animal inoculations from material obtained during life from splenic and hepatic punctures will be of the greatest value in further attempts to assign a place to this micro-organism in nature." In describing his discovery, Darling told an audience in Baltimore in 1907: "[The] New World disorder is bound to appear in Baltimore some day."[17] Little did he suspect then the ubiquity of histoplasmosis in the world.

The discovery of histoplasmosis would have sufficed to assure Darling a place in medical history. But it marked only the beginning for this industrious investigator. He dedicated six papers to record his observations on histoplasmosis; he would author hundreds of additional scientific communications on other tropical diseases that attracted his interest (see Appendix A: Bibliography of Publications by Samuel T. Darling).

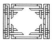

At the time of Darling's arrival in Panama, yellow fever was no longer the threat it had previously been. Instead, malaria became the leading tropical disease in Panama in terms of morbidity and mortality. During the year 1906, 21,739 cases of malaria were admitted to Canal Zone hospitals and 233 of these died.[19] Malaria became one of the leading causes of death among canal laborers, second only to pneumonia. During the period 1905 to 1914, 1,312 deaths were attributed to pneumonia and 734 to malaria.[20]

Except for Gorgas, who had personally treated 1,055 cases of malaria during a six-month period in the wards of Ancon Hospital, few were more aware than Darling regarding the devastating effects of malaria upon the Canal Zone laborers.[21] Darling performed most of the post-mortem examinations in the Canal Zone and signed out autopsy after autopsy with the pathological diagnosis of *EA Fever* (estivo-autumnal fever), the time-honored name for falciparum malaria.[22]

Estivo-autumnal fever (also called irregular intermittent type fever) had been recognized by early Roman observers as appearing predominantly in late summer and early fall.[23] This seasonal distribution was corroborated even in Baltimore, where out of 542 cases of malaria observed at Johns Hopkins Hospital by Hewetson and William Thayer, 188 were due to estivo-autumnal infection and all except five of these were seen during the second half of the year.[23] Thus, even prior to his arrival in Panama, Darling may have already been familiar with the clinical features and morbid anatomy of the malarial fevers. This experience was augmented by the alarming number of deaths from malaria seen at Ancon Hospital. A health problem of this magnitude must have preoccupied all those involved in the sanitation and health services of the isthmus. What was needed was a more scientific basis for improving the strategy to control malaria and its mosquito vector.

Darling approached the malaria problem systematically. He developed simple and effective methods of collecting, feeding, and breeding mosquito larvae in the laboratory.[24] Arrangements were made for sanitary inspectors along the isthmus to send daily to the laboratory bottles containing mosquito larvae and pupae. The latter were transferred to glass moist jars partly filled with fresh water. Anopheles larvae were transferred to feeding tanks containing algae and organic debris, and placed on a table in front of a window having an eastern exposure, so that they got direct sunlight for a few hours in the morning. The water in the breeding jars was kept fresh by passing a jet of air through it. A few *Lemna* plants were placed in the tank for shade and shelter. The temperature in the tanks ranged between 72 and 84° F. Pupae were culled in the morning and evening and placed in breeding-out tubes half-filled with water and plugged with cotton. Each morning the newly emerged mosquitoes were transferred to biting jars. After trying pickle jars and malted milk jars with "much impatience," jars made of lantern chimneys were used. These were covered on both ends with crinoline gauze, fastened with adhesive plaster, and a strong rubber band. Inside the jar was placed a circular ring platform of stiff paper, which many of the mosquitoes used as a resting place. About twenty mosquitoes would be placed in a jar over a small, slender dish containing water on a Petri dish cover with a raisin or a piece of date for food. The jar would then be placed on a shelf in a dimly lighted place and protected from ants by kerosene cups. Until the mosquitoes were used for biting they were fed with dates or raisins.[24]

Earlier biting experiments were conducted at about eight o'clock in the evening on the wards at Ancon Hospital. A jar with mosquitoes was placed on the patient's forearm and covered with a heavy towel to prevent the strong light from distracting the mosquitoes. Females a few days old fed on dates or raisins would usually bite greedily. When reluctant to bite, a few gentle puffs on the opposite end of the jar would induce them to do so. Later, biting experiments were carried out at a more convenient time, at four o'clock in the afternoon.[24]

Mosquitoes were prepared for dissection and microscopic examination after killing them with chloroform or cyanide. The latter was found to be more satisfactory since it caused mosquitoes to spread their wings, aiding in their classification. Examination of the salivary glands required removal of the distal half of the thorax and abdomen by a transverse clean cut. The proboscis (feeding tube) was then grasped with a small pair of forceps and the specimen laid on a drop of saline on a slender dish cover under the dissecting microscope. The chitinous (horny) covering of the thorax was carefully slit or torn and the muscle organ beneath loosened slightly, and then the salivary glands drawn out by pulling out the proboscis with a needle, separating them from the head with a small, very sharp knife or needle, and placed in saline solution, 10 percent formaldehyde, or on films for staining. Sporozoites (infective parasitic forms) were seen either free or in epithelial cells and in the duct of the salivary glands, appearing as thin, slightly curved, spindle-shaped bodies, placed side-by-side, frequently as though matted together.[24]

Examining for zygotes (cells derived from the union of a male and female germ cells) required withdrawal of the hind-gut, mid-gut, malphigian tubules, and ovaries by pulling carefully on the last abdominal segment with one needle and holding the first abdominal segment with another. Zygotes were then detected with a lower-power Zeiss microscope lens, sixteen millimeter (lens magnification power) objective, and eight and twelve oculars (eyepiece magnification power).[24]

The number of gametes (germ cells) per cubic millimeter (cu mm) in a patient's blood and the number of gametes ingested by the mosquito (usually in about one cu mm) were estimated by exacting weighing experiments. Mosquitoes were weighed before and after biting, and the amount of blood ingested estimated in this manner. The average weight of mosquitoes twenty-four hours old before biting was 0.0008 gram (g) and 0.0016 g after biting, yielding an average weight of ingested blood 0.0008 g. At the time of biting the patient, two or three blood films for staining were taken and differential counts of leucocytes as well as the proportion of gametes to leucocytes made the following morning. After correcting for the specific gravity of blood in "malarial fever with slight anemia" (1.050) and knowing the malarial patient's leucocyte count, the number of gametes ingested by a mosquito could then be calculated. For example, if there were twenty-two gametes per hundred leucocytes and the patient's leucocyte count was 6,500 leucocytes per cu mm, then $22 \times 65 = 1,430$ and corrected for amount of blood ingested (0.0008 g and a specific gravity of 1.050), yielded a total count of 1,088 gametes ingested, only an estimated but useful approximation of the number of malarial parasites in the biting mosquito.[24]

Another scientific but amusing observation by Darling was relative to the "musical note" emitted by mosquitoes. Contrary to the popular belief that this noise emanated from vibration of the wings, repeated observations in the laboratory (by cutting or immobilizing the wings) indicated that vibration of the proboscis was responsible for the characteristic high-pitched note or buzz of the mosquito.[25]

Darling identified eleven different species of anopheles mosquitoes collected in Panama over a period of eight years and described their morphological variations, relative distribution from season to season and from place to place, and conducted rigorous dissection and inoculation experiments on mosquitoes that had been allowed to feed on malarious patients to determine their susceptibility to transmit malaria.[24] Darling summarized the results of these elegant yet meticulous experiments:

> It is concluded from this series of experiments that *A[nopheles] albimanus*, the common, white hind-footed mosquito — an extremely hardy, rapid developing, adaptable mosquito, is the transmitter of estivo-autumnal and tertian malarial fever in the Canal Zone at this time. Specimens of this species infected with tertian parasites become infective between nine and eleven and one-half days after the first feeding. When infected by estivo-autumnal parasites, sporozoites appeared in the salivary glands as early as the eleventh day in some mosquitoes, and later than twelve and one-half days in others.[26]

Based on the results of his studies on malaria, Darling introduced the concept of *species-specific* control to Gorgas' sanitation program and ensured a more effective and economical plan for vector eradication. He also warned that latent malaria carriers formed an important reservoir for the continued transmission of malaria and advised against their too early dismissal from the hospital. He estimated that patients having as few as twelve gametes per cu mm of blood after treatment, still constituted a potential and dangerous source for the continued transmission of malaria by mosquitoes.[26] Although complete eradication, as had been achieved in the case of yellow fever, was never duplicated for malaria, better control measures resulted in a diminution in the rate of admissions from malaria from 821 to 82 per thousand employees by the time the canal was completed in 1914, a marked reduction of 90 per cent.[27]

Not content with the completion of his studies on the taxonomy (classification) of the different species of mosquitoes found in Panama and their susceptibility to transmit malaria, Darling carried out additional experiments designed to yield useful information for helping to control mosquitoes. Observations on the effect of sea-water, salt-water, and solutions of heavy metals on mosquito larvae indicated that adding sea-water to a fresh-water swamp, for example, only hastened the development of mosquitoes instead of reducing their numbers.[28] After a number of experiments, Darling developed a cheap and efficient larvicide preparation for killing mosquito larvae. A mixture of crude carbolic acid, common resin, and alkali yielded a soap with excellent toxic and diffusing power (readily mixing with water). The compound was capable of eliminating mosquito larvae within a few minutes at a dilution of 1:5,000 and cost only fourteen cents per gallon.[28] "Darling's larvacide [*sic*]" became widely known and accepted.[29,30] The efficacy of caustic soda, arsenic, copper sulfate, and Darling's larvicide was quantitated as possible destructive agents to control vegetation, grass, and algae where mosquitoes bred. Copper sulfate was found to be more efficient at killing algae when used at high dilutions.[31]

Other experiments measured the amount of pyrethrum required to fumigate effectively a small room (152 cubic feet), using mosquitoes placed in wire-gauze cylinders to facilitate detecting the death point.[31] Darling noticed that in the traditional method, pyrethrum was burned in iron pots and an underlying layer of powder was covered with ashes and failed to come in contact with oxygen necessary for it to be consumed. By placing a layer of sawdust underneath in the form of a crater and the pyrethrum laid on top, the ensuing ignition was most complete. Accordingly, Darling tested twelve different samples of pyrethrum and determined that mosquitoes were killed in two hours using less than one-third of the amount required by the United States Army, resulting in considerable savings.[31]

Two important factors in the selection of mesh for wire screening of dwellings were studied: size and composition.[32] Anopheles mosquitoes were unable to pass through sixteen-mesh (sixteen holes to an inch) screening. Smaller species (such as the yellow fever-transmitting Stegomyia) occasionally escaped (ten out of several hundred mosquitoes) so that this size mesh was practically safe but not absolutely so. With regard to composition, Darling tested samples of wire made of brass (an alloy of copper and zinc), copper, a phosphorus bronze (copper and tin) alloy, and galvanized iron (their chemical composition analyzed in his laboratories) and exposed these to salt-laden wind (near the sea) and salt-free hot and moist air. When exposed to the latter conditions, galvanized iron and bronze screening corroded rapidly, while copper and bronze screening "resisted deterioration admirably." Exposure to moist salt-air, on the other hand, resulted in bad corrosion of the galvanized iron, brass, and copper screening, while the bronze screening resisted these changes to a much greater degree. Darling concluded that screening intended for use in the tropics should have a high copper content, higher than brass, and be as free as possible from iron.[32]

Darling described the results of these experiments in a thirty-eight page monograph entitled, *Studies in Relation to Malaria.*[24] This publication was so well received that several editions were printed by the Isthmian Canal Commission Press and later by the United States Government Printing Office. The monograph established Darling as a meticulous scientific investigator and respected malariologist. His reputation transcended the confines of the isthmus and the Board of Health Laboratories became a mecca for serious students in the field. Physicians, scientists, and parasitologists came to Panama, attracted by this remarkable man and his admirable work, eager to learn from him about malaria and other tropical diseases.

A visiting physician remarked on the enthusiasm with which the battle against mosquitoes was carried out in Panama by Gorgas and his men:

> The most interesting medical subject on the Canal is the fight with the mosquitoes carried on by Dr. Samuel T. Darling and Mr. J. A. Le Prince under the leadership of Col. Gorgas, and it is difficult to tell who of them is the most enthusiastic, as all of them have that in their countenance that Alphonse Daudet describes as characteristic of men who love their work. . . . In talking to these mosquito hunters it is amusing to hear them unconsciously personify and speak of the mosquitoes' mental attitude as if they were human. The stegomyia, for instance, is shy and timid, while the anopheles albimanus, the malaria carrier, is predatory, fierce and has its own very decided ways of thinking. . . . She will make straight for you across the room. She will do even more, she will make straight for you against the wind across a field. . . . One cannot converse for half an hour with these men without becoming aware of the high minded enthusiasm, and with their

ISTHMIAN CANAL COMMISSION
Laboratory of the Board of Health, Department of Sanitation

STUDIES IN RELATION TO ᴄMALARIA

By

SAMUEL T. DARLING, ᴄM. D.
Chief of Laboratory

SECOND EDITION

I. C. C. PRESS
QUARTERMASTER'S DEPARTMENT
MOUNT HOPE, CANAL ZONE

7.4 Darling's monograph, *Studies in Relation to Malaria*, second edition, published in Mt. Hope, Canal Zone, by the Isthmian Canal Commission Press, circa 1910.

untiring industry in eliciting interesting and useful facts and adapting them to the work in hand.[33]

The importance of Darling's malaria studies in Panama cannot be over-estimated. By placing on a firm scientific basis Gorgas' malaria control program, Darling assured its rapid, effective, and economical implementation. In terms of saving human lives and making the isthmus a hospitable region, Darling's studies on malaria surpass all of his other contributions.

Darling's investigations on amebic dysentery have been considered by some, along with his malaria studies, as his most important work.[34] A review of his publications on the subject provides an interesting aspect of the scientist who has made careful observations and reaches the conclusion that generally accepted views are incorrect.

Darling's interest in the life cycle of entamoeba began when he identified *Entamoeba tetragena* in a case of dysentery in September 1911.[35] His subsequent observations of autopsy material, as well as from patients sent to him by two of the staff physicians at Ancon Hospital, allowed him to suspect that *Entamoeba histolytica*, as originally described, might not be responsible for amebic dysentery in Panama. It particularly bothered Darling that in Panama, with its cosmopolitan population and among which many tropical countries were represented, he had been unable to find forms of *Entamoeba histolytica*, only those of *Entamoeba tetragena*. In order to test this supposition, he diligently tried many forms of staining the protozoon, so as to identify those microscopic characteristics necessary for adequate species classification. He pointed out the many possible errors that could result from improper staining and preservation techniques. In addition, he was able to study the life cycle of the entamoeba found in Panama by rectal inoculation experiments in young kittens.[36] Having in this manner satisfied his scientific curiosity, he concluded:

> We have too long been biased by the posthumous influence of [Fritz] Schaudinn. We have used too carelessly the Romanowsky stain with dried-fixed films for the identification of entamoebas. We have been content to base our diagnosis on observations limited to the large trophozoite found in the stools in dysentery and pathological tissue and to call the trophozoite "E. histolytica."[37]

He further stated that "The description of the life cycle of *E. histolytica* by Schaudinn and [Charles] Craig, therefore, were in all likelihood those of a spurious species, having resulted from observations of pathological changes in senile races of *E. tetragena*."[38]

The rebuttal makes for interesting reading. Craig, who was present when Darling presented his paper at the 15th International Congress of Hygiene and Demography in September 1912, remarked:

> I would say that I am sure that such a mistake could not be made . . . I am quite sure that I know artifacts when I see them, and I am still more sure that Schaudinn did . . . Specimens of both histolytica and tetragena frequently occur in the same case, and this does not appear to be considered by Dr. Darling in his paper.[39]

Darling's reply to Craig was a model of courteous dissention:

> It is possible that my observations on the morphology of E. tetragena, and the observations recorded by Dr. Craig on the developmental phase of E. histolytica, in which spore formation by budding is described, may be harmonized. Unfortunately, at this time no observations tending to confirm this view have been made.[40]

Darling's studies prompted others to review the life cycle of *E. histolytica* as described by Schaudinn and Craig, and found it to be incorrect. On the following year Craig concluded, after reviewing some of the material sent to him from the Canal Zone, that *E. tetragena* and *E. histolytica* were identical.[41] However, priority dictated that the name *E. histolytica* should stand and *E. tetragena* be dropped.

In 1909 Darling was called to face a problem of economic importance to the Canal Zone. An outbreak of a fatal illness, locally known as *murrina* or *derrengadera*, occurred among horses that had recently been brought from the United States and pastured with native horses.[42] After becoming familiar with the manifestations of the disease and its pathologic anatomy, Darling proceeded to carry his work into the laboratory. He infected experimentally a large number of animals available to him, including dogs, raccoons, cats, monkeys, and opossums, and determined their susceptibility to infection. A detailed description of the morphology of the causative agent followed. He was able to differentiate it from two other trypanosomes, *T. equinum* and *T. equiperdum* and, supported by Laveran, who examined his preparations, described it as a new species, *Trypanosoma hippicum*.[42]

Noting that only work animals were affected and not saddle horses, he suspected that transmission of the parasite occurred primarily by mechanical means, probably by inoculation of cuts and abrasions by flies. He outlined a program to halt further transmission of the disease and the epidemic, which threatened to destroy several hundred mules and horses, was thus effectively controlled.[42]

In July 1908, Darling examined two biopsies of skeletal muscle from a Barbadian who suffered from fever, slight headache, and stiffness of the muscles and joints. The patient was suspected of having typhoid fever and trichinosis, and the latter was sought in muscle biopsies. Instead, Darling found under the microscope cysts containing hundreds of little oval vesicular bodies having a round nucleus at one end.[43] He was puzzled by the unusual appearance of this parasite. Recognizing certain important differences from previously reported cases, he nevertheless diagnosed this as the third known case of human sarcosporidiosis. To reconcile the discrepancies, he put forth the *blind alley theory*, which allowed for certain morphological alterations to occur when a parasite, whose customary habitat is one of the domestic animals or a still lower order of life, by chance parasitizes an unusual host such as man. To test this hypothesis, Darling conducted experiments in guinea pigs, feeding them sarcosporidia obtained from rats. Sacrificing the animals at subsequent intervals, he found cysts which resembled to a great extent those seen in the biopsy of skeletal muscle.[44] In further experiments, he injected sarcosporidia from an opossum into guinea pigs and, again, noted the occurrence of morphologic alterations.[45]

Unfortunately, Darling's experiments with guinea pigs were uncontrolled. Kean and Grocott reviewed the evidence in 1945 by examining sixty guinea pigs and found five of these parasitized naturally with what Darling had called sarcosporidia.[46] Based on these observations and on Darling's detailed descriptions and beautiful drawings, they concluded that the parasite in question resembled more *Toxoplasma gondii* than *Sarcocystis*. The issue could not be settled at the time in the absence of serological data, but it was suspected that Darling was actually describing the first instance of toxoplasmosis in man.[47] To further justify Darling's conclusion, it should be recalled that *T. gondii* was initially described in 1908 as occurring in rabbits and the gondi.[48] The first widely known report of toxoplasmosis in man did not appear until 1939, fourteen years after Darling's death.[49]

In August 1910, Darling discovered a case of Oriental sore (leishmaniasis) in a man who had been living in the bush on a rubber tree plantation outside the Canal Zone. Three additional cases were found later, and Darling reported these in the *Journal of Cutaneous Diseases* in December 1911.[50] The finding of autochthonous cases of cutaneous leishmaniasis in Panama was important, since until then Oriental sore had been known to occur only in the Old World and in Brazil.

Darling's knowledge of the subject is evident as he described the clinical features of the disease, its causative agent, mode of transmission, geographical distribution, climatological factors, immunity, diagnosis, and treatment.[50] By analogy of its distribution in the Old World, he predicted that it might be found when sought for in America between latitudes 40° S and 40° N, in localities having an average annual temperature of 17.6° C or more, and in which the average winter temperature is not lower than 6.3° C. Although not extending as far north as he theorized, the lesions of *Leishmania tropica* have been found in the Yucatan peninsula of southern Mexico.[50]

In May 1905, Darling performed an autopsy on a case of bubonic plague. He was injected at that time with 10 c.c. of Yersin's antipest serum.[51] Six years later, he performed another autopsy on a case of septicemic plague and again received ten c.c. of Yersin's antipest serum. The second injection was followed in six days by urticaria, which spread to almost all parts of the body above the knees. Later that day, Darling awoke with a feeling of "intense depression" as though fainting. No pulse could be detected at the wrist, but a few minutes later it was forty-six and he appeared ashen, with cold perspiration. Periods of intense tingling of the skin, with prostration and feeble pulse lasting fifteen minutes, recurred repeatedly. Dysphagia was experienced when he attempted to swallow water. During the following seven days he described pain and urticaria on various parts of his body. Finally, on the eighth day, a general feeling of well-being returned.[51]

In sharing this experience in the form of a case report, Darling wished to caution against the indiscriminate use of antiserum for the immunization of contacts. He considered the value of Yersin serum as doubtful in preventing or "absorbing" an attack of plague. He described his illness as "very disagreeable," particularly because of the "consequent loss of time from business."[51]

Darling's reports on rabies, leprosy, filariasis, relapsing fevers, verruca peruana, strongyloidiasis, tuberculosis, plague, anthrax, bilharziasis, piroplasmosis, typhus, pellagra, beriberi, and scurvy exemplify his unlimited scientific curiosity. Important laboratory notes dealt with the recovery of bacillus dysenteriae from blood, blood platelets in tropical anemia, special methods for detecting intestinal worms, cultivation of leprosy bacilli, staining of the capsule of pneumococcus, and the use of bismuth salts in media to detect formation of sulfur bodies of bacterial origin. The *Proceedings of the Canal Zone Medical Association*, published under the auspices of the American Medical Association, provide an interesting record of the medical activities of the staffs of Ancon and Colon Hospitals for this period (see Appendix C: Proceedings of the Canal Zone Medical Association). Darling's comments, which followed many of the papers presented by his colleagues at the meetings of the association, reflected his knowledge of the literature on a variety of subjects.

In addition to his clinical and research work in the laboratory, Darling was from time to time asked to investigate health problems in villages of the "interior" provinces of Panama, on the premise that these might have important consequences on residents of the Canal Zone and other workers of the Panama Canal. In 1910, for example, Gorgas directed Darling to investigate reports of an "alarming" infant mortality and outbreaks of smallpox and whooping cough in the villages of La Chorrera and Chame.[52]

Darling visited La Chorrera and isolated *Bacillus dysenteriae* from an eight-month old infant with diarrhea. The organism agglutinated with dilutions of 1:1,000 of polyvalent *B. dysenteriae* serum, thus confirming the presence of this important pathogen. Darling, with his customary thoroughness, then investigated the sources of drinking water and found these to be "from sub-soil seepage through three or four feet of sandy clay caught in shallow, uncovered wells" insufficiently protected from possible contamination.[52] He also tested samples of water for chlorine content, alkalinity, and presence of *Bacillus coli*, but found no evidence of "pollution." To prevent an epidemic occurrence of diarrhea among children and dysentery among adults, Darling recommended appropriate hygienic measures, such as boiling drinking water, proper cooking and preparation of food, and prevention of contamination of food by flies and contact with infected material, "as far as possible."[52] A "peculiar pustular eruption" on the body and limbs of one of the children yielded an acarid (mite) which was sent to the entomologist for further identification, although Darling thought this undoubtedly was a variety of mite from the genus *Liponyssus*. Not content with these observations, he actively sought anophelines from his sleeping quarters, and mosquito larvae from several puddles and pools, with negative results. He found large numbers of *Stegomyia* larvae in water barrels near the houses in the village. Finally, he identified ticks from dogs, horses, and cattle as *Amblyoma cajennens*, *Dermacentor nitens*, and *Margaropus annulatus*, variety *microphus*, the latter "known to convey Texas cattle fever."[52]

In Chame, Darling found many infants and children suffering from whooping cough and malaria, which he thought must contribute "very largely" to the death rate.[52] He examined the blood from sixteen children and found estivo-autumnal (falciparum) and tertian (vivax) malarial parasites in six. In addition, "the blood smears showed very marked eosinophilia and an increase in the small mononuclear elements. The first is an indication of uncinariasis, and the latter of whooping cough, which was widely prevalent."[52] Twenty-one mosquitoes taken from the sleeping quarters were all *Anopheles albimanus*, "the common invertebrate host of malaria for this region." Specimens of the common bed bug, *Cimex lectularius*, as well as both the house flea, *Pulex irritans*, and cat flea, *Ctenocephalus felis*, were easily "procured" from houses visited. "These fleas," Darling noted, "to a very slight extent in some localities, are concerned with the transmission of bubonic plague."[52]

A reported outbreak of smallpox in Chitré, in the province of Herrera, prompted Darling to visit schools, a number of houses, and to examine several persons in the villages of Chitré, Los Santos, and Guararé, in October 1910.[53] Darling found only two convalescent cases of smallpox and thought the disease was mild in type and not epidemic. However, he noted that a large number of children had not been vaccinated in recent years and recommended that a thorough vaccination program be implemented in Chitré, Los Santos, Guararé, Las Tablas, and Pedasí.[53]

Reports such as these were forwarded to Gorgas for his approval as Chief Sanitary Officer in charge of all health problems in the region. Furthermore, Darling's ascendancy in the hierarchy of the Department of Health, from interne to physician to pathologist and, finally, to chief of the Board of Health Laboratories, required the approval of Gorgas. At the time of his arrival in Panama, Gorgas had hoped that the laboratory work would develop "into a more general field of tropical investigation."[54] The abundance and quality of Darling's subsequent research publications must have pleased Gorgas. His high regard for Darling's knowledge and expertise was evident when he invited Darling to join the commission formed to study the health problems and high mortality among workers in the Rand Mines of South Africa in 1913.[55] For these reasons, it is suprising to find little mention of Darling's contributions in Gorgas' numerous publications about the health and sanitation in Panama.[56] A satisfactory explanation is not readily apparent for such an omission. No animosity is known to have existed between the two men. Both enjoyed each other's company and were often seen together walking the jungle paths and canoeing the streams of Panama.[14] It is possible that Darling preferred to work in relative anonymity and removed as much as possible from any unnecessary distractions and administrative duties.[2] If so, Gorgas would have surely respected his industrious colleague's wishes and allowed Darling's work to speak for itself.

Darling's laboratory was the undisputed center of research activity in Panama during the construction of the canal. Through his publications, Darling gained a worldwide reputation. His knowledge and experience were sought elsewhere in hopes that his accomplishments in Panama would be duplicated in other parts of the world. Having helped to solve most of the health problems of Panama, Darling accepted the challenge and left the isthmus to join the Rockefeller Foundation's International Health Board in 1915.[57,58]

8

Rand Mines, South Africa

In 1913, William Gorgas invited Darling and Major Robert E. Noble, U.S. Army, to accompany him as members of a commission on a trip to the Rand Mines in South Africa. The commission was asked to investigate the high mortality among diamond and gold mine workers in the Transvaal and Rhodesia, conduct a sanitary survey of the region, and render appropriate recommendations.[1,2]

The British government was concerned about a marked increase in the number of deaths from pneumonia noted in the autumn of 1913 among African workers on the Rand Mines.[3] Aware of Gorgas' sanitation work, the Transvaal Chamber of Mines sent to Panama a representative, Samuel Evans, to explore the possibility that Gorgas could help them solve such a serious health problem that threatened to close the mines.[3] Evans examined the canal health records and found that a similar problem had challenged the Americans in Panama as early as 1906. West Indian workers appeared to have diminished resistance to pneumonia and soon after their arrival began to die from it at a shocking rate.[3] Gorgas blamed crowded living conditions and applied common sanitation measures to correct this health problem. The solution rested on the principles of dispersion (building of less crowded living quarters separated by safe distances) and segregation (separation of pneumonia victims).[3] Within a few months, pneumonia as an epidemic illness disappeared from the isthmus. This "minor" sanitary achievement was overshadowed by the more spectacular triumphs over yellow fever and malaria.[3] Upon Evans' recommendation, a commission made up of Gorgas, Darling, and Noble, was employed by the Chamber of Mines to make a survey of the Rand region and to advise them about sanitary problems.[3]

After spending several days in New York collecting information, the members of the commission sailed for Plymouth, England, on the *Imperator*.[2] Additional time was spent in London collecting data and interviewing medical men familiar with the Rand.[3] Among the friends and notables that Gorgas visited in London was Sir Ronald Ross, winner of the Nobel Prize for discovering the transmission of malaria by mosquitoes. The group, including Marie Gorgas, Darling, and Noble, also had lunch with Sir William Osler at Oxford.[3]

On November 15, 1914, Gorgas, Darling, and Noble, sailed on the S.S. *Briton* of the Union-Castle Line to Cape Town.[4] After a pleasant and uneventful trip, the travelers reached their destination seventeen days later and immediately took the train for the two-day, 950-mile trip on the veldt to Johannesburg.[2,4] The commissioners established their offices at the Carlton Hotel and, after meeting with medical and administrative officials of the Rand and the Chamber of Mines, outlined a program for visiting and inspecting the region, including its more than fifty hospitals.[4]

A salient point of the investigation was the method of recruitment for the hundreds of thousands of laborers employed in the diamond and gold mines. Darling and Noble traveled to Inhambane in Portuguese East Africa (now Mozambique) to observe first-hand the sources of labor supply and the long journey that took them from there to the receiving compounds in South Africa.[5] Once enrolled in Inhambane, the workers were transported by ship and rail to Rossana Garcia and held there until twelve hundred were recruited. The unacclimatized lot then traveled by train from sea level to an elevation of 5,500 feet, scantily clad and in crowded conditions.[5] By the time of arrival to their destination, a few of the men were already ill from pneumonia and more became so in the receiving compound before transferred to the mines.[5] The contrast between the "very fine" climate in Johannesburg and Delagoa Bay in Portuguese South Africa was considerable, making the latter one of the hottest places on the map. Darling and Noble remained there only as long as necessary, avoiding as much as possible "champagne before breakfast" and "giraffe sausage and rhinoceros steaks on the menu."[6]

Darling described the work done by the miners as consisting of drilling and lashing.[7] Each miner handled a drill from three to five feet in length and most of the drilling was done by hand — a very laborious and slow process. The workers went down mine shafts as far as 4,000 feet, working from five to six a.m., taking a light meal beforehand of a little cocoa and bread, some taking a little corn-meal mush, and remained down all day, or until three or four in the afternoon.[7] The men were gathered in gangs of twenty to forty supervised by a white foreman. Living quarters consisted of single-story buildings made of brick, stone or *dargar*, in the form of a hollowed square open in the center. Men were confined to this enclosure, where they were allowed to cook, fight, and spend all their time when not at work. Each room in these buildings held anywhere from twenty to sixty laborers in three-tiered bunks.[7]

Among the 300,000 workers in the Transvaal district, the death rate

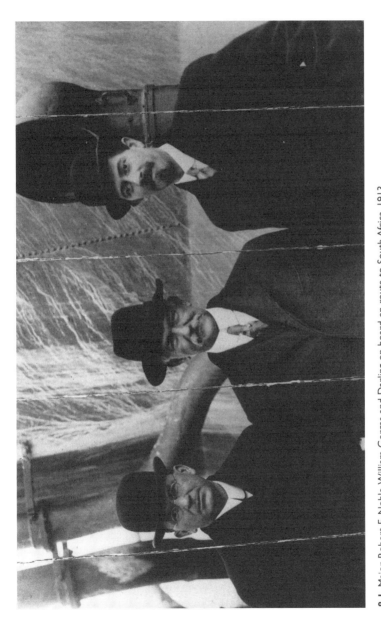

8.1 Major Robert E. Noble, William Gorgas and Darling on board en route to South Africa, 1913. Reproduced with permission, courtesy of Gerald L. Baum.

was found to be more than twice that experienced among Canal Zone employees (22.84 versus 10 per thousand, respectively, for the year 1912).[8] The four leading causes of death among mine workers were pneumonia, phthisis (tuberculosis), meningitis, and enteric fever. Epidemiological studies showed that two main factors contributed to the high mortality: (1) exposure to these diseases by new arrivals, presumed to have a low resistance to pneumococcus and other infectious agents, and (2) crowded living conditions. The most serious sanitary defect noticed was the crowded quarters, which allowed in general only 200 cubic feet of air-space and fourteen square feet of floor-space per worker. The close personal contact was blamed for the spread of infectious diseases, particularly of pneumonia, tuberculosis, and cerebro-spinal meningitis.[9]

Darling witnessed eleven autopsy studies performed in men who had died of lobar pneumonia, and the results showed that the actual cause of death in all cases was instead tuberculosis.[1] Both Gorgas and Darling were of the opinion that a considerable number of cases of death reported as occurring from pneumonia really resulted from tuberculosis.[9]

Examination of the diet disclosed that the two chief components of the daily ration for mine workers were two pounds of "mealy meal" and "five and 85/100 of meat" (compared to a soldier's ration in the British Army of sixteen ounces of bread and twelve ounces of meat).[10] Gorgas thought that this was too large a proportion of carbohydrates for men doing hard manual labor and recommended reducing the amount of mealy meal and increasing the meat portion. Darling observed that scurvy in South Africa was "very prevalent and fatal," and responsible for "horrible pathological conditions" at autopsy.[11] In every case inquired, scurvy was found to be associated with a dietary deficiency; it also occurred frequently in the dry season when there was little meat and no fresh vegetables.[11]

The medical services in the Rand were provided by about thirty-eight physicians among sixty-two hospitals, each duplicating pretty much what the other was doing. Gorgas advocated centralizing all these services into a first-class, well-equipped, and well-staffed hospital.[12]

The recommendations made by the commission to improve the sanitary conditions and reduce the death-rates among mine workers were direct and simple: (1) increase the floor-space to fifty square feet per worker; (2) improve the hospital system and care of the sick by creating a central hospital; and (3) establish a central sanitary system or department under the Chamber of Mines and a chief sanitary officer to represent the mines in all sanitary questions.[13]

Darling and Noble concluded their fact-finding trip in Inhambane and returned to Johannesburg in time to accompany Gorgas on a trip to Salisbury, the capital of Rhodesia. The government of Rhodesia was concerned about the large toll taken there by malaria and sought advise about malaria control methods. On January 25, Gorgas addressed about a thousand people at a theatre in Salisbury. Noble "presided over the slides" while Darling "took post at the back of the theatre" so as to let Gorgas know whether or not he was speaking sufficiently loud.[14] From Salisbury, the party left for Buluwayo, the principal town of Rhodesia, and from there visited the ruins of a prehistoric city thought to be Ophir, near the region from which Solomon and the king of Tyre obtained their gold, and Matapos Hill, where Cecil Rhodes was buried.[14]

After completing a report of their findings and submitting a set recommendations to the Transvaal Chamber of Mines, Gorgas and his two companions concluded their three-month stay in the *Witwatersrand* (the old name given by the Dutch to the region, meaning rim of white or clear waters) and sailed home from Cape Town on February 28, 1914.[2,14]

Gorgas made a wise decision when he selected Darling to accompany him as a member of the commission to the Rand Mines. Their friendship stemmed from a decade of professional interaction and together they enjoyed exploring by foot, horseback and canoe the jungle paths in Panama. Darling's experience as a pathologist was instrumental in identifying tuberculosis as a major cause of pneumonia and death among workers in the Rand Mines.

PART III

Rockefeller Years
1915–1925

9

Uncinariasis Commission
to the Far East

The International Health Board of the Rockefeller Foundation invited Darling in 1915 to head a commission assigned to study the incidence and control of hookworm in the Far East, more specifically in the Federated Malay States and Strait Settlements, Java, and Fiji.[1]

This initial step in the international expansion of a hookworm control program, which began in the southern states under the supervision of the Rockefeller Sanitary Commission, came about as the result of a series of fortuitous events.[2] By the turn of the century, John D. Rockefeller, Sr., had made donations to at least 800 different institutions and more than 670 individuals.[3] The senior Rockefeller decided to place his disparate philanthropic efforts under more able hands and appointed Frederick Gates, a former Baptist minister and a shrewd businessman, to administer this important aspect of his estate.[4] After reading William Osler's two-volume *Principles and Practice of Medicine*, Gates was impressed by Osler's lucid and informative style, but dismayed by how little was known about the causes and cures of diseases. He realized how "woefully neglected had been the scientific study of medicine in the United States."[4] Gates' enlightment turned the Rockefeller fortunes towards medicine.

In 1901, The Rockefeller Institute for Medical Research (and fore-runner of Rockefeller University) was incorporated for the purpose of conducting studies and investigations uninterrupted by the demands of clinical practice.[4] Eight years later, the Rockefeller Foundation was created with a more ambitious mandate, "to promote the well-being and to advance the civilization of the peoples of the United States and its terri-tories and possessions and of foreign lands in the acquisition and dissemination of knowledge, in the prevention and relief of suffering, and in the promotion of any and all of the elements of human progress."[4] All that was needed now were a few target diseases upon which to direct the Rockefeller Foundation's philanthropic efforts.

Gates believed that "disease was the supreme ill of human life and the main source of almost all other human ills such as poverty, crime, ignorance, vice, inefficiency, hereditary taints, and many other evils."[5] His evangelical zeal must have experienced another epiphanic revelation when he first heard about Charles Wardell Stiles, a zoologist and public health official of the U.S. Public Health and Marine-Hospital Service, who in 1902 had reported on the prevalence and geographic distribution of hookworm disease in the United States.[6] According to Stiles, hookworm was responsible for many, if not all, of the physical and mental deficiencies ascribed to minority populations in the South. And he was willing to sermonize about it to anyone who would listen about the "germ of laziness."[7] The opportunity came when he presented his ideas to members of the Rockefeller Foundation, including Gates. The impact was immediately felt and on October 26, 1909, John D. Rockefeller, Sr., addressed a letter to the twelve men selected to form the executive committee of the Rockefeller Commission for the Extermination of the Hookworm Disease, the greatest single cause of anemia and stagnation in the South affecting two million people.[7] Gates remained chairman of the commission for the five years of its existence, and appointed Wickliffe Rose, a professional educator and dean of the Peabody Normal School and of the University of Nashville, as executive secretary.[8,9] Rose differed from Gates in his approach and considered the campaign against hookworm disease as an essential wedge to stimulate local authorities to consider public health and hygiene as important components of a more lasting benefit than simply to control or eradicate vectors, parasites or microbes.[10] Eventually Rose, with his gentle patience, unfailing courtesy, and administrative flexibility, prevailed over the more abrasive and authoritative Gates.[8]

Convinced that hookworm disease was an ideal target for intervention, as it could be easily diagnosed and treated, the Rockefeller Foundation focused its resources on this scourge. Each sanitary inspector was equipped with a Bausch & Lomb collapsible microscope designed to fit in a saddlebag, a supply of medicine, popular literature for distribution among the curious, photographs and charts to illustrate day-time lectures, and a lantern with slides for evening demonstrations.[11] At the end of the five-year plan, the Rockefeller Sanitary Commission reported that over one million microscopic examinations had been done and almost half a million people had been treated for hookworm disease.[12] Despite the lack of controls and difficulties with follow-up data from a largely itinerant population, the foundation considered the fight against hookworm in the South a success and poised itself for a broader, international effort.

By May 1913, the Rockefeller Foundation had been chartered and its mission defined "to promote the well-being of mankind throughout the world."[13] A month later, the first major subdivision of the philanthropic empire, the International Health Commission, was established.[14] The third paragraph of the resolutions stated:

> Whereas the Commission has ascertained by diligent and extensive inquiry that Hookworm Disease prevails in a belt of territory encircling the earth for thirty degrees on each side of the equator, inhabited according to current estimates by more than a thousand million people; that the infection in some nations rises to nearly ninety percent of the entire population; that this disease has probably been an important factor in retarding the economic, social, intellectual and moral progress of mankind; that the infection is being spread by emigration; and that where it is most severe little or nothing is being done towards its arrest or prevention, therefore be it [r]esolved that this Foundation is prepared to extend to other countries and peoples the work of eradicating Hookworm disease as opportunity offers, and so far as practicable to follow up the treatment and cure of the disease with the establishment of agencies of the promotion of public sanitation and the spread of knowledge of scientific medicine.[14,15]

From the beginning, the International Health Board made it clear that these undertakings had to be a cooperative effort with the governments of the countries involved.[16] The Board provided the technical expertise and a portion of the expenditures, while the host countries facilitated the process and contributed in varying amounts. Once the project was assured completion and sufficient local personnel were adequately trained to continue the work, the Rockefeller team would gradually withdraw and place the responsibilities on local government and sanitary officials. This practice attempted to create good will, assure cooperation, and reduce any misperceived prominence for the visiting experts. Just as the Rockefeller Foundation's guiding words, "The well-being of mankind throughout the world," inspired its philanthropic activities, the slogan of the International Health Board, "A partner but not a patron," provided important guidelines to ensure the philanthropic investment survived into the future.[10,16]

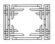

After a required check on his training, background, and personal traits that justified his membership on the commission to study the importance of hookworm in the Far East, and personal endorsements by William

Gorgas and Simon Flexner, Darling was offered the position to head the commission.[1,17,18] On January 7, 1915, he accepted the offer with "much pleasure," but was unable to leave Panama and report to duty in Washington until about February 8, on account of the illness of one of his children.[19] He added, enthusiastically:

> For eight years, as Chief of Laboratory here, I have been specially occupied in the study of parasitic diseases – malaria, trypanosomiasis, hookworm disease, yellow fever etc., and their control, so that I need hardly say how strongly the work appeals to me, which, it is understood, the International Health Commission contemplates undertaking in the tropics.[19]

Two other members of the Commission were selected by the International Health Board to accompany Darling: Marshall A. Barber from the Philippines and Henry P. Hacker from the Malay States field offices.[20] The purpose and object of the commission were stated in a memorandum of instructions prepared for the guidance of the Commission in the conduct of its investigations, more specifically "to determine to what degree [u]ncinariasis infection is a menace to the health and working efficiency of the people in the country under consideration." Darling was further instructed to conduct studies in such places and in such manner as might be deemed expedient.[20] The work of the commission was to be carried out under the auspices of the British Colonial Office and the Netherland Indies Health Department, and supported by the Rockefeller Foundation.[21]

Although the new position offered Darling no pecuniary advantage (his monthly salary would be $250, compared to his previous compensation of $375 as head of the Board of Health Laboratory in Panama), he readily accepted the challenge and made arrangements to leave Panama for his new post in February 1915.[1] However, one of the members of the commission (Barber) had to return to the United States on urgent personal business and Victor Heiser, director of the East for the International Health Board field staff, advised that Darling's employment be delayed until a later date.[1] Darling, however, cabled that the commission had previously urged for his availability in January and upon acceptance he had arranged with the Panama authorities to leave in February and could not delay his departure.[22]

By the time Darling departed for the Orient on the S.S. *Medina* (Peninsular & Oriental Navigation Company) in April 1915, he had requested the International Health Commission to obtain eighteen boxes of laboratory supplies needed to carry out the work assigned to him, including a number of books on parasitology, and had these packed by E. Leitz Wetzlar Company and shipped separately on the S.S. *Adriatic* to Singapore.[23] Upon his arrival in Liverpool, Darling took the precaution

to investigate the matter and, to his consternation, found that the shipment of supplies had been prepaid only to Liverpool and that the boxes
would have to be examined by the customs' officials, "entailing great
delay and breakage."[24] Although Darling accepted that the delay in the
shipment of the supplies was unavoidable considering the "Times" [of
war], he was able to find a responsible agent in charge of sending the
goods out on the next steamer from London on May 15. After he had left
London, Darling received a telegram from the agent requesting separate
packing lists for each box, which he did not have with himself. As no
"aerograms" were permitted to be sent from the ship, Darling had to wait
until he reached Gibraltar to wire for the needed papers. These were sent
to the American consul in Liverpool and, finally, the shipment of laboratory supplies went forward on the S.S. *Antilochus* to Singapore on May
22, 1915.[25] Despite all these hassles and concerns about the boxes of
supplies, Darling found time to visit the Colonial Office in London and
to obtain from Sir John Anderson, previous High Commissioner to the
Malay States, valuable letters of recommendation to various governors en
route as well as to officials in Malaya, which would facilitate implementation of the work of the commission.[24] If the International Health Board
had any doubts about Darling's abilities to work under difficult times and
to handle bureaucratic impediments in other countries, this experience
served to reassure them that indeed they had chosen the right person for
the job.

In Colombo, Darling met with Victor Heiser, director for the East field
staff, and spent a day discussing the proposed work.[26] The ship arrived in
Singapore on May 29, and the next three or four days were spent visiting
hospitals, medical school, quarantine station, water works, and learning
about the native people and their manner of living. After presenting his
credentials to Sir Arthur Young and enjoying lunch in the company of
Lady Evelyn at the Government House, Darling left Singapore for Kuala
Lumpur, where he arrived on June 2. There he called upon Sir Edward
Brockman, the Chief Secretary, and outlined to him their plans and
hopes.[26]

While waiting for the supply shipment to arrive, the members of the
commission used their time advantageously by visiting various points in
the states of Selangor, Negri Sembilan, and Perak, inspecting such places
as Port Swettenham, Seremban, Baru Gajah, Tanjong Malim, Ipoh, Kuala
Kangsar, and going north as far as Lenggong.[26] In this way a great deal
was learned about the various elements of the native population, their
customs, habits, manner of living, etc., and tentative plans were made for
prosecuting their work in the future.[26]

The commission decided to establish its headquarters in Kuala
Lumpur, the seat of government for the Federated Malay States, because
of its proximity to Port Swettenham, the entrepôt for Tamil coolies from

India, and its accessibility to other regions of interest, but most importantly, because of a large government hospital available there with a capacity for eight-hundred beds.[26] To facilitate the investigations on hookworm disease, the commission preferred to open its own ward of fifty beds and a connected laboratory at "a stone's throw from the hospital ward."[26] The hospital ward was opened on July 6 and cases were selected from each day's admissions to the hospital. The cases were then carefully studied, treated and "properly controlled."[26]

The commission received full cooperation from the government. Quarters and transport, including railway passes, were provided. A number of hospital assistants and assistant surgeons were also supplied by the hospital to aid the commission in their work.[26] However, the lack of properly trained laboratory assistants was viewed as somewhat of a hardship, as it took considerable time to train local personnel. Since the laboratory results were crucial for estimating the extent of parasitic involvement, Darling thought it would be wise in future expeditions to consider the advisability of including a trained assistant in the personnel of the commission.[26]

The members of the Board lived at a mess house on Tanglin Road and had a fine old wainscotted dining hall and a real punkah which they never used "for fear that it might fall with fatal results on one or more heads of the Board."[26] Darling found the climate pleasanter during the day than in Panama, but the nights were not so "salubrious" for there was very little breeze stirring.[26] Darling concluded this lengthy letter on an optimistic note: "The members of the Board are all in excellent health and spirits and keen on the work."[26] In addition to Darling, Barber and Hacker, the board added locally one assistant surgeon, a clerk, six laboratory assistants, three ward dressers, two scullions for the ward and the laboratory, for a total of sixteen personnel.[27]

An understandable complaint arose from the lengthy delays in exchanging mail and the lack of news engendered some concerns at the home office. Darling apologized for this and mentioned that it used to be so easy to get out reports and statements in Panama with the official service there, while now the mail service between New York and Malaya was getting "weaker and weaker." Heiser's last letter of August 19 had taken forty-seven days to get there.[28] Darling also informed the home office that most of the second-class mail arrived in very bad condition and suggested that this class of mail be more securely wrapped.[29]

Due to the war-time conditions, Darling's request for additional supplies was only incompletely filled. Stocks of chemicals and glassware were thoroughly depleted and impossible to supply as requested. Among scarce items were cover glasses (unable to obtain at all), a spectroscope for quantitative examination of oxyhemoglobin and urobilin, microscope slides (able to get only 1,800 instead of the fifty gross requested), Petri dishes, glass tubing, and rubber tubing.[30]

As the commission (also known as the Malaya Board) immersed itself in its investigations, Darling remarked: "The work is of great interest to me and reminds me so much of Panama in 1905–07. Malaria is the great plague. Diet and nutrition appear to play a tremendous part in the rate of recuperation from infections."[28] Already Darling was transgressing the Rockefeller Foundation's intentions of focusing on a single problem and disregarding other possible contributing factors (particularly social aspects).[31] He and his colleagues considered that both hookworm and malaria were responsible for anemia and lack of stamina in some of the populations they intended to study. The intimate relationship that existed between malaria and hookworm made it necessary for them to devote almost as much time and study to malaria as to hookworm disease.[20] Heiser had spent a few days with the Malaya Board going over all the features of their work to date and was impressed with the value of their observations and experiments. Heiser, however, did not wish to have any malarial research done by the Board at this time.[32] Darling appealed to Rose, recalling his great interest in the subject of malaria, saying that he regretted that decision more than he could express, knowing the number of unsolved problems in malaria, and now they would not have the opportunity to pursue the subject further. In making his final plea, Darling wrote to Rose:

> I am desirous of making myself useful to the commission on any matter within my powers but in considering the paramount importance of malaria in the [t]ropical and [s]ubtropical [w]orld and my familiarity with the subject I earnestly hope that I may be given an opportunity to carry out some investigations on this pest.[32]

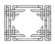

Strong opinions were commonly voiced about the poor reliability and low energy levels of certain ethnic groups, particularly the Tamils who emigrated from southern India to find work in Malaya.[33] Even though some of these social and physical characteristics could be ascribed to the parasitic infestations which the Board itself came to assess, the contempt for these groups because of their perceived laziness and inefficiency was expressed in derogatory terms: ignorant, superstitious, servile, unambitious, docile, and unstable.[33] On the other hand, Darling praised and expressed admiration for the Chinese. When he removed at autopsy the calvarium from a Chinese and noted the brachycephalic skull and its "wonderfully convoluted contents," he experienced a "profound respect" for the race and felt they deserved more of the East.[28] Yet, when he went into one of their pharmacies and inspected their therapeutic armamentarium, he could not help but think of them as conservative or backward with regard to disease and its causation.[28]

Heiser suggested that Darling visit the laboratory in Sumatra to observe what they were doing there. However, a "fierce jolt of dengue fever" held Darling fast, from which he expected to recover in a few days.[34] He described his symptoms as a fierce backache and a profuse eruption. He had long wanted to see a real case of dengue and now his curiosity was more than gratified, although he was disappointed because he didn't know whether he had been bitten by *Culex quinquefasciatus* or *Stegomyia scutellaris*.[35]

By August 1916, Darling had spent ten days in Sumatra visiting hospitals, laboratories and tobacco, rubber and tea estates.[36] He met with a number of health officials and obtained morbidity reports, learning what they had been doing and how much they knew about hookworm infection. Among a lot of "well-informed doctors," he found Baermann to have thought more deeply and truly into the whole hookworm subject than any other man he met. However, Baermann was having difficulty measuring the degree of soil pollution because of the problem of differentiating hookworm larvae from the many kinds of free-living nematodes inhabiting the soil. Darling kindly commiserated by saying that he had worked on the same problem enough to know how difficult it was.[36] Schüffner was very anxious to learn the anatomical features of anopheline larvae and Darling spent part of one morning with him on the subject. He was pleased and gratified of the way everyone had given up time to him, and said he was very glad that Heiser thought of him going to Sumatra.[36]

From Sumatra, Darling left for Java on August 4, 1916.[36] He welcomed the opportunity to study the effect of hookworm infestation on populations where malaria was less of a contributing factor than in Malaya. This would allow the Board to reach more solid conclusions about the relative contribution of hookworm to anemia.[37] Darling also was interested in applying comparative helminthology (the distribution of different parasites among different ethnic groups) as a means of explaining the currents of human migration in the world. The results of his observations in the Orient would germinate into an innovative presidential address to the American Society of Tropical Medicine nine years later entitled, "Comparative helminthology as an aid in the solution of ethnological problems."[38]

Darling had developed an admiration for the British and their colonial government, probably starting from the time he accompanied Gorgas to South Africa in 1913. In Kuala Lumpur he was brought into contact with a "fine lot of Englishmen" and this helped him to understand better what Thomas Macauley meant when he wrote about the "hereditary nobility of mankind."[39] He described the Dutch as continental in their manners and in their attitude toward the "big race problem." As far as he could see, only the English and the people of the Southern states had maintained a "proper" barrier against certain results of miscegenation.[39] During the trip to the Far East he had opportunity to strengthen these convictions. He found the Javanese to be servile everywhere except in Batavia (Jakarta), where they were "faintly indolent and ill-mannered."[39] The Malay, on the other hand, he described as possessing the graces and manner of gentlemen. Such strong opinions, although readily condemned today, reflect Darling's New England upbringing, his acceptance of colonialism, and the markedly segregated American enclave in the Panama Canal Zone.

The Java report was completed and submitted to the Rockefeller Foundation by December 1916.[40] However, Darling was still laboring over the extensive data accumulated on the hookworm studies in Malaya and a final report had not been sent to the expectant home office. He excused himself by saying that he had been disinclined to write much about the work and experiences for fear of conveying "incorrect and half-baked impressions."[39] It was only after seventeen months had passed that he felt he could speak with sufficient authority about the people and their diseases. The trips to Sumatra and Java had served as very important "correctives" to get a proper understanding of the natives' way of living.[39] The Malaya report was finally completed at the end of February 1917, and Darling was ready to start work in Fiji on the following month. He considered that the four months spent in Java had yielded information of the highest value. He was struck by the large amount of valuable work that had been done on cholera and plague in Java, but dismayed by the relative lack of information they possessed about malaria in their own country, and the usefulness in that Far-eastern part of the world of a consultant in anti-malarial problems.[41]

Darling was happy that Barber was going with him to Fiji, as this would shorten the time required to complete the work there. He thought that it would take about two months to finish the work in Fiji and estimated their final date of returning to New York in about September 1.[42] The day before sailing for Fiji, Sir Arthur Young and Lady Evelyn had them for dinner at the Government House and Sir Edward Brockman invited them for lunch. Darling was very pleased with the "splendid way" they had been treated during the entire period of their stay.[42] He thanked both gentlemen by "letter and the spoken word" and thought it would be appreciated if Rose would also write expressing their "sense of gratitude for the courtesies, hospitality and various arrangements made for our comfort and for furthering the progress of our work."[42]

On May 18, 1917, the members of the Malaya Board arrived in Fiji aboard the R.M.S. *Niagara*.[43] They soon were busy examining and treating indentured Indians from neighboring sugar estates, as well as

Fijians and "half-caste" children. Although 100 per cent of the adult Indians were found to be infected with hookworm, they showed little or no anemia. This permitted the Board to correlate more accurately the number of worms harbored with the hemoglobin measurements in residents of a country free from the plague of malaria. Darling seemed to be enjoying himself, as he found that he had excited the interest of the "entire population of Indians, Fijians, and even whites," with his hemoglobinometer.[44] A great rivalry developed among the white populations as to who would have the highest hemoglobin. He strongly recommended the use of a Dare hemoglobinometer in selected cases and places as a valuable means of exciting the interest of all people in such diseases as hookworm and malaria.[44] This brief moment of levity could be easily forgiven when taken in context of the arduous and onerous task of examining each night-soil sample for worms from almost four-thousand individuals.[45] Darling found that local assistants could not be trusted to make accurate reports and, therefore, in order to have reliable data on the number of worms after each treatment and purge, the stool examinations were exclusively done by the members of the Board or under their direct supervision. To avoid the danger of contamination from other pathogens such as cholera, dysentery, and amebiasis, the fecal samples were treated with a strong disinfectant. During thirteen years of tropical service, Darling had luckily remained free from helminthic infection although in Malay countries during malarial and hookworm surveys and stool washing operations he was exposed many times. However, just before leaving Fiji in August, he contracted amebic dysentery while doing a hookworm survey on the Rawa river.[46] On fecal examination, he found *Entamoeba dysenteriae* and trichuris (the latter a relatively harmless comensal).[46]

Unable to finish the investigations in Fiji by July, Darling wished to examine further the effect of chenopodium as a filaricide and felt confident that this could be demonstrated in time to complete the work and still be able to sail in August to Vancouver. The lengthy, hand-written, final report of the Uncinariasis Commission to the Far East was sent in advance to the Rockefeller Foundation and arrived ahead of the authors. The report was later published by the Rockefeller Foundation International Health Board in an abridged form consisting of 191 printed pages, 97 photographs, maps and graphs, and 54 tables.[47] Darling referred thereafter to the original report as the *magnum opus*.[48] This work deserved the qualification of *magnum* not only because of its length (over three hundred handwritten pages), but because it radically changed what was previously known about hookworm disease and offered a new approach to evaluation and treatment. Furthermore, it emphasized the importance of making a detailed *a priori* study of the social and cultural characteristics of the affected population and the danger of arriving at erroneous results unless other prevalent diseases were evaluated separately. Darling's meticulous and highly scientific work on hookworm disease revealed, as did his previous work on malaria in Panama, an innovative approach to the study of parasitic diseases of man.

In conducting its inquiry, the following plan of action was followed by the Uncinariasis Commission: (1) study by clinical and laboratory methods the cause of anemia among the patients who were admitted to a large general hospital; (2) examine at the detention (quarantine) camps at Port Swettenham and Singapore a large number of Tamil and Chinese immigrant coolies from Southern India and Southern China; (3) treat with chenopodium or some other vermicide, a considerable proportion of those who on examination showed evidence of hookworm infection; and (4) make every effort to trace the treated cases to the several estates and mines where they worked for the purpose of re-examining them in order to determine the consequent exposure to hookworm infection and malaria on their general health and working efficiency and, at the same time, estimate the relative effect of the two diseases in causing anemia and to determine the value of treatment.[49]

Stool specimens were examined for hookworm ova, either by the smear or centrifuge method, or by vermicidal treatment and the recovery of worms expelled. The latter was found to be more accurate. In the smear method, feces were diluted with water and dropped on two inch by three inch glass slides over an area delineated with a grease pencil, and combined with a mixture of equal parts of glycerine and saturated sodium chloride. The glycerine was used to clear the fecal material more rapidly, while the saturated saline solution allowed the ova to rise to the top, making it easier for the microscopist to detect these. In all cases, examination of the ova was done by an experienced microscopist and never entrusted to a subordinate.[50] In the centrifuge method, the fecal sample was mixed with water first and then placed in a test tube for centrifugation. After pouring the supernatant, a saturated solution of sodium chloride, with or without glycerine (if available), was added and the mixture centrifuged again. The floating ova were then removed with wisps of cotton and mounted on glass slides for examination. A modification of the centrifuge method used two or three drops of hot nutrient agar added to the test tube which, upon centrifugation, floated to the top and ova adhered to it. Once the agar solidified, it could be easily removed for microscopic examination. Although the smear method was the more accurate of the two, the centrifuge method was more expeditious and allowed for as many as thirty samples to be prepared in the course of an hour.[50]

The method of vermicidal treatment and recovery of worms was more

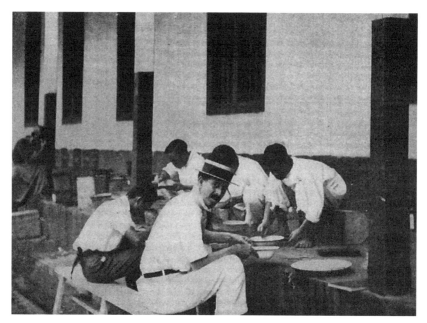

9.1 Darling and his assistants in Java washing fecal samples to detect hookworm larvae, circa 1915. Reproduced with permission, courtesy of Rockefeller Archive Center, Sleepy Hollow, New York.

9.2 Prisoners in Java jail and treatment squad changing "jerries" (receptacles for collecting feces), circa 1915. Reproduced with permission, courtesy of Rockefeller Archive Center, Sleepy Hollow, New York.

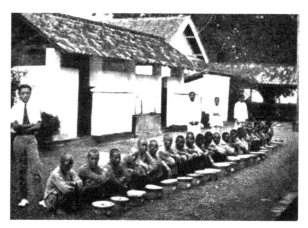

elaborate and required precautions to prevent inaccuracies. The individuals selected for this method were examined clinically and physically and selected on the basis of hemoglobin determinations. On the morning of the day previous to treatment, patients were allowed their usual diet. In the afternoon they were given some rice gruel and a half-pint of milk. At 5 p.m. a purgative was given (six drams or about three-quarters ounce) of a saturated solution of magnesium sulfate, or one ounce of sodium sulfate, or one ounce of castor oil. On the morning of treatment, all food was generally withheld, although in some cases a little milk was permitted. The first dose of the vermicide was given at 7 a.m.; the second and third doses were given at hourly intervals thereafter. Two hours after the last dose of the vermicide, a second purgative dose was administered, corresponding to the one given the night before. At 12:30 noon, the patients were allowed to drink milk, and in the afternoon they were given a little rice and curry, but vegetables with coarse fibers were prohibited because they interfered with the search for worms. A second treatment was given after an interval of from seven to ten days. The efficacy of treatment was determined by noting the percentage of total worms removed, careful search being made of four or more stools submitted by each case. This search for worms naturally proved to be a tedious and laborious process.[51]

Rigid "military" discipline was instituted to avoid any possible mixing of the samples from different cases.[52] In jails, where each person was confined to his own cell, it was comparatively easy to avoid confusion. In hospital wards, the patients and hospital attendants were instructed explicitly to avoid mistakes. In one series, the possibility of mixing samples was altogether eliminated by giving each patient at the time of treatment a dose of small glass beads.[52] The beads differed in color and size, and only one sort was given to each patient.

The stool samples were brought to the place of examination twice daily, at about 7 a.m., and again at about 2 p.m. The patients were checked for the numbers on their wrists to correspond with the numbers of the collection vessels. The samples were then washed either using a sink with running water or, more frequently, using a stream of water siphoned from a container placed several feet above the ground. The stream was regulated by a pinch-cock at the lower end of the hose to wash the samples placed on a large brass wire sieve with a mesh of fifty to an inch.[52] The washed stools were then distributed into photographic development trays, the dark brown ones found to furnish the best background for detecting the worms. The expelled worms were then picked up with needles or forceps and placed in properly numbered Petri (covered round glass) dishes containing normal saline. Finally, the excess salt solution was drained and the worms were killed by flooding the dishes with boiling alcohol. The worms, when scalded, became rigid and assumed shapes that were characteristic of the different species. Differentiation was thus rendered comparatively easy and the worms could be rapidly counted. The commission kept careful records of all the data obtained, including the number and sex of the different helminthic species expelled and recovered.[53] For example, in Java alone, altogether there were over 2,463 spleen examinations for malaria, 2,403 hemoglobin determinations, 447 blood examinations for malaria plasmodia and 394 persons treated, from whom 35,090 hookworms and 3,181 roundworms were recovered.[54]

The results of the investigation were summarized by Darling in a fifteen-page hand-written report which highlighted the most important findings.[21] The work disclosed that hookworm infection existed to a greater extent than was generally recognized. In most tropical communities where the majority worked in agriculture, practically one hundred per cent of adolescents and adults were infected. A positive correspondence was shown between the degree of infection (actual number of worms harbored) and the amount of blood loss or anemia suffered. It was estimated that about twelve hookworms were required to cause a loss of one per cent hemoglobin. Using rigorous methods of diagnosing cases of infection by the administration of vermifuge, instead of the less accurate method of microscopic examination of feces for ova, it was ascertained that a larger proportion of the inhabitants were infected with hookworms than was generally suspected. For example, where the microscopic examination revealed in the hands of the lay microscopist an incidence of 75 or 85 per cent infection, diagnosis by vermifuge revealed an incidence of 97 to 100 per cent. The usual method of diagnosis of hookworm infection by microscopic examination of stools for ova did not give any proper idea of the severity of the infections, i.e., the number of worms harbored by an individual and the degree of injury brought on the patient. In campaign work it was important to ascertain the number of worms being harbored for it was more desirable to institute campaigns for treatment in communities where the infections were heavy than where they were light. The therapeutics of several vermicides, more particularly of oil of chenopodium, were investigated by a method in which the efficiency of the drug was expressed by the percentage number of worms removed. Chenopodium was found to be more effective than thymol in expelling hookworms, but even more efficacious in removing ascaris and other helminths, such as oxyuria, trichuris, and flukes. Since toxic symptoms were elicited with all vermifuges at higher dosages, it was necessary to reduce the dose given to as small an amount as possible. Chenopodium retained its vermicidal efficiency upon reduction in dosage better than thymol. A dosage of one and one-half ml of oil of chenopodium was found to be highly efficient and only slightly toxic, sometimes only causing transient dizziness and vomiting. Two treatments of this dosage removed 90 per cent of the hookworms present. Treatment with one large dose of chenopodium compared with two broken doses showed no significant difference and the commission thought it was probably unnecessary to divide the dose as was customarily done. Although the ideal purgative to be used with chenopodium was yet to be found, magnesium sulfate answered the purpose very well at a dose of one-half to one ounce. Castor oil was found to increase toxic symptoms such as dizziness and deafness when administered with chenopodium, probably by enhancing the solubility and absorption of the vermifuge.[21]

Based on these findings, the commission outlined modifications to the present methods of intensive treatment and made the following recommendations:

An active campaign on an intensive plan rather than a passive dispensary programme must be prosecuted. All the people must be reached and the heavily infected ones treated without delay. Everyone should be treated for they are usually all infected with hookworm or other helminths. The incidence of infections was usually so high that the method of detecting infections by microscopic examination was, as ordinarily carried out, hardly necessary. Consequently, within the tropics and where as in mines and elsewhere a high incidence of infection prevailed, the population should be treated en masse by an intensive method and probably without the unnecessary preliminary examination of the stools for ova. Millions of people in India were waiting for treatment. The same was true of Brazil and other tropical places. The customary method of examining stools microscopically by a microscopist was found to be expensive, time consuming, and yielded untrustworthy results. Diagnosis by microscopic examination varied in accuracy depending on the skill, persistence, honesty and technique of the microscopist, and it probably yielded evidence of infection varying between 4 and 25 per cent less than actually existed. If the microscopist failed to detect this number of instances of infection before treatment they would probably make as great an error in the examination after treatment when the number of worms remaining were fewer. Consequently the "cures" based on the results of microscopic examinations made after treatment were not always valid. The infected persons whose infection the microscopist had failed to detect were not given an opportunity to receive treatment for hookworm, ascariasis, tenia, clonorchis or other helminths with which they could be infected. Moreover, they were given the impression that they were free from infection yet this large number of infected persons continued to seed their environment, thus leading to their own continued re-infection and to the re-infection of others, including those who had been treated. From a public health standpoint this could not be regarded in any other light than as unsatisfactory. The Public Health Officer wanted every last worm removed from everybody, but that was impossible of achievement. In every district a goodly number of persons escaped treatment, they happened to be ill, are absent, removed to another district or entered the district after the census had been taken. We may say, therefore, that 5 per cent of the population remained untreated. This number added to the number of positive cases which the microscopist failed to detect made a total of approximately 19 per cent of the total population which remained infected. This number of carriers the Public Health Officer did not get rid of by present methods.[21]

In the course of its investigations, the commission microscopically examined the fecal samples of 3,776 Tamils, Chinese, Malays, Bengalese, Singalese, and Eurasians, and found that of this number 87.8 per cent were positive for hookworm ova.[21] The work of the commission extended over a period of twenty-five months. Darling spent a month on the island of Sumatra investigating the methods of treating hookworm disease. Afterward, he visited the island of Java, and for four months studied hookworm infection both with and without malarial complications, among the natives in urban as well as rural sections. Then, for the purpose of checking up the findings of the commission in Java, Sumatra, and the Federated Malay States, Darling and Barber visited an island in the Fiji Archipielago (Viti Levu) known to be entirely free from malaria.[54]

In the Far East, members of the commission investigated malaria and hookworm at the same time. It was their practice to make a malarial survey for each estate visited. They were frequently of service to planters by being able to point out the breeding places of anopheline malarial carriers, and to advise them of the measures which might be taken against them. Nevertheless, not all the anemia encountered among the people was attributed to malaria or to hookworm. Underfeeding in rural communities played an important part in contributing to the general anemia and debility due to "these three hand-maidens of death" (hookworm, malaria and poor nutrition).[21] In Fiji, where there was no malaria, it was estimated that underfeeding resulted in a group of East Indians having 9.5 per cent lower hemoglobin than another well-fed group of the same race. Each group harbored the same number of hookworms. In the jail in Batavia, taking the 109 treated prisoners as a whole, their hemoglobin was 25.8 points per cent below normal (95 per cent). Darling estimated that 6.8 points loss was due to hookworm infection, 10.3 points to malaria and 8 points loss were due to hard labor.[21]

Wilson Smillie, who later worked on hookworm with Darling in Brazil, considered Darling a fortunate choice as head of the Uncinariasis Commission, since he was unhampered by traditional methods of procedure and routine:

At the time the commission began its work in the Orient, there was little scientific interest in hookworm disease. It was considered a dead subject. It was believed that everything concerning the life cycle of the worm was known, that the principles of prophylaxis and treatment were well understood, and the only things remaining to be worked out were minor and unimportant details in the prevention and treatment.[55]

Milford Barnes, who was assigned to assist Darling in Java, remarked that Darling's thoroughness and insistence upon first-hand information were characteristic of his work:

> If a question arose, such as if rice fields were breeding places for anopheline mosquitoes, he would know, and into the mud he plunged and wallowed about in it until he *did know*. Anyone who tried to dip larvae from such places with a dipper on the end of a long pole, or who sent a native boy to do the wallowing for him, was in Darling's opinion, simply a "pseudo" scientist.[56]

Sir Malcolm Watson was quoted by Barnes as saying that there was always a marked difference between what we knew before and after Darling had worked upon a subject. Before he had worked on it, we might *think* certain things to be true. After Darling had toiled over the subject, even though no new facts had been discovered, he would have so marshaled together the known facts and so fortified them with impressive data that our knowledge on that subject henceforth would be clear and definite instead of hazy.[56]

Several months before the Uncinariasis Commission completed its work in the Far East, Rose received a letter from Gorgas, now Surgeon General, anticipating that upon Darling's return he would like to send him, Juan Guiteras (a Cuban pathologist) and Henry Carter (of the U.S. Bureau of Public Health and Marine-Hospital Service), to Brazil to look into hookworm conditions there.[57] Gorgas expectantly concluded, "I do not see why they could not be doing investigative work down there while I am waiting to get rid of the German war."[57] Rose replied that the International Health Board also had designs for Darling, as they were thinking of him in connection with their malaria work and they were greatly in need of a man with his training.[58] There was a new proposition from Brazil which they thought might call for his particular ability. Rose invited Gorgas to talk this over in Washington later that week.[58]

By September 1917, Darling was back in Virginia and no doubt to the satisfaction of his wife, Nannyrle Darling, who had been repeatedly asking (as late as August 16) the home office for information about her husband's date of arrival in New York City from the Far East.[59] Once settled at home, Darling informed Rose that "Virginia was now covered

in every vacant lot and waste place with ragweed and chenopodium," and
that he had found a large clump of it growing right on the main street in
Charlottesville.[60] Despite these "homely" observations, Darling's
continued correspondence with the home office suggests that he was
already becoming restless and eager for a new assignment to see more of
the many wonders of the tropical world.

10

Institute of Hygiene, São Paulo, Brazil

The Rockefeller Foundation soon realized that one of the bottlenecks in accomplishing disease control campaigns on targeted diseases, mainly hookworm, malaria and yellow fever, was a lack of properly trained personnel.[1] A practical solution to this problem was the establishment of schools of hygiene, both at home and abroad. William Welch, not suprisingly, was asked to spearhead the establishment of a School of Hygiene and Public Health at Johns Hopkins, and he became its first director when the school opened its doors in October 1918.[1] Students were required to take courses which included bacteriology, biostatistics, epidemiology, sanitary engineering, and public health administration.[2] For the first time, thorough formal training was provided for the preparation of public health officers in the United States.[2] Similar efforts were made by the Rockefeller Foundation to create schools of hygiene in other parts of the world following the Baltimore model, that is, associated with a university to assure high quality training.[3,4]

On May 22, 1917, the International Health Board approved a plan of cooperation with the medical school in São Paulo, Brazil, to organize a department of hygiene.[5] Darling was nominated to serve as professor of hygiene and director of the laboratories of hygiene for a period of five years.[5] On September 17, 1917, Darling accepted the offer and Rose was much gratified, noting that the work Darling had done in the Far East had given him admirable preparation for attacking the two chief medical problems [hookworm and malaria] in the state of São Paulo and perhaps in Brazil as a whole.[6] On November 2, 1917, Darling wrote from Charlottesville, Virginia, saying that he had six cases of books, specimens, etc., ready for shipment to Brazil.[7]

Darling arrived in Rio in January 1918, and he was met there by Lewis

Hackett, director of the Rockefeller Foundation field operations in Brazil.[8] On the previous November, Darling had sent Hackett an outline of a cooperative plan of investigations between the school of hygiene and the field workers. This included mainly a continuation of the work previously carried out in the Far East on evaluation and treatment of hookworm disease.[9] In Santos, Darling was helped off the boat and through customs by an aide from the medical school and, although every box and trunk was opened, none of the contents were disturbed.[8] He spent the next two weeks visiting laboratories, doctors, and hospitals in São Paulo and found much to admire. He found that the people of Rio and São Paulo possessed a different culture but one with "interesting points of superiority."[8] The cleanliness of the streets and the general tidiness of both cities, surpassed anything he had ever seen.

The government had placed at his disposal a palace with about forty rooms, formerly owned by Baron Piracicaba and located at 45 Rua de Brigadeiro Tobias.[8] The old mansion had a garden and a grotto, classic figures on the roof and great, high iron fences and gate. Darling planned to use the upper floor and share the lower one with the Department of Experimental Pathology and Parasitology.[8]

A 29-year-old Brazilian, Geraldo de Paula Souza, was assigned as his first assistant.[8] Souza was a graduate of the school of medicine in Rio and had done considerable work at the Polytechnic Institute in São Paulo. He had studied also in Berne and Münich and was interested in water purification. Darling was pleased with his new assignment and commented that the climate was better than he expected. However, he longed for his family and added, "Now if I could only get my family safely here I would be very happy indeed!"[8]

The dean of the medical school, Arnaldo Vieira de Carvalho, was immediately impressed by Darling and commented that he had already conquered their sympathies by his fine manners and high scientific knowledge in all matters treated by him.[10] He further expounded that he expected that the help given by the American science, so well represented by Darling, would be of great benefit to the country. He guaranteed that everything possible would be done to facilitate the work of the "illustrious scientist."[10] Darling had not previously encountered — either in Panama or in the Far East — a strong anti-American sentiment hidden under superficial pleasantries. Only his uncompromising dedication to science helped him to weather the health, social, and political upheavals which later would threaten to undermine his work in Brazil.

The school of hygiene was scheduled to open in March 1918, in time for the start of classes in the medical school.[11] With the support promised by the local government, the remodeling of the building by painters and carpenters was making the laboratory "a thing of beauty" and Darling thought that "it will look better than my Portuguese will sound."[11] He found the language about as "difficult as Russian is said to be, and is as hard as Malay was easy."[11] Darling delivered the introductory lecture of the course on April 6 and this was followed by weekly lectures. To circumvent his difficulty with the language, Darling prepared the matter of the lecture and told it to his assistant Souza, who then delivered it in Portuguese "with true pedagogic frenzy even imitating the gestures and imaginary lines, diagrams and motions which I unconsciously made in the air while talking to him."[12] Eight months later he himself would deliver the lectures in Portuguese and was told that the students understood everything he said. "At any rate they have shown their good manners by not laughing at my pronunciation," was his final comment on the matter.[13]

Since Souza was scheduled to go to Baltimore for a course of hygiene at Johns Hopkins in September, Wilson Smillie, from the International Health Board field staff, was assigned to assist Darling during his absence.[8] More important for Darling, however, was the arrival of Mrs. Darling and the children to São Paulo in June. He acknowledged feeling "mightily relieved and overjoyed to find them undrowned, and looking so fresh and well-nourished. The presence of submarines off Barnegat [New Jersey] gave me such a scare that I lay awake nights seeing them."[12] The Darling family experienced bitter cold on their arrival in June and found an accumulation of one centimeter of ice in their suburb. Since homes were not provided with fireplaces, stoves or other heating devices, they attempted to keep warm with a kerosene heater, carrying it from room to room.[12] Mrs. Darling reminisced years later that life in São Paulo appealed greatly to the Darling family. They enjoyed a large home that was most adequate and had interesting and pleasant friends.[14]

Darling was well pleased with the design of the building provided by the government.[15] There was a lecture room, a library, a class laboratory, his personal laboratory, a bacteriological wing with five rooms, a "chemical wing" with seven rooms, and an office and a storeroom upstairs. Downstairs were four large rooms for the museum and other purposes and half a dozen rooms to be occupied by the Department of Experimental Pathology, besides other rooms used as dormitories for helpers and for fumigating experiments, animal houses in the backyard and a garden in front.[15] However, the workers were slow in getting things accomplished and he thought that perhaps he expected too much. He was unable to give any laboratory demonstrations until the supplies arrived, although he expected a consignment of these on one of the steamers that arrived that week.[15]

Even more disheartening was the tragic and unexpected loss of Wilson Smillie's wife, who died of puerperal fever four days after giving birth to a healthy little girl in São Paulo, under the care of a young American surgeon.[16] This loss was devastating to Smillie and hardly less to both Darling and Hackett, who tried to comfort him. Smillie blamed himself for not listening to the family's objection to taking his wife so far away from home and from all the advantages of good obstetrical care.[16]

Another calamity of more world-wide proportions was now arriving in Brazil. A severe epidemic of influenza (also called the Spanish flu, *hispaniola* or grippe) arrived in both Santos and Rio in early October.[17] Darling had been invited to read papers on hookworm and malaria at a medical congress in Rio, but when he arrived there the meeting had been "blighted" by the epidemic.[17] The entire city was "down, shops and banks were closed and means of transport much reduced."[17] The Santa Casa [hospital] was full, patients "lying in beds or mattresses on the floor, under the beds and in the aisles."[17] One of Darling's companions, Alex Pedroso, came down in 24 hours after arrival in Rio and became very ill, edematous and had albuminuria with delirium, great prostration and was still sick four weeks later. Darling took sick, had to go to bed on the following day, and returned to São Paulo feeling very weak.[17] In São Paulo the disease was increasing. Hospitals, soup kitchens and relief posts for the distribution of food and medical assistance were opened up by the various agencies working under government aid. The Boy Scouts were employed in conveying notices of new cases, discharges, and deaths to the Sanitary Office, in delivering medicines to houses, and in the telegraph service. Schools and cinemas were closed.[17] Hospitalization was the recommended mode of treatment, for the incidence was so high that whole families were struck down at once and there was much suffering from lack of sustenance.[17] Upon the outbreak of grippe in the city, Darling and his two colleagues, Smillie and Hydrick, offered their unreserved services to medical school dean de Carvalho, who was organizing the emergency hospital services. They were put in charge and gave their entire time to ward work in a 300-bed provisional hospital rapidly equipped and staffed at Mackenzie College by the Associacão Christã de Socorros Publicos (Christian Association of Public Aid).[18] Volunteer nurses were "mostly untrained but animated with a spirit of altruism."[18] Smillie soon came down with the grippe and was in bed for several days. Darling and Hydrick were able to stand up, presumably from enough immunity derived from their attack in Rio, but feeling "rotten."[17]

The suffering among the poor in the city, Darling reported, had been considerable. Each day some 7,000 new cases were reported and the deaths reached 250.[17] The predicted case mortality was 3 per cent and about 3,200 deaths were expected from the disease all told in the city. He concluded this ominous report of devastation: "Today came news of the signing of the armistice, but we were all so depressed from the 'Hespanhola' [*sic*] that there is hardly a shout or a cheer in the town."[17] The mortality predictions proved to be too conservative: out of a population of 450,000, the city of São Paulo suffered 5,500 deaths from the grippe.[18]

Smillie also wrote to Rose describing his own experiences with the influenza epidemic.[19] The Rockefeller team, consisting of Darling, Hydrick, and Smillie, volunteered to serve as staff for the recently opened Mackenzie temporary hospital. On the second day, the president of the State of São Paulo visited the hospital and volunteered to pay all expenses, allowing them to run a much bigger hospital than they could have with voluntary subscriptions. All nursing and executive work was done by volunteers and the hospital soon had the reputation of the best temporary hospital of more than thirty that were organized in the city.[19] The trio of volunteers experienced amusing incidents, as well as terrible ones. Darling was described as "a scream as a medical resident, for he is a therapeutic nihilist," while Hydrick and Smillie had "greatest faith in their own favorite remedies."[19] Smillie had almost all the losses first and came in for a good deal of "teasing," but he insisted that he had all the sickest patients. They needed all their courage, however, for whole families poured in and, in some instances, both father and mother died the same night, leaving a big family destitute.[19] Referring then to his own plight, Smillie left his own two motherless daughters under the care of a professor's wife who had been staying with him. They locked the gate to keep the servants in and Smillie stayed away, as he came down in the middle of it, "just when I was needed worst."[19] Fortunately, neither the professor's family nor Smillie's young children had the flu. The epidemic was now almost over, although still more than 200 deaths occurred every day. "No food was to be obtained, no cars were running, not even [enough] men to carry out and bury the dead."[19] Some of the old residents said that it reminded them of the yellow fever days, but from the awful stories he heard and the things he saw, Smillie was reminded more of the tales of the Black Death that swept through England. He concluded: "It was an experience of a lifetime, and I feel sure we did some good, and know that we stepped into the gap, which it would have been impossible to fill otherwise."[19]

Once the influenza epidemic was over, Darling returned to his duties at the school of hygiene, although the laboratory work was hampered by a delay in the delivery of needed supplies for almost a year.[20] Student microscopes were not available from the medical school and had to be ordered from the United States. Local supplies were "exorbitantly expensive."[20] A liter of formaldehyde, which in the United States was bought for 40 cents, here cost $5.30. Glycerine cost six-and-a-half times home prices. Even alcohol, which was made from local sugar cane and was a shade cheaper, was not nearly up to the grade expected.[20] They preferred to buy as many as possible of the articles available locally, even when these were more expensive, because of difficulties in procuring supplies from home due to the war and the incident delay to the passage of goods through local customs.[20] Darling noted that these conditions were peculiar to Brazil. The economic system seemed to be built on one staple crop – coffee. The wealthy planters and their families paid almost any price for what they required. There was no real estate tax and revenue of the country was largely derived from customs. While the South was developing industrially, particularly São Paulo, imported goods cost "like the mischief" and home-made articles were nearly as high, for they were protected by the customs' tariff.[20]

Part of the initial objectives for the cooperative agreement between the Rockefeller Foundation and the government of Brazil was to facilitate the training of young doctors in hygiene and public health by sending them to Baltimore. Following a site visit by Rockefeller officials in early 1919, a modification of plans was recommended, mainly to concentrate on the training of public health men in Darling's laboratory and to urge the establishment of a state school for health officers.[21] Another recommendation was to broaden the hookworm campaign to include work on malaria, Chagas' and other diseases, as in some districts these were of greater importance for purposes of the demonstration of the public health methods than hookworm disease.[21] Rose began to wonder if the Department of Hygiene and Public Health, which being started in a modest way at São Paulo, could be developed into a public health school sufficiently strong to train public health workers from other states.[22] Richard Pearce, director of the Division of Medical Education, responded that all agreed that Darling's department should be made a center for training health officers for Brazil.[23] Darling had already been asked by the secretary of the Interior to undertake the preliminary training of one of the school inspectors, in school hygiene.[24] At the official inauguration of the department on April 5, the governor of the state was reportedly amazed at the completeness of the department and most enthusiastic about its possibilities.[23] Pearce considered it now the best department of hygiene in Brazil, even superior to the Oswaldo Cruz Institute and Vital Brazil's Laboratory.[23] He expected Darling's laboratory to become eventually one of the show places of the town, to be visited by "all persons interested in public matters."[23] Darling's public health exhibits had already made an impression on the public and Pearce stated that he could "not express adequately my admiration of what Darling has already accomplished. It is all beyond my wildest dreams."[23]

The satisfaction derived from this milestone was soon tempered by the development of serious complications from the use of antihelminthic medication. Smillie reported on the death of an 8-year-old girl following a second treatment with oil of chenopodium.[25] She had received the first treatment two weeks before, at a customary dose of one-half ml of oil of chenopodium, without any symptoms whatsoever. Ten days later, she received a second course of treatment and became dizzy and, by the next morning, she was deaf but hungry and ate a lot of food given by her parents. The child collapsed unexpectedly on the second day and died.[25] A few weeks later, Hydrick lost another child from the same neighborhood and four additional deaths were reported by the local health authorities.[25] A new batch of oil of chenopodium, which appeared different in color, odor, and consistency, was suspected. Darling, who was accustomed to the pungent odor of the oil from his daily contact with it in the Far East, noted that the new oil was paler in color, of lower density, and more pungent and acrid than usual.[25] Darling hastily cabled to the home office: "Recent shipment chenopodium lacks characteristic odor, paler more pungent and toxic. Urge scientific investigation at source. Immediate inspection all home and field stocks, reduce children's dosage. Stop shipment atypical variety."[25] Both Hacker and Darling himself knew about the unacceptable toxicity of chenopodium when given with castor oil and this, of course, had been avoided by them. Darling considered chenopodium a valuable vermicide and thought that a scientific investigation of the whole subject, of its culture, preparation and properties, should be done.[24] He advocated a study of the botany of chenopodium and allied species that might be used to adulterate the product and of its chemistry and pharmacology.[25] He requested a quantity of seed of chenopodium from Maryland, sufficient for "sowing about a half acre."[26] He thought it would be "wrong" to condemn a drug before learning more about its composition, methods of manufacture and purification, and urged to be sent any information they could collect about its method of production, chemistry, and pharmacology.[26,27]

The lack of sufficient laboratory apparatus and supplies due to the war and customs restrictions precluded adequate laboratory instruction for classes and research for nearly a whole year. Despite this hardship, no time was lost and trips were made about the city and its suburbs, as well as into the interior of the state, inspecting water supplies, water purification plants, garbage and sewer disposal plants, to acquire familiarity with the public health status of the community.[18] In due time, some field work was begun in attempts to duplicate some of the experiments already made and reported by the Malaya Board and to test thoroughly the value of its recommendations. By the end of the first year, Darling found, as expected, that *Necator americanus* predominated over *Ancylostoma duodenale* among the population surveyed. Out of a total of hookworms expelled by treatment, 18,520 were identified as *Necator* and only 417 (or 2 per cent) as *Ancylostoma*.[18] This information was important for two reasons: *Necator* was less virulent and easier to remove than *Ancylostoma* and, therefore, higher doses of oil of chenopodium were not necessary for treatment.[18] Secondly, Darling was developing a hypothesis about the distribution of different species of hookworm among different ethnic groups. The autochtonous New World hookworm was undoubtedly *Necator americanus* and *Ancylostoma duodenale* had been introduced later by Mediterranean races and by the Japanese.[18] He was eager to further test this hypothesis by examining "uncontaminated" indigenous tribes.[18]

The Malaya Board had recommended a single one-and-a-half ml dose of chenopodium as sufficient to remove nearly all hookworms, instead of the customary three doses. This was now tested among 82 Brazilian males and, again, it was confirmed that two treatments removed 97.1 per cent of the total 10,886 worms expelled; in other words, a third treatment accomplished little more than removing less than 3 per cent of the total worm burden.[18] In this experiment Darling also confirmed his novel idea that the objective of a hookworm control or eradication campaign should not be to achieve a certain number of cures; instead, it should be *to remove as many worms from as many persons as possible*. Thus, in the series of 82 boys, only 28 per cent were "cured" by the first treatment, that is, had *all* their worms expelled; however, 90.8 per cent of the total worms were actually expelled after only one treatment.[18] He explained that it was not the few worms left after treatment in any individual that was important, but the millions who harbored 150 worms each left untreated. He advocated, therefore, *en masse* treatment of large affected populations such as existed, for example, in South India.[18]

Once again, the limited value of microscopic examination was demonstrated in a series of 81 young males. The incidence of infection was found to be 84 per cent by identification of ova by microscopists, but 98.7 per cent by the treatment method of expelled worms.[18] This affirmed Darling's previous recommendation that services of microscopists were unnecessary for purposes of conducting a hookworm control campaign since they missed 14 per cent or more of positive cases.[18]

In the course of the field work on hookworm infection, malaria surveys using the spleen rate method were carried out.[18] Severe malaria was encountered in one of the riverine villages. The spleen rate in that part of the village nearest the breeding places of suspected anopheline carriers was 73 per cent. They instructed the villagers on simple ditching and drainage operations to control the breeding and delimit the malaria present.[18]

Nearly all of the equipment requisitioned early in 1918 was received by June 1919 and regular class laboratory exercises were begun on the following month.[28] Twenty-seven lectures were given in the course of the year. In order to present the subjects clearly and comprehensively, the lectures were prepared in English and then translated into Portuguese. This entailed a great deal of personal and secretarial work, but it was believed that the students obtained a much more comprehensive notion of the subject presented than if the lectures had been delivered extemporaneously.[28] The lectures were well illustrated by charts, diagrams, lantern slides, models and microscopic preparations.[28]

During the second semester, laboratory exercises were held twice a week. Malaria, hookworm, water analysis, milk examination, disinfection, and fumigation were subjects treated. Field excursions were conducted in malaria and hookworm control, factory hygiene, anti-stegomyia (yellow fever and dengue), anti-fly, and anti-mosquito campaigns, demography, and sanitary inspection.[28] A program of school hygiene was now in operation under Darling's immediate control and supervision. A young woman was designated as school nurse and she was given some necessary preliminary training. One of the new school buildings with about 800 students was assigned by the government for purposes of demonstration under the charge of a Brazilian doctor.[28]

An active campaign of public health propaganda was pursued with the aid of a designer attached to the laboratory staff who prepared posters, placards, tables, diagrams, and charts. Literature of all kinds, such as circulars, posters, advertisements, etc., dealing with all phases of public health work were collected, catalogued, and card-indexed to be used for teaching and general reference.[28] Assistance was given to several students in preparing their graduating theses (necessary for obtaining a doctor's degree), including four of these dealing with public health subjects. Conferences were held with field directors and members of their staffs, with reference to anti-malarial measures and methods of hookworm treatment.[28]

A list of the research and other work accomplished included: field work on hookworm infection with special reference to devising methods for a more economical and scientific conduct of hookworm campaigns; isolation and cultivation of *Leptospira icterohemorrhagica* from São Paulo rats; study of a plague-like bacterial infection of city rats; bionomics of certain anopheline mosquitoes in São Paulo; study of the anatomical characters of anopheline larvae as a means of their rapid diagnosis in the field; study of the viability of culture of hookworm larvae; study of clinical cases of beta-naphthol (an anti-helminthic) poisoning; malarial survey of Paranagua; inspection of water supply of Rio de Janeiro, Ribeirão Preto and São Simão; inspection of the milk supply and methods of milk inspection in the city of Rio de Janeiro; preparation of papers on malaria and hookworm infection; and two laboratory bulletins dealing with malaria control in Malaya and work of the Malaya Board in hookworm infection: "Pesquizas Recentes sobre a Opilaçao na Indonesia," and "Sobre algunas Medidas Anti-Malaricas em Malaya."[28]

Field work was continued as time permitted, i.e., during vacation intervals from school work. Among the important problems investigated were the actual number of hookworms harbored by different classes of the population of São Paulo; the proper dosage and number of treatments required for treatment of hookworms infection; the effect of with-holding or permitting food when administering chenopodium; advantage or disadvantage of a preliminary purge given the night before administering treatment; and checks on the accuracy of field micro-scopists.[28] Plans and orders were submitted for the construction of a model for demonstrating water purification methods and for several types of latrines and septic tanks to be used to teach students and *fazen-deiros* or owners of coffee plantations about the different methods of preventing soil pollution.[28]

The results of field research on hookworm infection and treatment in Brazil was submitted by Darling to the International Health Board on May 24, 1920.[29] The seven-page report evidenced Darling's remarkable grasp of the scientific method. Darling's customary attention to important details and elegant experimental design allowed him to reach the following conclusions:

> "1. A preliminary purge does not add to the efficiency of the treat-ment of chenopodium, when the drug is given in two divided doses – 1 ½ c.c., being considered the adult dose.
> 2. A preliminary starvation period is not necessary in the treatment of hookworm disease with chenopodium in divided doses of 1 ½ c.c., on the contrary the efficiency of chenopodium is lessened.
> 3. A small amount of food given coincidently with the drug – when chenopodium is given in divided doses of 1 ½ c.c. in the treatment of hookworm disease – greatly diminishes the efficiency of the drug.
> 4. In the small doses of chenopodium that are given children, the decrease in the efficiency of chenopodium caused by the factors of preliminary purge, starvation period, and food, is much more striking than the full adult dosage of 1 ½ c.c."[29]

These studies, in collaboration with Smillie, were subsequently published by the Rockefeller Institute for Medical Research as two sepa-rate monographs in 1921 and 1922.[30,31]

Darling realized that, although the work accomplished by the International Health Board was satisfactory, it was not going nearly as far or fast enough to reach the millions of individuals affected. He esti-mated that among the agricultural population, hookworm infection as a cause of debility was manifest everywhere and that workers possessed only about 75 per cent of their normal working efficiency.[28] He suggested that a more popular and universal campaign which utilized a social service agency might be more practical.

The Institute was honored that year by a visit from President Altino Arantes and the Chief Sanitary Officer of the State of São Paulo, Arturo Neiva, as well as other prominent doctors and laymen from Argentina, Bahia, Minas Gerais, Rio de Janeiro, Matto Grosso, Paraná and São

Paulo.[28] Darling continued to acknowledge the courteous and "ungrudging" cooperation of the dean of the Medical School, Arnaldo Vieira de Carvalho; the Chief Sanitary Officer of São Paulo, Arturo Neiva; the able assistance of Smillie; and the cooperation of Hackett and Hydrick in the important field work performed.[28]

The following year of 1920 brought unexpected changes to Darling's projected five-year plan to develop an Institute of Hygiene in Brazil. Political turmoil and the death of the supportive dean of the medical school would jeopardize the scientific direction and future legacy of the Rockefeller philanthropic effort. For example, Darling's school hygiene program using an inspector and a nurse provided by the dean, was "simply dispensed" because the plans had not been authorized by congress.[32]

After having been recommended by Darling and receiving training for two years at the Johns Hopkins School of Hygiene and Public Health in Baltimore, Souza returned to São Paulo convinced of the soundness of American methods of sanitation but highly critical of Darling's plans and the direction for the Institute. Emulating the "morbid critical" (as he himself described) character of his compatriots, Souza superseded Darling's usually factual and concise twenty-page yearly report with an eighty-page diatribe mostly critical of what had been achieved during his absence.[33] He considered the development of the Institute of Hygiene as "too slow and misplaced." The bacteriology and parasitology sections were the only satisfactory departments for the course of hygiene, yet similar departments were already present and under competent directors, so that these did not constitute an innovation to the city or the medical school. Conversely, he complained that other needed departments had not been even equipped yet. Nothing was available for studies on statistics — not even a calculator, for epidemiological work, for nutrition and food supervision, for industrial hygiene or for sanitary engineering.[33] He also cautioned that the collaborative research done by Darling, Smillie, and Hackett should not constitute the principal aim of the Institute. He further admonished that such research should be based on a wider knowledge of the general needs of the country, obtained by means of the varied "social associations" of the members of the Institute.[33] He blamed both the government officials, as well as Darling and Smillie, for a lack of cooperation between the Institute and the Sanitary Service in Rio. "Outside of São Paulo," he wrote, "nobody knows that this Institute is anything but a simple chair of the Facultade de Medicina."[33]

Souza's motives for his scathing report to the Rockefeller Foundation are difficult to discern. Darling had selected him as the first Rockefeller trainee to be sent to Baltimore for training, practically anointing him as his successor when the original five-year plan for development of the Institute was completed.[34] The International Health Board had emphasized that any philanthropic effort must be made in collaboration with local government officials, so that the planted seed would germinate into a self-sustained health initiative.[35] Perhaps it was the bravado that sometimes clouds the judgment of recent graduates as they return to their native lands and proclaim themselves as more knowledgeable than anyone else. Years later (and perhaps somewhat wiser), Souza would write to the Rockefeller Foundation as director of the Institute of Hygiene, commemorating its twenty-fifth anniversary in the following terms: "This Institute keeps warm memories of the time when [the] Rockefeller [Foundation], collaborating with the State Government, did so much for its progress and for the development of hygiene among us, as well as the time when the sadly missed Dr. Darling and Dr. Smillie worked with us."[36]

Following Darling's unexpected return in April 1921 to the United States for health reasons, Smillie was named to replace him as acting director and Souza became his assistant.[37] Souza was now able to convince Smillie that what was really needed was an independent institute of hygiene devoted mainly to research. The director of the sanitary service in São Paulo, Pedroso (who had previously accompanied Darling to the ill-fated medical meeting in Rio) felt threatened by Souza and the Americans.[38] After meeting with Hackett and Smillie, Pedroso agreed that an institute was a good idea, but preferred that it be under the government's jurisdiction (sanitary service) and not as part of a medical school.[38] Smillie appeared to have been caught in the middle and he intimated to Rose that "the petty squarrels, and bickerings, jealousies and tiresome intrigues and inter-mural politics" placed the future of the medical school in jeopardy.[39,40] Souza's political influence eventually prevailed and he replaced Pedroso as director of the state's sanitary service and succeeded Smillie as director of the hygiene department.[41] Darling, who much preferred science to politics, must have been dismayed at these developments. Forced by failing health to return home and then moving to Baltimore during a period of convalescence, he may have felt fortunate to have escaped the political maelstrom that enveloped the institute he had started in São Paulo. The Rockefeller Foundation tried valiantly to support the institute despite the warring factions, but after more than a decade of frustrations, a decision was made in 1933 to finally pull out and stop all aid to the institute.[42] Future attempts to build schools of hygiene were thereafter wisely directed at sites where politics were unlikely to meddle with philanthropy.[41] This was a costly lesson for the International Health Board. As Farley aptly commented on the embarrassing events that followed Darling's departure from Brazil and the consequent change in policy by the Rockefeller Foundation, "Once bitten, twice shy."[42]

11

Darling's Paralysis

At the beginning of the third year of Darling's five-year assignment in São Paulo, the happiness and satisfaction that he and his family experienced living and working in Brazil were truncated by an unexpected health problem. In April 1920, Darling's left leg became paralyzed.[1] He immediately returned to Baltimore and was seen by Walter Dandy, a prominent neurosurgeon at Johns Hopkins, who diagnosed a brain tumor and advised rest over the summer prior to brain surgery.[1]

A detailed history of Darling's illness was obtained by the surgical resident, Dr. B. Noland Carter, on admission to the hospital on November 15, 1920:[1]

Onset of present illness in 1913 with sudden onset of a "queer feeling" [of his] left leg (paresthesia), accompanied by burning in [his] left hand and arm. There was no change in these periodic symptoms until 1915 when he noticed his slipper would fall off the left foot. In March, 1917 he noted after a tennis game and some intake of alcohol, a strong 'pull' in the left leg and thigh and twitching of the left abdominal muscles. This persisted until 1918 when he had influenza and was in bed for a week. Towards the end of this he was awakened by spasmodic contraction of the left calf which extended to the thigh. He expected cessation after a few seconds but it continued. Then the whole leg became rigid. Then his body felt stiff and rigid, his chest was so constricted that he could hardly breathe. Next he felt his arm swinging as if serving in a tennis game. Then he lost consciousness. A week later a similar attack [occurred] which left him dazed and sleepy.

The contractions continued one to two times a month. In September 1918 after working hard and having [a] gastro-intestinal upset he fainted but had no convulsion. Following this he was very weak, and unable to sit up straight. The next day he had a numb feeling along the back of his index finger and thumb and found that he could not control his pen while writing. For a week or so after he felt "used up" and his left hand and foot were difficult to control. His left leg showed clumsiness on strain or excitement.

By November, 1919 he began to get irritable and to feel that his health was giving out. By March, 1920 weakness and clumsiness in [his] left leg increased.[1]

Following Walter Dandy's advise, Darling rested at his wife's family estate in Virginia during the summer. He responded well but his left leg continued to feel weak and with tremor of the toes.[1] A mixture of nervous apprehension and comforting humor belied his correspondence with the Rockefeller Foundation:

> I went through Dr. Barber's clinic early last June and have been resting here in V[irgini]a ever since trying to reconcile myself to the rather disturbing news I received.
>
> The doctors seem to think I have a brain cyst on the surface of the right motor area (leg) the pressure of which is causing the symptoms. I feel that they are right. It may be *cysticercus* [a parasite] in origin.
>
> Dr. Barber wants me to take a perfect rest and return to him in October; an operation will no doubt be recommended at that time. At present I am carrying out Dr. Barber[']s instructions and have gained 23 pounds in weight! You would hardly know me I have fattened so, but am still slightly lame and a bit nervous at times.
>
> Most sources of worry and annoyance have been dismissed from my mind, but I cannot forget that Mrs. Darling and the children are still in Brazil where I had hoped to join them this fall. . . . [2]

He asked Mrs. Darling to return with the children in time to place them in school in September and to be on hand for his anticipated surgery in October.[2]

An examination on admission to Johns Hopkins disclosed weakness and lost joint position sense of the left foot, poor "stereognosis" (sense of position in space) of the left hand, a "drop" (weak) left foot, a positive left Babinski sign (indicative of right-sided brain injury), and abnormally hyperactive knee and biceps reflexes on the left. The pre-operative diagnosis was a "dural endothelioma near the falx cerebri" on the right side.[1] Three days later, on November 18, 1920, Dandy performed a craniotomy and removed a three-ounce tumor which was diagnosed pathologically as a "glio-sarcoma."[1]

The post-operative course was uncomplicated and for the next two months Darling remained convalescing at the Johns Hopkins Hospital in Baltimore. A regular correspondence ensued between Mrs. Darling and Wickliffe Rose, General Director of the International Health Board, conveying steady progress in her husband's neurological condition and a paternalistic and supportive response from the home office. Dandy reassured Mrs. Darling that "all felt that things will go well."[3] A week after surgery, she reported that Darling was wheeled every day out on the verandah to enjoy the fresh air. By Christmas, he was able to walk the length of a corridor "with the aid of his cane but otherwise unassisted."[4] A lengthy letter from Mrs. Darling punctuated the end of what had been a tumultous year for the Darlings:

> All the Doctors tell me Dr. [Darling's] progress is splendid. He can now walk from his bed to a chair absolutely alone and the use of his leg is returning faster than [his] arm – but he does not seem discouraged with it as we are assured the full use of his arm will return – but it will be some months before Dr. Darling is quite well and strong. We are only waiting for the paralysis to clear up a little more before leaving here as I could not manage Dr. Darling alone. I am thinking of taking him farther south as he dreads January and February here and from a surgical point of view Dr. Darling is no longer a surgical case. Dr. Darling wishes me to thank you very much for your many kindness[es] Dr. Rose and he wants you to know just as soon as he is able he will return to his field work.[5]

By now the International Health Board was aware that Darling's recovery was slow enough to preclude his returning to work soon. Before the end of the year, arrangements were made to send Wilson Smillie back to São Paulo to substitute for Darling as professor and director of the Institute of Hygiene.[6] Rose informed Darling about Smillie's trip to Brazil and admonished Mrs. Darling:

> It is altogether natural that he [Darling] should now begin to think about his work. I hope, however, that he will be able to dismiss this from his mind completely. The one thing in which we are interested now is his recovery: work will take care of itself by and by. For the present, he should make himself comfortable, keep himself entertained, and in a happy frame of mind.[7]

Darling was discharged from Johns Hopkins Hospital two months after surgery on January 21, 1921, and, as expected, moved south to convalesce in a more benevolent climate and where relatives and acquaintances awaited in Charlottesville, Virginia. Darling knew of no other form of entertainment than his work and, assisted by Mrs. Darling (he still was unable to write with his own hand), his personal correspondence resumed with frequent requests for books, reprints, and secretarial assistance with items related to his former activities, as well as updates of his condition:

> Thank you for forwarding the proof of the article on the Technic of Chenopodium Administration. . . . You might be interested in knowing that I *walked* out of the hospital Jan 27th something I never expected to do. Now I am steadily improving at home[;] a long, long period of convalescence ahead of me for the paralysis in my left and useful side will take some time to disappear.[8]

By the end of February, he was able to write clearly on his own a complete letter and proudly commented about it:

> I have just rescued the enclosed [manuscript] from my port-folio and the oblivion to which it might have fallen had I not had so good a diagnostician and surgeon as Dr. Dandy last June and November. . . . It is slow work getting well but I can note a little improvement each week. My left shoulder and arm are stubborn, but the muscles are slowly yielding. Fortunately I have my hitherto despised right and my hand-*righting* is not 'too bad' is it?[9]

Miss Miller replied admiringly:

> I could hardly believe my eyes when I saw your letter written in your own hand and when I think it was written with your right hand, which is the equivalent of my left it seemed to me perfectly remarkable and I don't think you need to be at all discouraged. I shouldn't be at all surprised to hear that you are actively at work again at any time.[10]

As spring arrived in Virginia, Darling was back in Esmont, Virginia, and he candidly wrote to Rose about his progress:

> Thank you for the notes in reference to hookworm specimens and the Lancet account of our Report. There are days when I yearn to get back into the midst of work once more. And then days, getting fewer in number and much farther apart, when I am not quite so keen about it. It is a matter now of building up and accumulating another supply of reserve nervous energy, and of waiting for a return of strength in atrophied muscle groups and of their old time coordinative powers. I am following the doctors orders to the letter. Each week I can note decided gains and no losses. My left shoulder girdle has been very stubborn but is now slowly yielding so that when I am fresh and rested I can elevate the elbow to the level of the shoulder and keep it there for a few seconds. I can go up stairs unassisted but require help to descend unless I go backwards, and in this case there must be a support on the right hand side (railing). The shoulder disability prevents me from being able to dress and undress myself, that is as to getting into sleeves on the left side. But now that the shoulder is loosening up I hope to rid myself of this annoyance in a few weeks.

I am walking now over a mile a day and sit around and go about at intervals from 8 a.m. to 8 p.m. without fatigue – a big advance the past week.

I am writing this with my right hand for my left is still rebellious to command and owing to weakness in the shoulder and pectoralis major. But this disability will soon be gone for I can now write a dozen words or so before fatigue sets in.[11]

The despondency that Darling felt at the beginning of his ordeal, when he noted the progressive worsening of his symptoms from paresthesias to localized seizures with secondary generalization and culminating in paralysis of his left side, particularly as he saw his inability to continue his work, must have initially filled him and his family with a sense of desperation and impending doom. The success of the operation at the hands of a prominent neurosurgeon and in a famous hospital, leaving him with only a residual weakness of the left arm and leg, filled him with joy and a sense of "rebirth."[1] Darling confided in his sister, Ruth Ann, and bubbled with optimistim about his recovery:

I do wish you could be here this beautiful afternoon. The front lawn is getting green and the grass is short enough for golf practice. I spent half an hour this morning with my golf sticks trying to loosen up my left shoulder. There is distinct improvement in my condition which I can note each week. Yesterday I washed my face and hands man-fashion for the first time since Nov. 18. I can go every where without a cane, though my gait is pretty one-sided. With a cane I can romp along fairly fast. My only serious obstacle to complete autonomy is in dressing and un-dressing. I cannot get into and out of my clothes without Nan's help. That means of course that I must always be in a good humour with her, particularly at dressing time. Oh it's so galling and aggravating to have to be under obligations to any one even your wife. Dear old Nan is sticking to me like a brick – kind of a mixed pickle metaphor that! And I am trying hard to get back to "normalcy". . . . You are very much like me – as I was from my 25– to 30th year, when I was becoming morbid from too much introspection and solitary living. I got normal by being dragged out of my shell – it was very easy and now I am so glad.[12]

While two of the children (Jinny and Buck) stayed with his sister in New Jersey, Mickey accompanied his parents in Virginia. Darling observed proudly: "Mickey is a great little man, he tries so hard to do everything man-fashion. Every morning he helps Grandpa feed the horses, gets the wood and chips in, gathers the sage, and assists as *1st asst* in each and every operation on the farm, agricultural and culinary."[12]

Three months later, Darling was back in Baltimore visiting the School of Hygiene and having tea with William Welch at Johns Hopkins.[1] He further described his progress:

> Mrs. Darling has turned me loose, saying that she is off on another case!. . . . I am arranging to work for a few hours each day at the Laboratory, and see how I get on. Next week I shall meet Dr. Dandy and Dr. Barber and have them tell me what I should be able to do for the summer. My lameness makes stair climbing (with balusters on left side or without them) a bit hazardous or impossible as yet. I fear that some degree of lameness will be permanent, but then, to that extent I shall be in Pasteur's class, will I not?[13]

No doubt with the approval and encouragement of his doctors, Darling moved by the end of June from Esmont to Baltimore. He began to spend more and more time each day at the Johns Hopkins School of Hygiene, taking care of unfinished business and projects interrupted by his illness. On July 11, he was able to examine for the first time since his operation a sample of mosquitoes from Puerto Rico given to him a year before for identification. He reported to Rose that the specimens were *Anopheles albimanus* and added, "Perhaps you can guess how happy I felt at being able to look through a 'scope at my old friend *A. albimanus.* I am feeling tip top every day."[14]

In addition to the use of the microscope, Darling considered using for the first time a typewriter "for correspondence and to exercise my disabled arm" while at the School of Hygiene in Baltimore.[15] The International Health Board promptly obliged by sending him a Corona typewriter from their stock. His comments about the typewriter are interspersed with the customary wit:

> I have always been opposed to operating a type-writer for I preferred to spend my time over a microscope, and typewriting requires more precision in the use of capitals and commas than long hand – orthographical equivocation too, certainly comes harder with the machine – but I am becoming a typist just as I have become a seamster (for the winter only I hope).[16]

On August 24, 1921, he replied to a request for follow-up information that some disability of the left arm and leg still persisted, but that he could go everywhere and could write now with his left hand.[1] "All the joys of life have returned and my old enthusiasms for work are as keen as ever. . . . I have become reconciled to my motor limitations – no more tennis or swimming – and am glad to be alive and happy once more."[1]

This state of happiness reached almost a state of euphoria, as can be deduced from a letter sent to his sister, after he had visited her in Pawtuckett, Rhode Island, and helped her to learn a poem she had to recite in school while suffering from a head cold:[17]

Baldibore, Baryland, Ogd. 26.

By dear liddle Jude Bride:

Sabby has a dew tdoy id dthe shabe ad forb of a dybe-wrider the whigh he borrowed from Brider Rogefeller, godzguedly you will have infligted od you adother sprig poeb – ad ud seaodable wod however.

"The withered badders of the gord are still,
Ad gathered fieldz are growig stragely wad,
While death boetic death with handz thad color whad they tough,
Weaves iddo the audueb woodz ids dapeedries of browed ad gold."

Well, little one, how are you and Alfredo? Happy I am sure. Tell Alf I met and old class-mate of his in Washington last week, Chapin by name. It was at a meeting of the Helminthological Society of Wash. I have never seen so many wormy men and women together in my life. Cobb – a free-living nematode, Cort of Colorado who has been counting hook-worm larvae in Trinidad the past summer, Chapin, Cooper Curtice and old enemy of Haemonchus contortus, Miss Cram, Hall, Hassall, Ransom and a few others. From an alphabetical standpoint the C's had it all to themselves.
I am feeling bully.
    Best love to you both,
        Affectionately, Sam"[17]

Darling became a Fellow by Courtesy at the Johns Hopkins University School of Hygiene (directed by William H. Welch) in Baltimore, with the blessings of the International Health Board.[18] For the next two years he channeled his enthusiasm and energy teaching students and publishing from the vast quantity of material he had collected in Panama, the Orient, and South America. He worked in a crowded office located in the first floor of the old biological laboratory at the corner of Eutaw Street and Druid Hill Avenue.[18] Those who came in contact with him were impressed with his vast knowedge and expertise. His associates were two graduate students, Shulamite Ben-Harel, a young woman from Palestine, and a young man from Japan.[1,19]
Periodically he would receive pathological specimens and parasite samples sent to the International Health Board for diagnosis or proper identification. He also took advantage of the Rockefeller facilities to distribute and publish samples of his work. Occasionally, a controversial matter would come his way, as when C. F. Craig took exception to certain statements he made in an article "The tertian characters of quotidian aestivo-autumnal fever," published in the *American Journal of Tropical Medicine*.[20] Darling confided his feelings about such encounters in these terms:

> I have been expecting to hear from him [C. F. Craig] and had asked the men here to keep a look-out for me. Of course I feel that Dr. Craig is dead wrong, others think so too. If I reply it may act as a breath of wind to dying embers. If I remain quite quiet his quotidian plasmodium may fade peacefully away into limbus where all discarded terms which have been reduced to the synonomy are confined. I am interested in reducing it to the synonomy – never have cared for polemics. It is a good plan sometimes to let the other fellow or the other girl have the last word. . . . [21]

Darling experienced one of his "slumps" in the early spring of 1922 and he traveled to Jersey City, where his wife and children were staying, to seek comfort and their company. He was able to take some of the responsibilities "which Mrs. Darling was bearing, and can stand any amount of noise and romping with the children without nervousness."[22] Realizing perhaps that togetherness was an important component of his complete recovery, a decision was made to buy a home and settle the family in Baltimore "until the children were educated."[23] On August 23, 1921, the Darlings moved into a two-story bungalow home at 2711 Elsinore Avenue in northwest Baltimore, within walking distance to the Johns Hopkins School of Hygiene.[24] The previous owner had also been paralyzed and the first floor was designed to facilitate mobility of a handicapped person.[25] The home was spacious enough to allow Darling to have separate rooms for his study and laboratory. The upstairs plan included three bedrooms; one for Mrs. Darling, one for "Jinny," and one for "Buck and Mickie [*sic*]," in addition to a library and children's study.[25] Darling was quite pleased with this arrangement: "You will see that I can shoo the family upstairs and can lock myself in for solitude," he wrote to his sister Ruth Ann, and added, "The automatic gas steam heater and hot water heater are treasures – no coal, no ashes, no dust, no waste."[25]

By November, he reported to Miss Miller:

> The children have "found" themselves at school and are doing well. I am enjoying work at the School immensely. This year my health and strength permit me to take up more fully interests in the work of the Dept. of Med[ical]. Zool[ogy]. I had always thought of myself as a pathologist but I find that they regard me as a medical zoologist. There is a very fine atmosphere here in the med. zool. dept. and it seems to be one of the bright particular stars in the hygienic galaxy.[26]

His immediate chief, Robert Hegner, tried to make his connection with the School of Hygiene a more permanent one. But Darling had recuperated sufficiently two years after surgery and was beginning to feel once more the "call of the tropics."[18] He was eager to return to the field and resume his studies on tropical diseases.

12

Station for Field Studies in Malaria, Leesburg, Georgia

The International Health Board scheduled a meeting for January 19 and 20, 1923, in Baltimore, and invited Darling, Dr. King from the United States Bureau of Entomology, members of the board and others interested, to review "what had been done, what should be undertaken, how and by whom" in malarial field studies.[1]

John Ferrell, director for the United States at the International Health Board, asked Darling regarding the possibility of conducting field studies in malaria control in one of the southern states during the present year, if he "still felt equal from a physical standpoint to the task," and if the work was of the type he would prefer.[1] The answer from Darling must have been affirmative on both counts, since within two weeks a tentative itinerary was made to observe field conditions in Virginia, North Carolina, South Carolina, Georgia, and Alabama. By March 21, Darling sent a three-page list of supplies to be obtained from A. H. Thomas and Co., and forwarded to his new address at Leesburg, Georgia.[2] Some of the requested items were required urgently, since the "season is opening for anophelines and we shall miss some important observations unless we are able to have the items sent to us at once."[2] In a whimsical note, Darling requested that all his mail be sent to Leesburg, and remarked: "I am now definitely on the spot trying as hard as I can to think like a mosquito. To avoid being bitten by an infected one is my fervent prayer. Oh, how I shall pray this next year!"[3] Darling was surely aware that prayer would be insufficient to protect him from malaria, as time would later prove.

Darling arrived in Leesburg on March 27, 1923, and was soon busy getting acquainted with people and places.[4] He was looking for a suitable location to use as a laboratory and thought he had found a good one in a school building. The hotel where he was planning to stay was very poorly protected against mosquitoes. It was screened but in the usual "imperfect" way with holes under the door and in the floor. Francis O'Connor, who was assigned to assist Darling at the station, was already busy catching larvae and pupae through the ice.[4] The timing of their arrival couldn't have been better: the first recently emerged adult anophelines were detected on March 29.

While anxiously waiting for the supplies and equipment requested, Darling asked the foundation for an advance for $250 to buy a Ford car, which he needed to conduct surveys and mobilize himself, to be deducted in two monthly payments from his salary.[5] Since his arrival, Darling spent a good deal of time in the field making preliminary surveys for the establishment of observation stations. He rented three rooms for the laboratory and started to make mosquito dissections. He thought Leesburg was going to be a good place to study malaria.[6] Spring was rapidly advancing in Georgia and "dogwood was in bloom, magnolia buds were swelling, fields were pink with peach blossoms, and mosquitoes too were on the wing."[7]

Leesburg had been selected partly because of the severity of malaria there, for Darling desired to become thoroughly familiar with certain fundamentals first and it was felt this could be done better where the malaria was severe than where it was mild, as it appeared to be in many other places inspected.[8] The country was flat and dotted with swamps, pools, and limestone sinks, which were ideal breeding grounds for mosquitoes. The river margins were wide and represented by many transient and permanent pools. Furthermore, the soil had peculiarities in that the absorption and seepage of rains was poor and the run-off slow. The water table was high and differences in elevation were slight. Darling requested for the services of an engineer who could determine in three to six months some elevations and let him know whether the ponds could be connected with one another and these with creeks and rivers.[8]

Although Darling requested that the two microscopes he needed be sent to him on loan from those available at the foundation, these were ordered from Bausch & Lomb at a cost of $219.69, and his supplies budget of $500 was soon exhausted.[9] His request for mosquito bars from Abercrombie and Fitch, entomological supplies from Ward's Natural Science Establishment, a hydrogen-ion comparator from LaMotte Chemical Company, and a reference text on the microscopy of drinking water, were temporarily put on hold.[9]

In April, the International Health Board asked Darling if he would be interested in a request from the New York State Board of Health to visit Wappingers Falls and Cornwall, in the Hudson Valley.[10] Some malaria had been detected in that area and the board needed an outline of procedure and estimate of the cost of carrying out the work. Darling replied that he would like very much to outline a plan of procedure and could easily dedicate a few days to this work.[11]

In May, two weeks were devoted to taking new "stills" (photographs) showing severe cases of hookworm and mass treatment of school children, and to the completion of a malaria film in which most of the scenes were selected by Darling to illustrate special points in malaria control.[12] These included preparations of ova, larvae, and adult mosquitoes, as well as predatory larvae and fish. The photographer thought that it would be necessary to hire professional actors from New Orleans to re-enact cases of malaria with chills and fever, but Darling was able to "secure some good native dramatic talent for these scenes among members of the local school board."[12]

The International Health Board was now considering Darling's proposal to help men in training and others interested in malarial surveys by sending them to him for preliminary instruction. He was very desirous of helping men to an understanding of malarial field work, in so far as his "experience and the opportunities there could be utilized."[13] The length of time spent at the station would depend on the circumstances. Two or three weeks would be sufficient except in the case of men for special malarial duty to be assigned to the Orient. In those countries a detailed knowledge of the anopheline larvae was important because of the importance in control work, and it would be imperative to give them special instruction in this subject.[13] The Georgia State Board of Health also was interested in sending their county health officers to Leesburg for instruction in malaria. Darling promised to take two county health officers at a time for three or four days and show them some of the more important features of their work, such as anopheline surveys, method of obtaining the spleen and blood index and laboratory features, so long as they came "equipped with a Ford car and a microscope."[14]

Complying with a request for a statement of the way he handled the students or men passing through the malaria station in Leesburg, Darling clarified that his aim was to try and have the men learn by *doing*.[15] The visitors understood that they were not to be mere observers but actual members of the staff and that the work assigned to them must be carefully and conscientiously done. The men were required to visit the stations established on some of the plantations regularly and to make collections of adult mosquitoes and to "dip for larvae."[15] They examined spleens of the children on various locations and had assigned to them certain children infected with malaria whom they were required to visit regularly and whose blood and spleens were to be examined regularly as well. A certain amount of laboratory work was required of them as, for example, testing larvicides, analyzing malarial data cards, identifying larvae, etc. The men were required to supply themselves with field clothing so that they could crawl under houses for mosquitoes and wade into water for larvae and get wet. An effort was made to "provoke rivalry" among them to see who could return to the station with best evidence of having made a satisfactory inspection. He endeavored to suggest to the men that they take rooms at the hotel where he lived so that not only in the laboratory but after the day's work he would always be accessible to them and so that they could have informal conferences and "wherever necessary criticism."[15] The main precepts, he summarized, were: punctuality, learning by doing, taking pain to show the men how, and then setting them to do it themselves, filling each day full of accomplishment, accessibility on the part of the director with frequent informal conferences on the verandah.[15] When some of the visitors complained directly to headquarters about the uncomfortable accommodations, unpalatable food, and discourteous service at the Magnolia Hotel in Leesburg, Darling responded that all of this was true, but that this was a small price to pay for the benefits obtained from being close to the laboratory and the opportunity to discuss after dinner any topic of interest on the hotel verandah.

Replicating his ability to attract students as well as experts in the field of malariology while in Panama, the Station for Field Studies in Malaria at Leesburg also became a mecca for malariologists and health officers from the United States and the rest of the world (see Appendix F: Visitors and Workers, Field Station for Studies in Malaria, Leesburg, Georgia). Darling named a few of these in a letter to his sister, Ruth Ann:

> Some 40 persons will have passed through the station at the end of the month. Walch and his wife from Holland and Sumatra, he is already an authority on malaria. Mrs.W is thin as a plate and crawled under the houses like a ferret. Pantaleoni of the L[eague] of Nations and Italy was here, Drensky from Bulgaria and his wife. Bailey from San Salvador. Kendrick from Ceylon, Cumpayon from Australia, Hops from the Malay Settlements, Lessa from Brazil. Wu Lien The from China. Kudo from Japan and Ill. Leach from the Philippines no Phillipines (without looking at the dictionary). Besides several men who have been sent by State Boards of Health too.[16]

Eager to interest medical students in careers in public health, Darling visited Emory Medical College and suggested to the dean that both junior and senior students be permitted to hear his talk on mosquitoes and malaria.[17] The proposal was not received with enthusiasm and, even less, his suggestion for an evening illustrated lecture on hookworm and malaria. "Apparently the Emory students, like many children in South Georgia, are not coerced into the paths of discipline," was Darling's wry comment.[17] The next day he lectured to half of the junior class and found an opportunity to mention the needs of the International Health Board for a "good type of man" to whom a career in public health might be

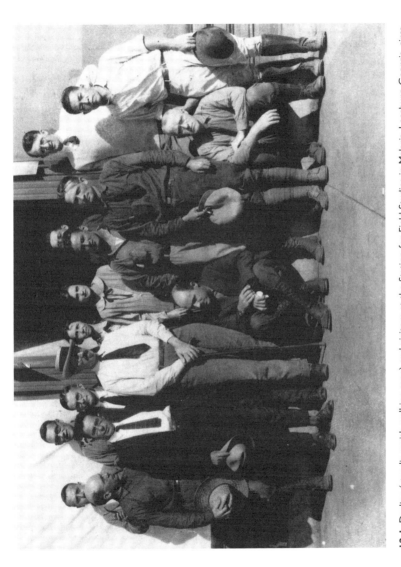

12.1 Darling (standing with walking cane) and visitors at the Station for Field Studies in Malaria, Leesburg, Georgia, circa 1924. Reproduced with permission, courtesy of Rockefeller Archive Center, Sleepy Hollow, New York.

welcome and attractive.[17] After the lecture, the students were invited to descend from the amphitheater, gathered around Darling at the blackboard, and inspected eggs, larvae and adult mosquitoes "with critical acumen."[17]

The importance of establishing a "rather intimate" relationship with the families studied by the doctor or those conducting the survey was emphasized by Darling.[18] He had been impressed in house-to-house visits in south Georgia with the necessity of gaining the confidence of the people in making health surveys. This took some time in "backward" communities. A survey could not yield trustworthy results if the people remained suspicious and "in-cooperative" as when surveyors ran rapidly through a community without really getting acquainted.[18]

In October, Darling attended a state-wide conference on public health in Savannah by invitation of Abercrombie and the president of the Georgia Medical Society.[19] He found himself on the program as one of the principal speakers, along with Assistant Surgeon General Lumsden, Robert L. Mattox, a former mayor of Atlanta and president of the American Bankers Association, and the honorable J. A. Holloman of Savannah. Darling spoke on the effect of hookworm and malaria in lowering the efficiency of the laborer using figures derived from his experiences in Brazil and the Orient.[19] He assured the audience that there was severe malaria in Georgia and suggested the necessity of further investigation. He was told later that he had presented some "good stuff" and he derived the impression from several of those present that his talk had been "not altogether uninteresting."[19]

By the end of the year, Darling was thinking along the possibility of limiting the propagation of anopheline larvae by affecting the food supply of the larvae.[20] The species of anophelines varied with the seasons and, presumably, with the quantity and character of the food of the larvae which, in turn, depended on sunlight, rainfall, shade, soil, aeration, etc. He requested the board to provide him with the services of a plant physiologist, preferably a person trained as a biologist or zoologist, and one who could perform water analyses and study the plankton of anopheline breeding places and the food of anopheline larvae as it is selected from the plankton during the changing seasons.[20]

A request for additional supplies included a list of books: Dorland's *Medical Dictionary*, Brumpt's *Précis de Parasitologie*, Manson's *Tropical Diseases*, Stitt's *Bacteriology and Parasitology*, Craig's *The Malarial Fevers*, and *Practical Land Drainage*.[21] Also requested was an inexpensive surgeon's or obstetrical bag, square-shaped opening with two lids at the top, suitable for carrying materials for taking blood specimens.[21] Although Russell thought that the library in Leesburg was very meager, Darling remarked that he had his own collection of reprints, which were available to all for use. What they lacked were current entomological and malarial periodicals but they had recently received on loan several volumes from the Surgeon General's library.[22] Darling's preferences for malaria reference material included Byam and Archibald's *Practice of Medicine in the Tropics* and James' *Malaria at Home and Abroad*.[23] Their chapters on malaria and mosquitoes were undoubtedly the best on malaria in English at the present time, according to Darling.[23]

At times Darling would ask the home office to obtain unusual samples and materials for investigative purposes. He recalled that in the East Indies natives used a poison to "stupefy" fish.[24] They would dam a stream, make a "decoction" of the plant in a pool beside the river and then run the poison downstream. The decoction would stun the fish temporarily and then these were easily caught. He thought the poison was commercially known as "derris" and asked for a quantity to perform larvicidal tests at the Station.[24] He also learned from an entomologist that there was a South American fish poison which could be a good larvicidal agent against mosquitoes.[24] The poison was a dried root or woody shrub known as "Cube" or "Barrasco." Darling requested a shipment of fifty to one hundred pounds of this material, ground to a coarse powder by a drug miller in New York, sealed in tin canisters, and sent to the Station for trial as a larvicide.[25]

The International Health Board utilized Darling's expertise in tropical pathology to good advantage by sending him a steady number of inquiries and specimens received from all over the world. Pathological material came from a patient in the hospital for the insane in Sandy Gallop, Australia.[26] He critically reviewed a report by Docherty on the value of carbon tetrachloride as an antihelminthic, pointing that no reference to the species of worms expelled had been made.[27] On reviewing the correspondence between the foundation and the Alaska River Fox Farms, he thought that the cause of death of the silver foxes was due to carbon tetrachloride poisoning, since this was characterized by "liver necrosis and defective fibrinogen formation resulting in hemorrhage due to insufficient coagulation, the clot lacking body and toughness, a condition which favors even capillary hemorrhage," as found by the government veterinarian in the dead animals.[28] Tissue from a Javanese woman who died at Moengo, Surinam, of blackwater fever showed that the hemoglobinuria had cleared before death and that it was, therefore, not a "pronounced" case of blackwater fever.[29] In theorizing whether a member of the crew of the steamer *Burnjam* was a case of yellow fever or malaria from Sierra Leone and Surinam, Darling vented his frustration at the lack of suitable pathological material from such cases. He asked if it would not be feasible to circulate a notice among all health and quarantine officers in America, West Africa and elsewhere, about the importance of saving tissue from the liver, preferably in Zenker solution or at any rate in formalin for all suspected cases of yellow fever.[29] The apparent gross tissue resemblance of blackwater fever to yellow fever was noticed only by the unpracticed observer and he thought that the two conditions were quite distinct to the experienced eye.[29] Sections of tissue from an Italian merchant who died at Warri Hospital of suspected yellow fever from Nigeria had no characteristic lesions of yellow fever.[30] Another case of suspected yellow fever from Nigeria also had none of the characteristic changes of yellow fever, but the pigmentation and bile staining of malaria.[31] Darling was suspicious that some, if not all, of the suspected cases of yellow fever sent from West Africa were instead due to malaria. Referring to an article on the value of "melaniferous leucocytes" in the diagnosis of malaria, he commented that pigmented mononuclear leucocytes were encountered more commonly in the sub-tertian or estivo-autumnal types, but that this was only a subsidiary sign of infection since plasmodia usually were found if the search was sufficiently prolonged.[31] Hookworms received from Rabaul, New Guinea, presented no public health problem, since the specimens closely resembled a nematode taken from pigs in Fiji and India.[32] In a case of suspected yellow fever from Colima, Mexico, he was unable to find "the fat existing in the minute intracellular droplets usually seen in yellow fever," and, instead, found abundant evidence for biliary cirrhosis.[33] He thought it impractical to utilize microsporidian parasites to control mosquito breeding, as suggested by Kudo, and did not think that a very large sum of money should be granted by the Foundation for this purpose.[34] He found little support for the common view that a special kind of mosquito transmits malignant malaria.[35] His experiments in Panama had shown that *Anopheles albimanus* were readily infected with both tertian and subtertian parasites. Other representatives of the *Anopheles* group tended to utilize common breeding places such as ground pools, stream margins, the grassy margins of ponds, ditches and other natural collections of water with grass, vegetation and algae, except those very swiftly flowing.[35] He thought it would be impossible to concentrate efforts on one representative of this group without affecting all the others representatives of the group. Examination of hookworms received from the Solomon Islands confirmed his suspicion that *Necator americanus* was the predominant hookworm in that population.[36] Tissue sections of two cases of suspected yellow fever from Piedacuesta and Onzaga, Colombia, revealed hepatic necrosis and typical changes of yellow fever only in the first one.[37] His critical comments of an article on the use of fish for mosquito control resulted in a list of forty-one pertinent observations and corrections demonstrating the difficulties in applying this method.[38] He was also interested in the treatment of syphilis by inoculation of malaria and commented that wherever he had been and inquired about this, it had seemed as though the natives of the tropics rarely or never developed paresis (syphilitic general paresis of the insane).[39] Since acute cases of malaria were available at all times of the year in the region, it would be easy in the summer to infect mosquitoes and he would like very much to cooperate with anyone interested in the problem.[39] A batch of hookworms found in dogs, cats, and hogs from Puerto Rico were readily identified by Darling as *Ancylostoma braziliense*, *Ancylostoma caninum*, and *Necator suillus*, respectively.[40]

Possible introduction of yellow fever into the East after the opening of the Panama Canal had concerned the British government in India and, particularly, the Indian Medical Service.[41] While in Panama, Darling had become interested in this problem and had ova of *Stegomyia scutellaris*, the Indian mosquito that breeds inland, sent from India to Panama.[41] He found that ova survived for several months in the dry state and remained viable. Since for safety reasons he had destroyed immediately all specimens as they emerged, he was unable to conduct further experiments to determine if this species could act as a vector for yellow fever. But he cautioned that if *scutellaris* proved to be an efficient carrier, then upon the introduction of yellow fever into India, the disease could spread into the interior far beyond the littoral where *Aedes egypti* was distributed and usually confined.[41]

Darling was of the opinion that Boyce's observations on yellow fever in West Africa were based on insufficient and erroneous observations, and had expressed himself in those terms to the Yellow Fever Commission of the Colonial Office in London in 1914.[42] This evidently coincided with Sir Ronald Ross' assessment of Boyce's competence. However, Darling thought that Sir Ronald was a "a very hard-headed Scot" who "went about constantly equipped with a logic-chopper."[42] It was very difficult to make a statement on any subject without "being knocked down with that instrument," Darling concluded.[42]

As a confirmed therapeutic nihilist, Darling recalled that none of the cases of yellow fever treated at Ancon Hospital or quarantined in Panama received the "Sternberg bichloride treatment."[43] General Gorgas, he further recalled, believed in making the yellow fever patients as comfortable as possible. Darling had no doubts that Gorgas had tried a number of different medicaments when treating cases at Havana, but at Ancon Hospital about the only utilized medication he recalled, outside of quinine for malaria, was "a small quantity of iced champagne."[43]

Based on his experience with yellow fever cases, Darling "felt disinclined" to make any comments on histories or post-mortem reports made by others on yellow fever and then sent to him from time to time by the International Health Board.[44] He considered that these represented to some extent observations made by others "with the best intentions in the world by usually inexperienced observers who misinterpreted what they saw."[44] The presence of black material in the stomach, for example, required examination under the "scope" or spread in a thin layer to recognize its true nature. In his experience, black vomit of yellow fever was "always somewhat reddish in thin layers."[44] The black material seen in septic processes was derived from bile and never had this reddish color. He was neither impressed with bleeding gums, since these were common enough among blacks, Chinese, and other natives. In his experience, jaundice in yellow fever sometimes was hardly perceptible until after death, and marked or deep jaundice was only exceptionally seen.[44] Markedly jaundiced cases thought to be yellow fever were always something else, usually long-standing malaria. He recalled that among the commonest causes of jaundice found among laborers in Panama in 1905, 1906 and 1907, was pneumococcal infection.[44] Pain over the liver and jaundice practically always meant lobar pneumonia. Yellow fever urine rarely, if ever, was bile stained and in fatal cases was "highly albuminous."[44] The scientist prevailed over the speculative clinician as he concluded in one particular instance: "Considering the sections of tissue and the meager and unconvincing histories and autopsy report I would not feel justified in calling these cases yellow fever."[44]

After reading Darling's remarks about post-mortem findings in yellow fever, Henry Carter, who had the privilege of first interviewing and offering Darling a position to work under Gorgas in Panama almost twenty years before, not only agreed but added a few comments of his own: "If a piece of linen, such as one's handkerchief, be dipped in the black vomit of yellow fever and held so light can shine through it, the tint is red or purplish, never green (as described by Henry Warren, about 1750)."[45] Carter noted that it was important to determine how long after death the autopsy was made. If a reasonable time had elapsed (6 to 10 hours) the incision, as usually made, was extremely dry; if the autopsy was done very soon after death, the incision may, and generally would, be normally bloody. Although he agreed with Darling that jaundice was seldom very deep in yellow fever cases, Carter recalled "one of Dutralau's aphorisms" that "the dead are always yellow," and that this became more apparent with time after death, "because the blood after death drains from the front of the body to the back as it lies and thus renders the yellow color more apparent than it was in life."[45] Carter regarded with "some doubt" a case in which no free black vomit was found in the stomach (unless the patient had vomited shortly before death). He recalled that he and Darling had differed on this same point, regarding the "supposedly" last case of yellow fever reported on the isthmus of Panama on May 16, 1906.[45] Thus, this famous last case of yellow fever, which marked the eradication of the dreaded yellow scourge and assured a successful completion of the isthmian canal by the Americans, was marred by a controversy over the interpretation of the pathological findings. The deciding vote about the correct diagnosis was most likely cast by Gorgas, based on his vast clinical experience with yellow fever patients in Texas, Cuba, and Panama.

Darling was appreciative that a good attempt at species sanitation was being made in Panama, better than was ever made by the "old timers."[46] He recalled that *Aedes taeniorhyncus* was very annoying in Ancon for several years and that his children were badly bitten from playing about in the damp grass where these mosquitoes rested during the day. Those who were in Panama from the early days feared to spend much time out of doors and were not brought in contact so much with *taeniorhynchus*.[46]

When asked if Dr. Chagas' plan to fumigate houses in Brazil every eight days to control anopheline mosquitoes was scientifically sound, Darling advised that it would be wise to precede such fumigation by an investigation of mosquito habits dealing with the length of time mosquitoes remain in habitations after a blood meal.[47] In the Far East, the tropics, and in Leesburg, adult mosquitoes were known to spend a considerable time inside habitations. They were ready to oviposit (lay eggs) two and one-half days after a blood meal and five days after they emerged. However, this could not be confirmed by laboratory experiments and there was much uncertainty about how long mosquitoes remained inside houses and how frequently it would be necessary to fumigate houses in order to destroy all infected anophelines.[47]

When consulted about the utility of a black-painted mosquito catcher used by the Italians, Darling replied that he had two catchers painted black around the funnel and tried them at the station with unsatisfactory results when compared to the results obtained by the unpainted glass mosquito catchers equipped with a rubber bulb, such as those regularly used at the station.[48] He also believed that anophelines were not "negatively heliotropic" in an absolute sense, since they did not swarm about lighted lamps but seemed to be attracted towards lighted places. He recalled that in Panama, when he was conducting "incriminating" experiments, he used to feed the mosquitoes on ward patients about eight o'clock in the evening when the ward was usually dark. He would turn on a light at one end of the ward and conduct the biting experiment at the other end. He found that by holding the lantern chimney with the biting area pointing toward the light, all the anophelines would take up a position facing toward the light rather than away from it. He would then interpose the patient's arm, placing it against the gauze on the biting surface of the jar and if hungry they would all proceed to feed.[48]

Darling's inventiveness and ability to improvise as situations demanded were evident when he decided to demonstrate in his talks to schools and small groups of laymen, mosquito eggs, larvae and hookworms, as well as slides with drawings of malarial parasites. He advised the home office that he needed a small, hand-illuminated stand and, if none of the sort could be found in the market, he recommended that one be constructed for his use.[49] The accompanying diagram showed a regular $3.75, two-battery-powered flashlight, topped with a sleeve attachment composed of a frosted glass holding a removable slide and glass cell, and a lens magnifying 10 to 25 diameters for viewing the mounted specimens or slides.[49]

Favorable comments by Darling on S. M. Lambert's hookworm work in Fiji, prompted a grateful response from Lambert:

> It is especially pleasing to receive such a commendation from a man of Dr. Darling's calibre, on whom I look as the grand daddy of us all when it comes to tropical diseases and the hookworm game. Years ago he wrote almost completely about things that I am still finding out myself and then discovering that he knew all about them before.[50]

After reviewing a set of slides of liver and kidney from a case of carbon tetrachloride poisoning from Jamaica, Darling was interested in the statement from a government pathologist that "the microscopic appearances are practically identical with those that occur in cases of the so called vomiting sickness."[51] Darling was familiar with the "rather long" history of the vomiting sickness of Jamaica, already told by a number of investigators. At first, it was formerly thought to be "a kind of yellow fever." Later it was said to be caused by the meningococcus, and still later, ascribed to eating the "bruised fruit" of the ackee plant (*Blighia sapida*).[51] He couldn't see how it could be yellow fever, but considered of great importance to know whether fatal cases diagnosed as vomiting sickness, presented lesions of central zone necrosis "such as are seen in carbon tetrachloride poisoning and yellow fever," and wanted very much the opportunity to examine slides and tissues from undoubted cases of vomiting sickness.[51] Four months later, Darling was able to examine slides of cases of Jamaica vomiting sickness obtained from Harold Scott in Jamaica and concluded that he could see no resemblance between ackee poisoning on the one hand, and yellow fever or carbon tetrachloride poisoning on the other.[52] Darling's curiosity about the pathology of Jamaica vomiting sickness antedated by four decades a similar interest which resurfaced in 1963, when Douglas Reye described in Australia a new catastrophic illness in children which he named encephalopathy and fatty degeneration of the viscera.[53] As a result, comparisons were made between Reye syndrome and Jamaica vomiting disease.

Invitations to talk to doctors and laymen about malaria were received from time to time. In January 1924, Darling addressed the medical students in Augusta, the Kiwanis club, the Albany Board of Health, doctors of the district, and laymen.[54] He also had invitations to address the Women's Club and the Lions' Club at Macon. Darling and a colleague "motored the entire way" so that he could acquaint himself with the topography and mosquito breeding places. He added: "Four hundred and sixty miles were covered within five days and I never felt the slightest fatigue or ill effects from the trip, although there were heavy rains, and the roads the entire way were soft and muddy and we had to use chains the entire distance."[55] In these talks he took the standpoint of the investigator and emphasized the importance of making surveys and of getting definite information first. People seemed interested in the subject of malaria and the work they were doing, and he was sure "that much good will come from it."[54] Although he didn't mind giving these talks, he confessed that "public speaking is not my forte, and never will be."[55]

In mid-June, Darling left Leesburg for Tennessee, where he planned to make a rapid malarial survey in the neighborhood of Humboldt, followed by a trip to Washington and Baltimore for a few days, and expecting to be back at the station about June 26.[56] On June 13 he visited Gibson county and made a rapid malarial survey, finding splenic enlargement in the river bottom lands and adult *Anopheles quadrimaculatus* in houses where the County Health Officer had failed to find them.[57]

On June 19, he arrived in Baltimore and visited the School of Hygiene, consulted the library, and shipped personal papers and specimens on malaria to Leesburg.[57] Somehow, he found time to examine for spleen enlargement children in Mercy and Hebrew Hospitals. Five days later he had a "sharp attack" of estivo-autumnal (falciparum) malaria which was treated immediately on microscopic diagnosis by thirty grains of quinine bisulfate in solution daily given in morning hours before noon with bromides "to control deafness."[57] This dosage was continued for eight days and thereafter about twelve grains every day for two months.[57] On July 1 he felt well enough to report in his own handwriting (his faithful Corona typewriter had been left behind) that he was "on the mend" after a sharp attack of malaria, which he believed was acquired in Leesburg. His temperature had reached 104° F and some fever had persisted for four days. He had walked slowly for the first time that morning.[57] He was anxious to return to the station but was advised to remain in Baltimore for a few days until fully recovered.[58] He finally returned to Leesburg on July 9.

In July, Paul Russell and C. B. Blaisdell undertook a survey of anophelines in southeastern Georgia in the piney woods country between Albany, Brunswick, and Savannah. Russell had been working for the past year on identification of the anopheline species based on their larval characteristics.[57] By September, Russell had perfected the method of identifying the three species of anophelines (*quadrimaculatus*, *punctipennis*, and *crucians*) using their larval "characters."[57] Darling checked Russell's work and was convinced of its accuracy. According to Darling, such identification would obviate to a great extent the necessity of laboriously breeding out the larvae and waiting for the emergence of the adult. Another rapid survey was conducted in Seminole, Decatur, Miller, and Calhoun counties on August 31. In this region there was an abundance of limesinks and, due to the drought, there were residual pools which harboured *quadrimaculatus* larvae. Adult mosquitoes were found in a number of the homes and enlarged spleens were encountered among children. The topography and results of the survey indicated that that region in southwestern Georgia corresponded closely with the conditions in Lee County, all of which favored malarial endemicity.[57]

As the end of the year approached, Darling felt that they had become much better informed about the distribution of the three targeted species of mosquitoes in relation to topography and geology.[57] He thought that a clearer notion was emerging of the fundamental nature of the malarial problem on "what might be called the physical and biological sides."[57]

Darling was named to the sub-committee on Medical Research of the National Malaria Committee, along with C. C. Bass (Tulane University), M. A. Barber (U.S. Public Health Service), W. E. Deeks (United Fruit Company), and R. W. Hegner (Johns Hopkins).[59] By July 1924, he was notified of his election as president of the American Society of Tropical Medicine.[60] He replied: "My head is so swelled from quinine and election to the presidency of the American Society of Tropical Medicine that it will be difficult for me to believe that I might have been regarded as an afterthought."[61]

By September, Darling had been at the Leesburg station nearly eighteen months. He seemed quite content with his new lease on life and satisfied with his work, as he acknowledged to his younger sister, Ruth Ann, in a letter from "Fleeburg" (as he jokingly called Leesburg):

> You ask about happiness and whether any one is ever satisfied with their lot. I believe that I have almost attained to that state of mind. It is funny almost tragic I suppose everybody feels, that one can be happy down here in the swamps of Georgia. You saw the place dirty and cold, cobwebs and all. But in summer it glows with interest. The verandah is crowded every warm night. We have a lantern and I talk about my travels with lantern slides to illustrate the words. Interesting conversations take place between the visitors and myself during which all the subjects under the sun are discussed. At 8 a.m. we start off for the job of the day, visiting the malarial stations examining spleens of children suffering from malaria, taking hemoglobins and blood specimens for malaria. Hunting for anopheline larvae and adult mosquitoes. The men and women too for we had two of the latter sex here this summer and crawl houses and in stables and under bridges to find where the malarial mosquitoes hide. Then we return to the lab and hotel where we eat a country dinner and talk after it on the porch. In the afternoon we have various studies under way bearing on the habits of the malarial mosquito and how best to blot her out.[62]

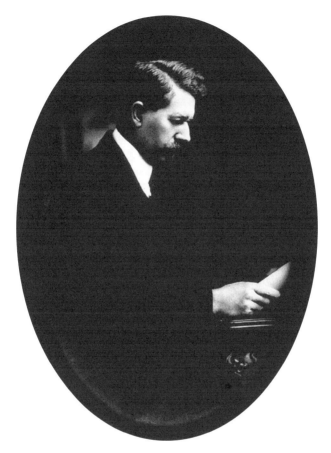

12.2 Darling sitting at a desk, undated. Reproduced with permission, courtesy of Mr. Sam Darling, British Columbia.

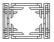

Darling noted a scalp swelling on the neurosurgical site and immediately left Leesburg for Baltimore on October 2, quite despondent and certain that his brain tumor had recurred.[63] Mrs. Darling heard his cane on the walk outside their home one evening, as he arrived unannounced. She greeted him at the door and he answered by stating that he had come home to die.[63] Although he wanted to see Walter Dandy, his neurosurgeon, immediately, he was persuaded to wait till morning. At the crack of dawn he and his wife took a taxi to see Dandy, who received him warmly and compassionately. A careful examination revealed a simple local infection in the old incision, which was rapidly and effectively treated. He got into a cab as soon as he could and went directly to the train station without his bags or tickets and boarded a train back to Georgia.[63] Afterwards, he recalled that "a two minute conversation with Dr. Dandy was sufficient to satisfy me that I had nothing whatever to worry about."[64] Russell had initially hoped that Darling's illness was nothing more than a "little bit too much work and that a rest at home will improve the condition immediately."[65] Darling reassured him that "it was not that I was overtaxed but that I was overconcerned about a circumstance which had no pathological significance whatever so far as my health was concerned. Symptoms which were purely nervous in origin immediately vanished and I returned at once to Leesburg."[64]

This health interlude had come at an inopportune time for Darling and the Foundation, since several important visitors and guests were scheduled to arrive at the station in Leesburg. Professor Émile Brumpt, an eminent French parasitologist; Thorvald Madsen, president of the Health Committee of the League of Nations; Vernon Kellogg and F. F. Russell, both members of the International Health Board, were all scheduled to arrive on October 26.[66] To everyone's relief, Darling was able to return on time and spent "two very strenuous but thoroughly interesting days with the group of distinguished visitors brought here by Colonel Russell."[67]

As an eventful and busy 1924 was coming to an end, an attractive opportunity was presented to Darling by the Rockefeller Foundation to attend an International Congress in Malaria to be held in Rome in the following spring.[68] Should he be disposed to go, the International Health Board would appoint him as a representative and expected for him to stay in Europe long enough to visit Lewis Hackett in Italy, and "perhaps visit certain other points with members of the Malaria Committee of the Health Section of the League of Nations."[68] Darling replied enthusiastically that he would be glad to have the opportunity of attending the congress, go over the malaria situation in Italy with Hackett, and he earnestly hoped that he would have the opportunity for visiting with members of the malaria committee of the Health Section of the League of Nations, and other points where malaria was a problem.[69] Since he had an important engagement in Washington as president of the American Society of Tropical Medicine, Darling would like to return home by May 25, and thought that if he left the station by the middle of March there would be sufficient time to accomplish all his objectives.[69] No one could have foreseen the tragic consequences of that trip when it was initially proposed to Darling in December 1924.

13

Malaria Commission, League of Nations

The *Baltimore Sun* reported on March 26, 1925, that Darling would be sailing Saturday from New York City to Europe.[1] This would be his fifth "scientific expedition" and on this trip he was scheduled to visit Switzerland, Italy, Greece, Palestine, Egypt, and Morocco. The newspaper noted that on this occasion, Mrs. Darling and their children would not accompany him, as they had done previously on his trips to Panama, Malay Archipelago, Brazil, and Georgia.[1]

Departure plans were slightly altered when the intended steamship was found to be completely booked. Alternate reservation was made for him to board instead the *Conte Rosso* (Lloyd Sabaudo Line), sailing from New York to Naples on March 21.[2] He needed a new passport and visas from Italy, France, Great Britain — the latter covering his proposed visits to Palestine, Syria, Turkey, and Spain.[2] Darling's travel arrangements were all taken care of by the International Health Board, including his brief stay in New York City at the McAlpin Hotel, on Broadway and Thirty-fourth Street, before sailing for Europe.

The specific plans were for Darling to spend one month in Italy, accompanied by his friend and colleague, Lewis Hackett. In Palestine, Syria, and Turkey, he would be joined by Paul Carley, and in Spain by Dr. Bailey. On his return trip he was scheduled to stop in Paris to see Professors Selskar Gunn and Émile Brumpt, and in London to visit Andrew Balfour. An option also was offered for Darling to see Professor Swellengrebel in Amsterdam, and perhaps a short visit to Yugoslavia with Hackett. Altogether the scientific expedition was expected to take between three and four months.[3]

Despite strong protests from Darling that his work on quinine and other experiments at the malaria station in Leesburg would suffer from an early departure, and a Western Union telegram in which he insisted "URGE SAILING DUILIO MARCH TWENTY SIX . . . NOT EARLIER . . . ," Darling had little choice but to accept the March 21 departure date.[4] To partly assuage his disappointment, accommodations aboard the *Conte Rosso* were upgraded to a single-berth, outside room located on D deck, and he was assured that he would be "most comfortable while en route."[5] Rockefeller personnel kindly informed Mrs. Darling that her husband "was looking well and vigorous before he sailed."[6]

Darling's arrival in Naples was expected to be soon after April 1.[7] On April 3, he was met in Rome by Lewis Hackett, director of the International Health Board field office in Italy. Hackett, who had known Darling and watched him evolve throughout his career, accompanied him to see the sights and obtained a valuable insight of his companion from that experience:

> The Darling I met in Rome . . . was at the height of his mental power — not at all the wiry enthusiast I had known in Panama, brilliant and temperamental, not the harassed teacher of Brazil, doggedly working out a great constructive program . . . , not the restive 'chief' of Leesburg . . . , with his white days and black days. . . .
>
> "Here was a new man in Rome – a little stouter than I had ever seen him . . . — but with the keen, handsome, expressive countenance which commanded the attention of utter strangers. His manner was carefree, eager, and self-confident. He was enjoying the maturity of a vast experience and the zest and power of a miraculously recaptured youth.
>
> . . . His mind always ranged beyond the particulars of the medical sciences toward the philosophical aspects and social significance of the phenomena which he observed and analyzed. He was a thoughtful and imaginative scientist with plenty of common sense to govern the speed and versatility of his mental processes.
>
> . . . Then there was also that piercing quality of intelligence which, when stimulated by a pertinacious curiosity and backed by a diversified experience, a splendid memory, and the power of rapid analysis, always gives us the feeling that we are in the presence of genius.
>
> . . . Darling had a certain robustness of thought and of humor, but he was at the same time keenly sensitive to all kinds of beauty. He had "moments," as he called them, of great joy and stimulation in Italy. In the Protestant cemetery in Rome he lingered beside the graves of Keats and Shelley, and full of emotion he said, with the touch of extravagance so characteristic of him, "don't think I care to see anything else in Rome," but later went twice to the Colosseum at night. In Florence we had a delightful afternoon driving about in a carriage and there his "moment" came when he saw by chance a tablet on a wall recalling Elizabeth Barrett Browning and "Sonnets

from the Portuguese"' the beauty of which had greatly appealed to
him at one period in his life. In Venice we happened to enter the cathedral on the day of St. Mark in the late afternoon during the
celebration of high mass. The ancient and mosaic-covered walls were
illuminated only by candles, and the ceremony was entirely choral. A
hundred strong voices of men and boys filled the enormous cathedral
with the beautiful chants of religious exaltation. In Milan, in the dim
enormous aisles, he lost himself in the absorption of beautiful distant
singing. I pulled at him a little – "We shall lose our train" – "We
mustn't lose this moment," he replied, with a little smile."[8]

Darling was preoccupied during his first few days following his arrival
in Rome with his presidential address to the American Society of Tropical
Medicine in May. He used Hackett as "a sparring partner" to try out his
ideas, arguments, and conclusions. Almost six weeks after his arrival in
Europe, Darling finally completed the manuscript for his presidential
address and sent it to the home office.

> There has been so much to do since I arrived, that I have not had time
> to finish properly my address to the meeting of the Am. Soc. Trop.
> Medicine. I shall be eternally obliged if you will have the ms [manu-
> script] enclosed shaped up typed and a copy sent to Dr. Ransom
> Secretary Am. Soc. Trop. Med. Washington in time for the meeting
> May 26 or 5. Am sending this off from a ... little old Calabrian village
> near the toe of Italy. . . . Am well, feeling bully, seeing a lot, but saying
> nothing, slept under two blankets and an overcoat last night . . . As
> Buck [son] says, "Love to all." Sincerely, S. T. Darling.[9]

This would be his last communication to the International Health
Board and the last letter Mrs. Darling would see from her husband.

14

Death Near Beirut

On May 22, 1925, Sir Eric Drummond, Secretary General of the League of Nations, dispatched an urgent message from Geneva, through the French Telegraph Cable Company, to George Vincent, president of the Rockefeller Foundation:

> DEEPLY REGRET INFORM YOU DRS SAMUEL DARLING AND NORMAN LOTHIAN MET WITH FATAL AUTOMOBILE ACCIDENT WHILE TRAVELLING AS MEMBERS LEAGUE OF NATIONS MALARIA COMMISSION NEAR BEYROUTH YESTERDAY HAVE SENT OFFICIAL NOTIFICATION SECRETARY STATE WASHINGTON ASKING THEM TO INFORM RELATIVES.[1]

As the news of the tragedy spread throughout the world, messages from friends and scientific colleagues began to pour into the stunned Rockefeller Foundation and International Health Board offices, expressing their sympathy to his family and grieving for what was considered to be a great loss to the scientific world (see Appendix G: Obituaries and Condolences).

Details of the accident were given by survivors and by Paul Carley and Lewis Harkness, from the Department of Health in Jerusalem, who inspected and took photographs of the accident site.[2] Following is a reconstruction of the details of the accident, taken from this report and from an account of the accident in the newspaper *La Syrie* of May 23:[3]

> On Thursday, May 21st, 1925, the members of the Malaria Commission of the League of Nations paid a visit to the General High Commissioner and the Governor of Great Lebanon. After an executive meeting in Beyrouth [sic], they proceeded at once by two motor cars to Brumana, a summer resort, where they visited the sanatoria and were given a lunch in their honor.

After about three o'clock, the Commission separated into two groups, the first taking the Bikfaya–Antelias road to Beyrouth, and the other the Beit Mary road. The latter party consisted of Dr. Ottolenghi [Acting President of the Commission], Dr. N. V. Lothian, of the Secretariat of the League of Nations, Dr. Swellengrebel, of Amsterdam, Dr. Ludwig Anigstein of Warsaw, Dr. S. T. Darling of the U.S.A., Mlle. Besson, the typist of the Commission, Colonel Delmas, Director of Health for Syria, and Madame Delmas.

After lunch Madame Delmas wished to return to Beyrouth in advance of the others. A return party was made up of Drs. Lothian, Darling and Swellengrebel, who also wished to return early to Beyrouth, Mlle Besson and Madame Delmas.

They left Brumana about 2:30 p.m. in a seven-seater French car [assigned by the government to Colonel Delmas], driven by an experienced French military chauffer. The top of the car was put down at Dr. Lothian's request, in order that the occupants might get a better view of the surroundings. The front seats were occupied by the chauffer and Dr. Lothian, the middle seats by Dr. Swellengrebel and Mlle. Besson, and the back seat by Madame Delmas and Dr. Darling (on the left).

The car passed through Beit Mary about 2:45 p.m. Past Beit Mary, some two kilometres, is a gently curving stretch of road about 1/2 kilometre long. There is sufficient gradient in this stretch of the road to permit the attainment of considerable speed by a car which is free-wheeling. [However, the car was found to be in "second speed" and "running along normally" by investigators later.] After passing Beit Mary and the fork in the road for Ainbou Debs and Caroubier, there is at the end of this gently curving stretch of road a sudden sharp "S" bend before reaching the spot known as Khaimett and Mara. It is not possible to see the beginning of this bend until one is some 100 metres from it. To one unfamiliar with the road the logical assumption is that the road turns to the right rather than to the left. It is also possible that direct rays of the sun caused reflections in the mirrors, so that the chauffer did not notice the turn, but kept right on . . . into empty space.

The car continued its downward course and went over the embankment of the turn, in a due west direction. . . . The car lighted on all four wheels, having dropped about 7 feet. . . . There is a rather sloping plateau here, extending about 40 metres in the direction in which the car was travelling [*sic*]. The ground is covered with rocks of various sizes. The impact of the car striking the ground was sufficient to throw all passengers out except the driver. The car continued upright for about 20 metres, turned to the left (south) and stopped. Dr. Swellengrebel recalls being thrown into the air and striking the ground twice. . . . Finding that he was but slightly injured and hearing his name called he went to Dr. Lothian . . . Dr. Lothian, whose chest was crushed but was in full control of his mind said that he was "done for". Dr. Swellengrebel then went to Dr. Darling who was lying on his side with his knees drawn up with his fractured head against a loose rock. He was vomiting blood stained gastric contents and moaning slightly. . . . Dr. Swellengrebel was about to start in search of help when Dr. Lothian called him again. Dr. Swellengrebel went back to Dr. Lothian and Dr. Lothian gave him certain information concerning the affairs of the Commission, charged Dr. Swellengrebel with giving certain messages to his family and his fiancee and died in Dr. Swellengrebel's arms. Realizing that Dr. Lothian was dead Dr. Swellengrebel went over to Dr. Darling who moaned slightly. Dr. Darling was pulseless. He died in a very short time (five minutes).

Other victims were Mlle. Besson, who died shortly thereafter from a crushed liver. Madame Delmas suffered a severe skull fracture in the naso-orbital region and a fracture of the right humerus near its head. She was taken to Brumana hospital and later that evening underwent trephanation [*sic*] by Dr. Baur at St. John's Hospital in Beyrouth.

General Sarrail, High Commissioner, the moment he learned of the accident, sent ambulances and trucks and delegated Colonel Bureau, Chief of the Military Cabinet, together with another French Army officer, to spend the night at the spot.

"The bodies of Drs. Darling and Lothian and Mlle. Besson were taken to the Hospital and prepared for burial. The Consul General of the U.S.A., His Britannic Majesty's Consul General and the Consul General of France were present when the bodies were sealed in zinc caskets.

On Sunday, May 24th, 1925, at 9.15 a.m. a funeral service was read by an American Clergyman over Dr. Darling, a Church of England service over Dr. Lothian and Roman Catholic Service over Mlle. Besson. All Departments of the French Government were represented, certain orations read by representative of the High Commissioner for Syria, the Governor General of the Grand Liban, a representative of the Department of Health, and Dr. Ottolenghi on behalf of the League of Nations. The representative Consul Generals then thanked the representatives of [the] Government of Syria. The President of the Arabic Medical Association of Beirut decorated all three caskets with the Order of Merit of Lebanon. Under full military escort, the procession moved to the Port Offices where the bodies were placed in a room awaiting disposition.[2]

Carley's report concluded:

I then went into the instructions which had been cabled me. Dr. Darling's personal effects were counted and sealed in a box by the American Consul. Cremation of Dr. Darling's body was impossible in Beyrouth. On Friday, May 29th, in company with the American Vice Consul, I saw the casket placed in another box. He sealed it with the Consular seal and put aboard the S/S Sinaia, and with it the box of personal effects, all papers, bills of lading, etc. were handed by the American Consul to the Captain of the ship for delivery to the authorized member of the Rockefeller Foundation staff who will meet the body in New York.[2]

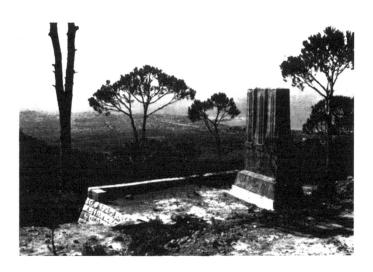

14.1 Monument erected by the Syrian government at the site of the fatal motor car accident near Beirut. Reproduced with permission, from *Man's Mastery of Malaria* by Paul F. Russell, courtesy of Oxford University Press, New York.

On May 22, Russell wrote to Mrs. Darling describing how he "was staggered by the news which greeted me on my arrival at the office this morning in the cable from Sir Eric Drummond." Russell communicated with Welch by telephone as soon as he could reach him and asked him to see Mrs. Darling. In the meantime, Miss Florence Read, Assistant Secretary to the International Health Board, was sent to comfort Mrs. Darling at her side. "Miss Read is going to Baltimore to find out personally if there is any way in which we can be of service to you," Russell wrote Mrs. Darling. He added: "I need not tell you, I am sure, what a staggering blow this is to all of us. Dr. Darling's past accomplishments have given him a unique place in the scientific world and we were all building great hopes on his work for the next years."[4]

On the following day details of the accident and about Darling's scientific contributions appeared in *The New York Times* and in the Paris edition of the *New York Herald*. Condolence messages poured in at the Rockefeller Foundation headquarters at 61 Broadway in New York City.[5]

Among the notable expressions of sympathy were those from Sir Eric Drummond, Secretary-General of the League of Nations in Geneva:

> That Dr. Darling should have been willing to bring his great knowledge and experience to the help of the Malaria Sub-Committee of the League's Health Organisation, and that your Foundation should have been ready not only to lend his services but also to bear the expense involved thereby – these facts were of great encouragement to those concerned in pressing forward with their plans. It is the more tragic that this collaboration should have ended in so terrible a disaster.[6]

From J. Kligler, of the Malaria Research Unit, Department of Health in Haifa:

> I saw a good deal of Darling during his visit here. And he saw a great deal of the work. His penetrating eye saw far deeper than any of the other members of the Commission. He saw what was not shown as well as the things that were. He was head and shoulders above the others. He always tried to get down to the root of things. I urged him to linger a while for a more intensive study, but he felt with regret that he had to move on. . . . He stood the strain of the journey remarkably well. He often suffered a good deal but he would not miss a single thing. His mind was always alert and there was a twinkle in his eye whenever he caught something new. Towards the evening he showed fatigue and on two or three occasion suffered from neuralgic pains. He disliked the methods of the English here. He seemed to think that there was too much loafing and coffee drinking. . . . He resented coffee drinking as a waste of time and an interruption of work. . . . His questions always suggested something that might have been done or done differently or done better. His loss leaves a vacuum that will not easily be filled. No other member of the Commission combined the scientific approach, the splendid training, the vast experience in a degree that Darling did. Nocht was the practitioner above all else. James saw everything with the skeptic eye of an unsuccessful Indian experience. Swellengraebel's interests centered almost solely in the types of mosquitoes. But Darling embraced all these. He had his specific interest – the spleen. But he was keen on the habits of the native mosquitoes. He was anxious to note anything new relating to methods of control. The question of cost was constantly in his mind. His interest covered the whole field.[7]

Dr. Paul F. Russell wrote from Penang, Malaya:

> This sudden passing of "S.T.D." is a loss to me that could only be second to a death in my immediate family. For during our months together in Georgia I came to love him as a friend and mentor, besides

having a very great respect for him as a scientist, a scholar and a gentleman. We had many intimate associations at the Station and on various tours of duty and he came to have a very large place in my world.

Many were the talks we had about Malaya and countless already have been the things out here that have recalled him to my mind, that have been noted as facts that he would be interested in or that have been recorded to be discussed at our next meeting. When the news of his death came it suddenly seemed as though my very reason for being here ceased to exist and I have not yet been able to recapture the enthusiasm for the work that I owe in such large measure to my association with Dr. Darling.

From the day I arrived at the Station on September 26th 1923 when Dr. Darling spent an hour showing me things of interest in the laboratory, until the very last of my stay in Leesburg in December 1924 when on a Sunday morning he took me over to the laboratory to show me the differences between the three species of hookworms he knew I would find here in Malaya, he never spared himself to teach me from his vast store of information about tropical medicine and parasitology.

I saw him with the visitors who came to the Station last summer to be taught malariology. I should like to record that I never at any time saw him impatient in the matter of teaching. True, I have seen him irritated in a human way by some stupidity or other in the connection of the routine of the office or field work but never, I use the word candidly, never did I see him impatient or irritable when teaching. A relatively small matter but one that was very characteristic of his patience is the fact that no doubt a hundred times he was asked for an opinion as to whether or not a blood platelet lying on a red cell were a malaria parasite or not. A hundred times he looked carefully at what must have been obvious immediately to him; a hundred times he explained without impatience why the platelet was not a parasite.

He denied himself the ordinary comforts of life that he might be closer to his work but he always surrounded himself with mental pleasures. One of the chief reasons why he lived in Leesburg rather than in Albany where he might have had many conveniences and palatable food was that he might have the evenings on the "Magnolia" porch with his guests at the Station.

Dr. Darling deliberately chose to live in the most malarious county he could find. This was logical of course but nevertheless courageous. He was indefatigable in his labors and had no patience with slackers. He was busy day and night, thoroughly happy in his researches, insatiable in his curiosity, tremendously eager to find out the real facts behind malaria. It was never too hot or too cold. It never rained too heavily. The roads were never impassable with Albert driving. The distances were never too far. It was never too late. Failure had no place in his life and many a man learned in no uncertain terms his unfavorable opinion of an excuse. A thing to be done was to be done as expeditiously as possible regardless of the circumstances.

All phases of life interested him. On the porch after lunch and in the evening he has talked of such diverse matters as the orientation of the Egyptian tombs; tuberculosis in South Africa; newspapers of New York in the late 19th century; the political situation in England and the United States; hookworm disease in Malaya, in the Dutch Indies, in Brazil; Thomas Hardy; the fate of the white race; the medical history of Panama; the story of yellow fever; every phase of malariology; quaint foodstuffs of the Orient; religion; philosophy; metaphysics. He was a genial, fluent conversationalist but never trivial. His wit was ready and his sense of humor keen.

Darling frequently said that he didn't believe in mixing business with pleasure and yet I found it a pleasure to do the work of the day with him.

He never wanted to make hotel reservations because he said he might lose an adventure if things were carefully prepared beforehand. In his researches he never neglected to explore the new paths that opened up before him but he never got lost.

Dr. Darling's death leaves a gap in the scientific world difficult to fill; a gap in my world impossible to fill.[8]

Upon a motion by William Welch, the International Health Board appointed a committee to draft a statement of appreciation to be read on the minutes of the Board and presented at its November 1925 meeting.[9]

Darling's body and personal effects aboard the Fabre Line S.S. *Sinaia* were scheduled to arrive in New York on about June 20. Floyd Harned, from the Transportation Department of the Rockefeller Foundation, was authorized by Mrs. Darling to receive these upon arrival of the steamship. After a visit from Walter Dandy, Mrs. Darling gave permission to the neurosurgeon to perform "a head section" to determine if the brain tumor had recurred.[10] Dandy made arrangements to perform the autopsy at the facilities of the New York City Department of Health on July 1 at 9:30 a.m.[11] A few days later Dandy asked if it would be possible to prepare for a necropsy on Darling at the Rockefeller Institute autopsy room instead.[12] Despite all these preparations, the post-mortem examination could not be performed, as it was found that Darling's body had not been embalmed, despite statements to the contrary from Beirut. This unfortunate situation may have stemmed from confusion about disposition of his remains immediately after the accident. Both Darling and Mrs. Darling had expressed their preference for cremation after death. However, since no facilities were found for this in Beirut (as erroneously reported), authorities in charge elected to ship the body instead to New York for cremation.

In the confusion surrounding the disposition of the body, it is possible that embalming was either poorly done or omitted altogether. A representative of the Rockefeller Foundation received Darling's body when it arrived at Pier 61 at the foot of Thirty-first and Brooklyn streets in New York.

Mrs. Darling took a train from Baltimore scheduled to leave at 8:23 a.m. and to arrive in New York at 12:30 a.m. on June 27. She stayed at the McAlpin Hotel, the same hotel where her husband had stayed before embarking on his last trip three months earlier. Funeral services were scheduled to be held at Leffert's Place Chapel, 86 Leffert's Place, on July 1 at three o'clock. The Episcopal service was presided by Reverend Powers. After the service, the body was taken to the Fresh Pond Crematory for cremation. The bronze urn was simply inscribed: *Samuel Taylor Darling, M.D., 1872 1925*.[13]

In the resolution of the International Health Board, written by William Welch and Edwin Jordan, and presented to the Rockefeller Board as a tribute to Darling, a paragraph referred to his qualifications as a scientist:

> Dr. Darling possessed in eminent degree the qualities of the successful scientific investigator — joy in the exploration of nature and the search for truth, command of methods and ingenuity in technique, knowledge of the literature of his subject, the scientific imagination combined with a critical analytic type of mind, judicious selection of problems as presented by circumstances of time and place, and the most rewarding lines of attack upon these problems. His own example, his attractive personal qualities, and his generosity secured the enthusiastic loyalty and devotion of his assistants and fellow workers.[14]

William Welch, a towering figure and respected dean of American medicine, had been a guiding force in Darling's career. It was Welch (himself a pathologist) who first saw in the young medical student and pathology resident in Baltimore the potential for greatness, and who recommended him to Gorgas in 1905 for the post of intern at Ancon Hospital in Panama. It was also Welch who knew closely about Darling's career at the Rockefeller International Health Board and of his contributions to tropical medicine from investigations in the Far East, Brazil, and Georgia. What Darling had accomplished in his brief twenty-year career surpassed the productivity of other investigators during a lifetime of work twice that long. Darling would have appreciated this candid evaluation of his work by a man who, among his many distinctions, had an uncanny ability to judge the future potential of young prospects, opened the first teaching pathology laboratory in an American medical school, chaired the governing board of the Rockefeller Foundation for three decades, and published the first scientific journal in the United States.

Darling and Welch had striking similarities and glaring differences.

Both had been enamored of the science of pathology and both had begun their work in the laboratory. Both were staunch defenders of the scientific method. Both loved to teach and to train young men in their respective disciplines. But Welch was seldom on time for his lectures, while Darling expected punctuality from others. Darling did not seek administrative posts or memberships in committees. He avoided the limelight and disliked public speaking. Although Welch started by teaching pathology and bacteriology in the laboratory, his administrative skills promptly resulted in exchanging the laboratory for an office. Darling, on the other hand, preferred to be in the laboratory, relatively unencumbered by administrative duties.

Darling was also unencumbered by any social aspirations or material gains. He accepted positions to work in Panama and in the Far East despite substantial reductions in salary. In Leesburg, he preferred uncomfortable accommodations and unpalatable food in exchange for proximity to the laboratory and the opportunity to partake of his knowledge and experience with his students and colleagues at the verandah of the Magnolia Hotel after dinner.

On a visit to his home in Baltimore, at 2711 Elsinore Avenue, Florence Read, an assistant administrative secretary who was sent by the Rockefeller Foundation to comfort and accompany Mrs. Darling at the news of her husband's death, found the following quote from Rudyard Kipling copied by Darling and displayed on the wall above his desk:

> Money dominates everybody except the man who does not want money. You may meet that man in your farm, in your village, in your legislature. But be sure that, whenever and wherever you meet him, as soon as it comes to a direct issue between you, his little finger will be thicker than your loin. You will go in fear of him; he will not go in fear of you. You will do what he wants; he will not do what you want. You will find that you have no weapon in your armory with which you can attack him; no argument which you can appeal to him. Whatever you gain, he will gain more. If your wealth is necessary for you, for purposes not your own, use your left hand to acquire it, but keep your right hand for your proper work in life.[15]

Andrew Balfour, first director of the London School of Hygiene and Tropical Medicine and president of the Royal Society of Tropical Medicine and Hygiene at the time of Darling's death, aptly summarized his colleague's accomplishments:

> Darling was a brilliant and versatile man, as someone has said, "always scientific, careful, imaginative and honest.". . . . He was the outstanding tropical parasitologist and pathologist of the United States, and by his work and character has given a fine example, not

only to his countrymen, but to all who are concerned with those problems which he spent his life in trying to solve and in the solving of
which he lost it.[16]

Appendix A
Bibliography of Publications by Samuel Taylor Darling

The author–date (Harvard) style of citation is used in this bibliography. Darling's publications are listed in chronological order to facilitate search for specific references. The bibliography is divided into eight categories:

I. Original articles published in the *Proceedings of the Canal Zone Medical Association/Proceedings of the Isthmian Canal Zone Medical Association.*
II. Pathological reports and laboratory notes.
III. Discussions following paper presentations.
IV. Original articles published in other journals (other than *Proceedings of the Canal Zone Medical Association/Proceedings of the Isthmian Canal Zone Medical Association*).
V. Papers presented at meetings.
VI. Monographs.
VII. Letters to the Editor.
VIII. Abstracts.

Papers published in more than one journal are indicated by an asterisk (*). (Multiple publications for an article was not uncommon practice at the time, particularly if the initial publication was in a local journal of lesser circulation, such as the *Proceedings*.)

A list of abbreviated and complete names of periodicals cited, as well as the number of publications by Darling in each journal, is given at the end of this appendix.

I. **Original articles published in the *Proceedings of the Canal Zone Medical Association*.** (This periodical changed its name to *Proceedings of the Medical Association of the Isthmian Canal Zone* starting with volume V, Part 2, which covered the period from October 1912 to March 1913.)

1.* 1908a. The relapsing fever of Panama. *Proc. Canal Zone Med. Assoc.* 1: 3–38.
2. 1908b. Rabies: an account of the disease and its incidence in Panama. *Proc. Canal Zone Med. Assoc.* 1: 77–89.
3. 1908c. Preliminary report on the varieties of anopheles mosquitoes which transmit malaria. *Proc. Canal Zone Med. Assoc.* 1: 138–140.
4.* 1908d. Sarcosporidiosis: with report of a case in man. *Proc. Canal Zone Med. Assoc.* 1: 141–152.
5. 1908e. Filariasis and elephantiasis. *Proc. Canal Zone Med. Assoc.* 1: 175–178.
6.* 1909a. Transmission of malarial fever in the Canal Zone by anopheles mosquitoes. *Proc. Canal Zone Med. Assoc.* 2: 34–38.
7.* 1909b. Experimental sarcosporidiosis in the guinea-pig and its relation to a case of sarcosporidiosis in man. *Proc. Canal Zone Med. Assoc.* 2: 104–110.
8.* 1910a. Oriental sore in Panama. *Proc. Canal Zone Med. Assoc.* 3 (Part 2): 7–20.
9.* 1910b. Bacillus dysenteriae recovered from peripheral blood and stools of cases in Panama. *Proc. Canal Zone Med. Assoc.* 3 (Part 2): 42–46. (With Lewis B. Bates)
10.* 1910c. Murrina, a trypanosomal disease of equines in Panama. *Proc. Canal Zone Med. Assoc.* 3 (Part 2): 47–64.
11.* 1911a. Blood platelets in tropical and other forms of anemia. *Proc. Canal Zone Med. Assoc.* 4 (Part 1): 7–20.
12.* 1911b. The intestinal worms of three hundred insane patients detected by special methods. *Proc. Canal Zone Med. Assoc.* 4 (Part 1): 41–48.
13. 1911c. Observations on the factors concerned in the cultivation of leprosy bacilli and on the development of a therapy. *Proc. Canal Zone Med. Assoc.* 4 (Part 1): 122–131.
14.* 1911d. A case of oriental sore (dermal leishmaniosis) in a native Columbian. *Proc. Canal Zone Med. Assoc.* 4 (Part 1): 154–155. (With R. C. Connor)
15.* 1911e. Oriental sore. *Proc. Canal Zone Med. Assoc.* 4 (Part 1): 177–187.
16.* 1911f. Verruca peruana. *Proc. Canal Zone Med. Assoc.* 4 (Part 1): 203–213.
17.* 1911g. Strongyloides infections in man and animals in the isthmian Canal Zone. *Proc. Canal Zone Med. Assoc.* 4 (Part 1): 214–234.
18.* 1911h. The probable mode of infection and the methods used in controlling an outbreak of equine trypanosomiasis "murrina" in the Panama Canal Zone. *Proc. Canal Zone Med. Assoc.* 4 (Part 1): 235–238.
19.* 1911i. Chronic proliferative tuberculosis — an unusual type of the disease. *Proc. Canal Zone Med. Assoc.* 4 (Part 2): 7–10. (With H. C. Clark)
20.* 1911j. *Linguatula serrata* (larva) in a native Central American. *Proc. Canal Zone Med. Assoc.* 4 (Part 2): 11–14.
21. 1911k. A method of staining the capsule of the pneumococcus. *Proc. Canal Zone Med. Assoc.* 4 (Part 2): 15.
22. 1911l. Observations on the laboratory diagnosis of plague. *Proc. Canal Zone Med. Assoc.* 4 (Part 2): 68–79.
23. 1911m. Notes on *Entamoeba tetragena*. *Proc. Canal Zone Med. Assoc.* 4 (Part 2): 81–82.

24. 1911n. Notes on transmission of *Tr. hippicum* by means of *Musca domestica*. *Proc. Canal Zone Med. Assoc.* 4 (Part 2): 82.
25. 1912a. Status lymphaticus with report of a fatal case. *Proc. Canal Zone Med. Assoc.* 4 (Part 2): 83–97. (With H. C. Clark)
26. 1912b. Note on the infection of mules by *Tr. hippicum* through mucous membranes. *Proc. Canal Zone Med. Assoc.* 4 (Part 2): 106.
27. 1912c. Observations on amoebae and entamoebae in Panama. *Proc. Canal Zone Med. Assoc.* 4 (Part 2): 122–131.
28.* 1912d. Two cases on anaphylactic serum disease over six years after the primary injection of horse serum (Yersin's antipest serum). *Proc. Canal Zone Med. Assoc.* 5 (Part 1): 37–45.
29.* 1912e. Notes on the life history and viability of *E. tetragena*. *Proc. Canal Zone Med. Assoc.* 5 (Part 1): 67–71.
30.* 1912f. Anthrax of animals in Panama with a note on its probable mode of transmission by buzzards. *Proc. Canal Zone Med. Assoc.* 5 (Part 1): 103–107. (With Lewis B. Bates)
31.* 1912g. The pathological features of a case of bilharziasis of the large bowel in a Martiniquan. *Proc. Canal Zone Med. Assoc.* 5 (Part 2): 52–54.
32. 1913a. Report of a case of glio-sarcoma of the retina in a Jamaican two years old. *Proc. Canal Zone Med. Assoc.* 6 (Part 1): 48–54. (With Dennis F. Reeder)
33. 1913b. Equine piroplasmosis in Panama. *Proc. Med. Assoc. Isthmian Canal Zone* 6 (Part 1): 55–59.
34. 1913c. Entamoebic dysentery in the dog. *Proc. Med. Assoc. Isthmian Canal Zone* 6 (Part 1): 60–62.
35.* 1914a. South Africa. *Proc. Med. Assoc. Isthmian Canal Zone* 7: 7–15.
36.* 1914b. The endotrypanum of Hoffman's sloth. *Proc. Med. Assoc. Isthmian Canal_Zone* 7 (Part 1): 80–87.
37.* 1914c. The pathological affinities of beriberi and scurvy. *Proc. Med. Assoc. Isthmian Canal Zone* 7 (Part 1): 88–103.
38. 1914d. Anatomical distribution of *Strongyloides stercolaris*. *Proc. Med. Assoc. Isthmian Canal Zone* 7 (Part 1): 104–106.
39. 1914e. A note on typhus fever. *Proc. Med. Assoc. Isthmian Canal Zone* 7 (Part 1): 152–163.

II.   Pathological reports and laboratory notes.

1. 1908a. A case of arterio-venous aneurysm of the arch of the aorta; pathological report. *Proc. Canal Zone Med. Assoc.* 1: 163–165. (With W. E. Deeks)
2. 1908b. A case of anesthetic leprosy; pathological report. *Proc. Canal Zone Med. Assoc.* 1: 169–171. (With W. M. James)
3. 1909a. Laboratory Notes: The Rose-Bradford kidney. *Proc. Canal Zone Med. Assoc.* 2: 119–120.
4. 1909b. Laboratory Notes: An infection by *Lamblia intestinalis* in an American child. *Proc. Canal Zone Med. Assoc.* 2: 120.
5. 1909c. Laboratory Notes: A fatal case of pellagra. *Proc. Canal Zone Med. Assoc.* 2: 120–121.

6.   1911. A description of ainhum with report of interesting cases occurring in one family; pathological report. *Proc. Canal Zone Med. Assoc.* 4: 118–121. (With Henry Weinstein)

7.   1914. A case of acute lymphatic leukemia; pathological report. *Proc. Med. Assoc. Isthmian Canal Zone* 7 (Part 1): 111–115. (With Herbert C. Clark)

III. Discussions.

1.   1908a. Deeks WE. Pneumonia on the isthmus of Panama. *Proc. Canal Zone Med. Assoc.* 1: 62–70. (pp. 72–73)

2.   1908b. Brem WV. Tuberculosis in Panama: incidence and association with pleural adhesions. *Proc. Canal Zone Med. Assoc.* 1: 90–95. (pp. 96–98)

3.   1908c. Connor ME. Sanitation. *Proc. Canal Zone Med. Assoc.* 1: 115–121. (pp.124–126)

4.   1909a. Brayton ND. Bilharziasis in the new world. *Proc. Canal Zone Med. Assoc.* 2: 7–13. (p. 14)

5.   1909b. Herrick AB. The surgical treatment of very severe and late cases of amebic dysentery. *Proc. Canal Zone Med. Assoc.* 2: 71–74. (pp. 77–78)

6.   1909c. Connor RC. Hemoglobinuric fever on the C.Z., observations with special reference to treatment on 80 cases occurring in European laborers admitted to Ancon Hospital. *Proc. Canal Zone Med. Assoc.* 2: 83–90. (pp. 90–92, 94)

7.   1909d. Williamson NE. A study of the liver in necropsies at Colon Hospital. *Proc. Canal Zone Med. Assoc.* 2: 113–116. (pp. 117–119)

8.   1910a. Brem WV. Studies of malaria in Panama. *Proc. Canal Zone Med. Assoc.* 3 (Part 1): 7–24. (p. 27)

9.   1910b. James WM. Quartan malaria and its parasite. *Proc.Canal Zone Med. Assoc.* 3 (Part 1): 29–55. (pp. 56–57)

10.   1910c. Deeks WE. The carbohydrate diathesis. *Proc. Canal Zone Med. Assoc.* 3 (Part 1): 77–88. (pp. 92–93)

11.   1910d. Brem W. Treatment of blackwater fever. *Proc. Canal Zone Med Assoc.* 3 (Part 1): 95–111. (pp. 116–117)

12.   1910e. Herrick AB, Earhart TW. The value of trophic bone changes in the diagnosis of leprosy. *Proc. Canal Zone Med. Assoc.* 3 (Part 2): 26–33. (p. 33)

13.   1911a. Dutrow HV. Diseases of the faucial tonsils, with special reference to tonsillectomy. *Proc. Canal Zone Med. Assoc.* 3 (Part 2): 93–109. (p. 113)

14.   1911b. James WM. Practical value of the Ross "thick film" method in the diagnosis of malaria. *Proc. Canal Zone Med. Assoc.* 4 (Part 1): 49–70. (p. 71)

15.   1911c. Deeks WE. Four cases of pellagra. *Proc. Canal Zone Med. Assoc.* 4 (Part 2): 55–56. (pp. 58–59)

16.   1912a. Hill RB. A possible relationship of bacilli of the colon group to pellagra with report of 2 cases. *Proc. Canal Zone Med. Assoc.* 4 (Part 1): 98–101. (pp. 103–104)

17.   1912b. James WM. Discussion of Dr. Darling's observations on amoebae and entamoebae the previous meeting. *Proc. Canal Zone Med. Assoc.* 4 (Part 2): 147–148. (pp. 148–152)

18. 1912c. James WM. Report of a case of infection with *Entamoeba tetragena*. *Proc. Canal Zone Med. Assoc.* 5 (Part 1): 46–52. (pp. 52–53)

19. 1912d. Noland L. Report of a case of stab wound of the heart: Operation and recovery. *Proc. Canal Zone Med. Assoc.* 5 (Part 1): 72–73. (p. 73)

20. 1913. Deeks WE, Baetz WG. An analysis of 500 medical cases in the tropics with the clinical diagnosis in the light of autopsy findings. *Proc. Med. Assoc. Isthmian Canal Zone* 6: 14–36. (p. 37)

21. 1914a. Baetz WG. Syphilis in colored canal laborers — a resume of 500 consecutive medical cases. *Proc.Med. Assoc. Isthmian Canal Zone* 7 (Part 1): 17–29. (pp. 30–31)

22. 1914b. Levy WV. A case of Hodgkins disease in a West Indian negro. *Proc. Med Assoc. Isthmian Canal* 7 (Part 1): 116–124. (pp. 124–125)

23. 1914c. Clark HC. Two rare manifestations of tuberculosis. *Proc. Med. Assoc. Isthmian Canal Zone* 7 (Part 2): 7–10. (pp. 10–11)

24. 1914d. Runyan RW. Report of a case presenting accessory collections of thyroid tissue. *Proc. Med. Assoc. Isthmian Canal Zone* 7 (Part 2): 12–14. (p. 14)

25. 1914e. Clark HC, Drennan LM. A case of primary carcinoma of the vermiform appendix. *Proc. Med. Assoc. Isthmian Canal Zone* 7 (Part 2): 15–17. (p.18)

26. 1914f. Asburn PM. Observations bearing on the control of malaria. *Proc. Med. Assoc. Isthmian Canal Zone* 7 (Part 2): 32–37. (pp. 37–38)

27. 1915a. Jacob JE. A discussion of emulsions of crude carbolic acid, with special reference to their bactericidal action. *Proc. Med. Assoc. Isthmian Canal Zone* 7 (Part 2): 57–62. (pp. 63–64)

28. 1915b. Clark HC. Preliminary notes on neoplasms found in inhabitants of Panama Canal Zone, with special reference to their occurrence in the negro and mestizo. *Proc. Med. Assoc. Isthmian Canal Zone* 7 (Part 2): 65–84. (pp. 84–85)

29 1925. Fricks LD. Training facilities for malaria personnel. *South. Med. J.* 18: 460–461. (pp. 461–462)

IV. **Original articles published in other journals.** Those articles which were published initially in the *Proceedings of the Canal Zone Medical Association* are indicated.by an asterisk (*).

1. 1904. Typhoid orchitis. *Maryland Med. J.* 47: 292–295.

2. 1906a. A protozoan general infection: *Histoplasma capsulatum*, producing pseudotubercles in the lungs and focal necrosis in the liver, spleen, and lymph nodes. *J. Am. Med. Assoc.* 46: 1283–1285.

3. 1906b. The accessory nasal sinuses and pneumoccal infections; a preliminary communication. *J. Am. Med. Assoc.* 47: 1561–1563.

4. 1906c. New organism discovered (*Histoplasma capsulata*). *J. Am. Med. Assoc.* 47: 2098.

5. 1907a. A new world tropical infection. *J. Alumni Assoc. Coll. Phys. Surg.* (Baltimore) 9: 97–102.

6. 1907b. Notes on histoplasmosis — a fatal disorder met with in tropical America. *Maryland Med. J.* 50: 125–129.

7.   1908. Histoplasmosis: a fatal infectious disease resembling kala azar found among natives of tropical America. *Arch. Intern. Med.* 2: 107–123.

8.* 1909a. The relapsing fever of Panama. *Arch. Intern. Med.* 4: 150–185.

9.* 1909b. Sarcosporidiosis, with report of a case in man. *Arch. Intern. Med.* 4: 150–185.

10. 1909c. The morphology of the parasite (*Histoplasma capsulatum*) and the lesions of histoplasmosis, a fatal disease of tropical America. *J. Exp. Med.* 11: 515–531.

11.* 1909d. Transmission of malarial fever in the Canal Zone by anopheles mosquitoes. *J. Am. Med. Assoc.* 53: 2051–2053.

12.* 1910a. Experimental sarcosporidiosis in the guinea-pig and its relation to a case of sarcosporidiosis in man. *J. Exp. Med.* 12: 19–28. (Also published in *J. Trop. Vet. Sci.* 5: 470–480.)

13. 1910b. Factors in the transmission and prevention of malaria in the Panama Canal Zone. *Ann. Trop. Med. Parasitol.* 4: 179–223.

14. 1910c. Panama ticks. *J. Econ. Entomol.* 3: 222.

15. 1910d. Equine trypanosomiasis in the Canal Zone. *Bull. Soc. Pathol. Exot.* 3: 381–385. (Also published in *J. Trop. Vet. Sci.* 6: 55–58, 1911)

16. 1910e. Sarcosporidiosis in the opossum and its experimental production in the guinea-pig by the intra-muscular injection of sporozoites. *Bull. Soc. Pathol. Exot.* 3: 513–518.

17.* 1911a. Oriental sore in Panama. *Arch. Intern. Med.* 7: 581–587.

18.* 1911b. Murrina, a trypanosomal disease of equines in Panama. *J. Infect. Dis.* 8: 467–485.

19.* 1911c. Blood platelets in tropical and other forms of anemia. *Trans. R. Soc. Trop Med. Hyg.* 5: 46–57.

20.* 1911d. The intestinal worms of three hundred insane patients detected by special methods. *Bull. Soc. Pathol. Exot.* 4: 334–341.

21.* 1911e. A case of oriental sore (dermal leishmaniasis) in a native Colombian. *J. Am. Med. Assoc.* 56: 1257–1258. (With Roland C. Connor)

22.* 1911f. Oriental sore. *J. Cutan. Dis. Syphil.* 29: 617–627.

23.* 1911g. Verruca peruana. *J. Am. Med. Assoc.* 57: 2071–2074.

24.* 1911h. Strongyloides infections in man and animals in the isthmian Canal Zone. *J. Exp. Med.* 14: 1–24.

25. 1911i. The probable mode of infection and the methods used in controlling an outbreak of equine trypanosomiasis (murrina) in the Panama Canal Zone. *Parasitology* 4: 83–86.

26.* 1912a. Bacillus dysenteriae recovered from the peripheral blood and stools of cases in Panama. *Am. J. Med. Sci.* 143: 36–40. (With Lewis B. Bates)

27.* 1912b. *Linguatula serrata* (larva) in a native Central American. *Arch. Intern. Med.* 9: 401–405. (With Herbert C. Clark)

28.* 1912c. Notes on transmission of *Tr. hippicum* by means of *Musca domestica*. *J. Exp. Med.* 15: 365.

29. 1912d. The examination of the stools for cysts of *Entamoeba tetragena*. *J. Trop. Med. Hyg.* 15: 257–259.

30. 1912e. A mosquito larvacide-disinfectant and the methods of its standardization. *Am. J. Public Health* 2: 89–92.

31. 1912f. Some blood parasites (Haemoproteus and Haemogregarina). *Bull. Soc. Pathol. Exot.* 5: 71–73.

32. 1912g. A note on the presence of *Linguatula serrata*, Frohlich 1789, in man in Central America. *Bull. Soc. Pathol. Exot.* 5: 118–119.

33. 1912h. Reduction of virulence in a strain of *Trypanosoma hippicum* selected from a guinea-pig. *Bull. Soc. Pathol. Exot.* 5: 184–187.

34. 1912i. Two cases of anaphylactic serum disease over six years after the primary injection of horse serum (Yersin' s antipest serum). *Arch. Intern. Med.* 10: 440–444.

35. 1912j. Essential features of the lesions caused by *Trypanosoma hippicum*. *C. R. Soc. Biol.* (Paris) 72: 150–152.

36 1912k. Experimental infection of the mule with *Trypanosoma hippicum* by means of *Musca domestica*. *J. Exp. Med.* 15: 365–366.

37. 1912l. Infection of mules with *Trypanosoma hippicum* through mucous membranes. *J. Exp. Med.* 15: 367–369.

38.* 1912m. Anthrax of animals in Panama with a note on its probable mode of transmission by buzzards. *Am. Vet. Rev.* 42: 70–75. (With Lewis B. Bates)

39. 1913a. The use of bismuth salts in media to detect the formation of sulphur bodies of bacterial origin; a preliminary note. *Am. J. Public Health* 3: 233–235.

40. 1913b. Observations on the cysts of *Entamoeba tetragena. Arch. Intern. Med.* 11: 1–14.

41. 1913c. Budding and other changes described by Schaudinn for *E. histolytica* seen in a race of *E. tetragena. Trans. R. Soc. Trop. Med. Hyg.* 6: 171–173.

42. 1913d. Budding and other forms in trophozoites of *Entamoeba tetragena* simulating the "spore cyst" forms attributed to "*Entamoeba histolytica.*" *Arch. Intern. Med.* 11: 495–506.

43. 1913e. The immunization of large animals to a pathogenic trypanosome (*Trypanosoma hippicum* (Darling)) by means of an avirulent strain. *J. Exp. Med.* 17: 582–586.

44. 1913f. The rectal inoculation of kittens as an aid in determining the identity of pathogenic entamoebae. *Bull. Soc. Pathol. Exot.* 6: 149–153. (Also published in *South. Med. J.* 6: 509–511).

45.* 1913g. Equine piroplasmosis in Panama. *J. Infect. Dis.* 13: 197–202.

46.* 1914a. The endotrypanum of Hoffman's sloth. *J. Med. Res.* 31: 195–203.

47.* 1914b. The pathological affinities of beriberi and scurvy. *J. Am. Med. Assoc.* 63: 1290–1294.

48. 1915a. Arteritis syphilitica obliterans; a pathological report of several cases of complete occlusion of large arteries — aorta, carotid, and subclavian in which syphilis was the causative factor. *J. Med. Res.* 32: 1–26. (With Herbert C. Clark)

49. 1915b. Sarcosporidia encountered in Panama. *J. Parasitol.* 1: 113–120.

50.* 1916a. South Africa. *Hosp. Bull. Univ. Maryland* 12: 55–59.

51. 1916b. Murrina. *Ref. Handbook Med. Sci.* 6: 552–554.

52. 1917. Relapsing fevers. *Ref. Handbook Med. Sci.* 7: 508–523.

53. 1918a. The treatment of hookworm infection. *J. Amer. Med. Assoc.* 70: 499–507. (With Marshall A. Barber and H. P. Hacker)

54   1918b. Sobre algunas medidas antimalaricas en Malaya. *Med. Cirug.* (São Paulo) 9: 265–274.

55.   1919a. Pesquizas recentes sobre a opilacao no Indonesia. *An. Paulist. Med. Cirug.* (São Paulo) 10: 25–38. (Also published in *Inst. Hyg.* (São Paulo) 2: 25–38.)

56.   1919b. Recent researches on hookworm infection in Indonesia. *Indian Med. Gaz.* 54: 446–453.

57.   1919c. Sarcosporidiosis in an East Indian. *J. Parasitol.* 6:9 8–101.

58.   1920a. Suggestions for the mass treatment of hookworm infection. *Lancet* 2: 69–72.

59.   1920b. The teaching of vital statistics to medical students in Brazil. *J. Am. Med. Assoc.* 75: 337–339. (With Wilson G. Smillie)

60.   1920c. Observations on the geographical and ethnological distribution of hookworms. *Parasitology* (London) 12: 217–233.

61.   1920d. Experimental inoculation of malaria by means of *Anopheles ludlowi*. *J. Exp. Med.* 32: 313–329.

62.   1921a. The technic of chenopodium administration in hookworm disease. *J. Am. Med. Assoc.* 87: 419–420. (With Wilson G. Smillie)

63.   1921b. The distribution of hookworms in the zoologic regions. *Science* 53: 323–324.

64.   1921c. The tertian characters of quotidian aestivo-autumnal fever. *Am. J. Trop. Med.* 1: 397–408.

65.   1922a. Health conditions in Brazil. *Estudante Brasileiro* 1: 15–17.

66.   1922b. The rat as a disseminator of the relapsing fever of Panama. *J. Am. Med. Assoc.* 79: 810–812.

67.   1922c. The hookworm index and mass treatment. *Am. J. Trop. Med.* 2: 397–447.

68.   1922d. Hookworm disease. *Nelson Loose-Leaf Medicine*, Ch. 6.

69.   1923a. Ascertaining the splenic index and the mosquito focus from school-children. *J. Am. Med. Assoc.* 80: 740–743.

70.   1923b. The occurrence of *Ancylostoma braziliense*, de Faria 1910 in the Philippine Islands. *J. Parasitol.* 9: 234–235.

71.   1924. *Ancylostoma braziliense* de Faria 1910 and its occurrence in man and animals. *Am. J. Hyg.* 4: 416–448.

72.   1925a. The spleen index in malaria (Editorial). *Boston Med. Surg. J.* 192: 90–91.

73.   1925b. Comparative helminthology as an aid in the solution of ethnological problems. *Am. J. Trop Med.* 5: 323–337.

74.   1925c. Medical research in malaria. *South. Med. J.* 18: 440–444.

75.   1925d. Entomological research in malaria. *South. Med. J.* 18: 446–449.

76.   1925e. Discussion on relative importance in transmitting malaria of Anopheles quadrimaculatus, punctipennis, and crucians, and the advisability of differentiating between these species in applying control measures. *South. Med. J.* 18: 452–458.

77.   1926a. Splenic enlargement as a measure of malaria. *Ann. Clin. Med.* 4: 695–712.

78   1926b. Mosquito species control of malaria. *Am. J. Trop. Med.* 6: 167–179.

V. Papers presented at meetings.

1. 1911. Verruca peruana. Read at the American Medical Association Section of Pathology and Physiology, 62nd Annual Session, Los Angeles, June 1911.

2. 1912a. The part played by flies and other insects in the spread of infectious diseases in the tropics with special reference to ants and to the transmission of *Tr. hippicum* by *Musca domestica*. Read at the 15th International Congress of Hygiene and Demography, Washington D.C., September 1912.

3. 1912b. Murrina, a trypanosomal disease of horses in Panama, and the means used in controlling an outbreak. Read at the 15th International Congress of Hygiene and Demography, Washington, D.C., September 1912.

4. 1912c. The identification of the pathogenic entamoeba of Panama. Read at the 15th International Congress of Hygiene and Demography, Washington, D.C., September 1912.

5. 1913. Relapsing fever in Panama. Read at the 17th International Congress of Medicine, Section XXI Tropical Medicine and Hygiene, London, 1913.

6. 1922. The hookworm index and mass treatment. Read at the 18th Annual Meeting American Society of Tropical Medicine, Washington, D.C., May 1922.

7. 1923. The spleen index in malaria. Read at the National Malaria Committee Conference on Malaria, meeting conjointly with the Southern Medical Association, Washington, D.C., November 1923.

VI. Monographs

1. 1910. *Studies in Relation to Malaria*. Laboratory of the Board of Health, Department of Sanitation. Isthmian Canal Commission. Mount Hope, Canal Zone. 1st edition, 38 pp; 2nd edition, 42 pp.

2. 1920. *Hookworm and Malaria Research in Malaya, Java, and the Fiji Islands. Report of Uncinariasis Commission to the Orient, 1915–1917.* International Board of Health (Rockefeller Foundation), Publication No. 9, 191 pp. (With M. A. Barber and H. P. Hacker)

3. 1921. *Studies on Hookworm Infection in Brazil*. Rockefeller Institute Medical Research Monograph No. 14, 41 pp. (With W. G. Smillie)

VII. Letters to the editor.

1. 1910. The trypanosome *T. hippicus*, nsp. *Am. Vet. Rev.* 37: 375–379.

2. 1912a. Romanowsky stain for entamoeba. *J. Am. Med. Assoc.* 59: 292.

3. 1912b. The staining of Protozoa. *Science* 37: 58–59.

4. 1912c. Oriental sore (cutaneous leishmaniasis) in the United States. *J. Am. Med. Assoc.* 80: 1260–1261.

VIII. Abstracts

1. 1911. Factors in the transmission and prevention of malaria in the Panama Canal Zone. *South. Med. J.* 4: 125–129.

2. 1912. The examination of the stools for cysts of *Entamoeba tetragena*. *Trop. Dis. Bull.* 1: 180.

3. 1913a. Verruca peruana. *Trop. Dis. Bull.* 2: 165.

4. 1913b. The identification of the pathogenic entamoeba of Panama. *Trop. Dis. Bull.* 2: 165.

5. 1913c. Two cases of anaphylactic serum disease over six years after the primary injection of horse serum (Yersin's antipest serum). *Trop. Dis Bull.* 1: 316–317.

6. 1913d. Budding and other changes described by Schaudinn for *E. histolytica* seen in a race of *E. tetragena*. *Trop. Dis. Bull.* 2: 720–722.

7. 1913e. Budding and other forms in trophozoites of *Entamoeba tetragena* simulating the "spore cyst" forms attributed to "*Entamoeba histolytica.*" *Trop. Dis. Bull.* 2: 165.

8. 1913f. The immunization of large animals to a pathogenic trypanosome (*Trypanosoma hippicum* (Darling)) by means of an avirulent strain. *Trop. Dis. Bull.* 2: 136.

9. 1913g. The rectal inoculation of kittens as an aid in determining the identity of pathogenic entamoeba. *Trop. Dis. Bull.* 1: 720–722 and 2: 389.

10. 1913h. Observations on the cysts of Entamoeba tetragena. *Trop. Dis. Bull.* 1: 462–463.

11. 1914a. Darling's larvicide. *Trop. Dis. Bull.* 4: 199–200.

12. 1914b. Notes on the life history and viability of *E. tetragena*. *Trop. Dis. Bull.* 3: 456.

13. 1914c. Relapsing fever in Panama. *Trop. Dis. Bull.* 4: 242.

14. 1914d. Studies in relation to malaria. *Trop. Dis. Bull.* 4: 78–82.

15. 1915a. The pathological features of a case of bilharziasis of the large bowel in a Martiniquan. *Trop. Dis. Bull.* 6: 229.

16. 1915b. The endotrypanum of Hoffman's sloth. *Trop. Dis. Bull.* 5: 104–105.

17. 1915c. The pathological affinities of beriberi and scurvy. *Trop. Dis. Bull.* 5: 107–109.

18. 1915d. Sarcosporidia encountered in Panama. *Trop. Dis. Bull.* 6: 200–201.

19. 1918. The treatment of hookworm infection. *Trop. Dis. Bull.* 12:1 85–186. (With M. A. Barber and H. P. Hacker)

20. 1919. Sobre algunas medidas antimalaricas en Malaya. *Inst. Hyg.* (São Paulo) 1: 12.

21. 1920. Sarcosporidiosis in an East Indian. *Trop. Dis. Bull.* 16: 96.

22. 1921a. Suggestions for the mass treatment of hookworm infection. *Trop. Dis. Bull.* 17: 77.

23. 1921b. Experimental inoculation of malaria by means of *Anopheles ludlowi*. *Trop. Dis. Bull.* 17: 144–145.

24. 1921c. Hookworm and malaria research in Malaya, Java, and the Fiji Islands. *Trop. Dis. Bull.* 18: 117–119.

25. 1922a Studies on hookworm infection in Brazil. *Trop. Dis. Bull.* 19: 247–248.

26. 1922b. The technic of chenopodium administration in hookworm disease. *Trop. Dis. Bull.* 19: 249. (With W. G. Smillie)

27. 1922c. The tertian characters of quotidian aestivo-autumnal fever. *Trop. Dis. Bull.* 19: 288–289.

28. 1923a. The rat as a disseminator of the relapsing fever of Panama. *Trop. Dis. Bull.* 20: 132.

29. 1923b. The hookworm index and mass treatment. *Trop. Dis. Bull.* 20:254–255 and Suppl. 1: 29–30.
30. 1923c. Ascertaining the splenic index and the mosquito focus from school-children. *Trop. Dis. Bull.* 20: 551–553.
31. 1924a. The occurrence of *Ancylostoma braziliense* de Faria 1910 in the Philippine Islands. *Trop. Dis. Bull.* 21: 236.
32. 1924b. *Ancylostoma braziliense* de Faria, 1910, and its occurrence in man and animals. *Trop. Dis. Bull.* 21: 969.
33. 1925a. The spleen index in malaria. *Trop. Dis. Bull.* 22: 342.
34. 1925b. Discussion on relative importance in transmitting malaria of anopheles quadrimaculatus, punctipennis and crucians, and the advisability of differentiating between these species in applying control measures. *Trop. Dis. Bull.* 22: 803.
35. 1926a. Comparative helminthology as an aid in the solution of ethnological problems. *Trop. Dis. Bull.* 23: 771.
36. 1926b. Splenic enlargement as a measure of malaria. *Trop. Dis. Bull.* 23: 813.
37. 1926c. Mosquito species control of malaria. *Trop. Dis. Bull.* 23: 831.

List of complete and abbreviated journal names in which Darling's publications appeared. The number of publications by Darling in each periodical is shown in parentheses.

1. *American Journal of Hygiene (Am. J. Hyg.)* (1)
2. *American Journal of Medical Sciences (Am. J. Med. Sci.)* (1)
3. *American Journal of Public Health (Am. J. Public Health)* (2)
4. *American Journal of Tropical Medicine (Am. J. Trop. Med.)* (4)
5. *American Veterinary Review (Am. Vet. Rev.)* (2)
6. *Annals of Clinical Medicine (Ann. Clin. Med.)* (1)
7. *Anaes Paulistas de Medicina e Cirugia (An. Paul. Med. Cir.) (São Paulo)* (1)
8. *Annals of Tropical Medicine and Parasitology (Ann. Trop. Med. Parasitol.)* (1)
9. *Archives of Internal Medicine (Arch. Intern. Med.)* (8)
10. *Boston Medical and Surgical Journal (Boston Med. Surg. J.)* (1)
11. *Bulletin de la Société de Pathologie Exotique (Bull. Soc. Pathol. Exot.)* (7)
12. *Comtes Rendus de la Société Biologique (C. R. Soc. Biol.)* (1)
13. *Estudante Brasileiro* (1)
14. *Hospital Bulletin of the University of Maryland (Hosp. Bull. Univ. Maryland)* (1)
15. *Indian Medical Gazette (Indian Med. Gaz.)* (1)
16. *Instituto de Hygiene (Inst. Hyg.) (São Paulo)* (2)
17. *Journal of the Alumni Association of the College of Physicians and Surgeons (J. Alumni Assoc. Coll. Phys. Surg.) (Baltimore)* (1)
18. *Journal of the American Medical Association (J. Am. Med. Assoc.)* (14)
19. *Journal of Cutaneous Diseases and Syphilology (J. Cutan. Dis. Syphil.)* (1)
20. *Journal of Economical Entomology (J. Econ. Entomol.)* (1)
21. *Journal of Experimental Medicine (J. Exp. Med.)* (8)
22. *Journal of Infectious Diseases (J. Infect. Dis.)* (2)

23 *Journal of Medical Research (J. Med. Res.)* (2)
24 *Journal of Parasitology (J. Parasitol.)* (3)
25 *Journal of Tropical Medicine and Hygiene (J. Trop. Med. Hyg.)* (1)
26 *Journal of Tropical Veterinary Science (J. Trop. Vet. Sci.)* (2)
27 *Lancet* (1)
28 *Maryland Medical Journal (Maryland Med. J.)* (2)
29 *Medicina e Cirugia (Med. Cirug.) (São Paulo)* (1)
30 *Nelson Loose-Leaf Medicine* (1)
31 *Parasitology* (2)
32 *Proceedings of the Canal Zone Medical Association* (also known as *Proceedings of the Medical Association of the Isthmian Canal Zone) (Proc. Canal Zone Med. Assoc./Proc. Med. Assoc. Isthmian Canal Zone)* (75)
33 *Reference Handbook Medical Sciences (Ref. Handbook Med. Sci.)* (2)
34 *Science* (2)
35 *Southern Medical Journal (South. Med. J.)* (6)
36 *Transactions of the Royal Society of Tropical Medicine and Hygiene (Trans. R. Soc. Trop. Med. Hyg.)* (2)
37 *Tropical Diseases Bulletin (Trop. Dis. Bull.)* (36)

Appendix B
Faculty, Class Schedules, Registration, and Grades, College of Physicians and Surgeons of Baltimore
Faculty Listed at Commencement Exercises, 1903[1]

Professors

Abram B. Arnold (emeritus); Harvey G. Beck (Clinical Medicine and demonstrator in Clinical Laboratory); Edward N. Brush (Psychiatry); George W. Dobbin (Obstetrics); Harry Friedenwald (Ophthalmology and Otology); Julius Friedenwald (clinical professor of Diseases of the Stomach and director of the Clinical Laboratory); C. Hampson Jones (Hygiene, Public Health and Clinical Medicine); N. G. Keirle (Medical Jurisprudence and director of the Pasteur Institute); William F. Lockwood (Materia Medica, Therapeutics and Clinical Medicine); Thomas Opie (dean); George J. Preston (Physiology and Diseases of the Nervous System); John Rurah (clinical professor of Diseases of Children); Frank Dyer Sanger (clinical professor of Nose, Throat and Chest); B. Holly Smith (principles and practice of Dental Surgery as applied to medicine); William Royal Stokes (Pathology and Bacteriology); Isaac R. Trimble (Anatomy and Clinical Surgery).

Associate Professors

Daniel Base (Chemistry); Harvey G. Beck (Clinical Medicine and demonstrator in Clinical Laboratory); Charles F. Blake (Surgery and clinical professor of Diseases of the Rectum); Charles E. Brack (Obstetrics); Thomas R. Brown (Clinical Medicine); Albertus Cotton (Orthopedic Surgery); Samuel J. Fort (Materia Medica and Pharmacology); Cary B. Gamble, Jr. (Clinical Medicine); William S. Gardner (Gynecology); Archibald C. Harrison (Anatomy and demonstrator of Anatomy); H. H. Hayden (Human and Comparative Anatomy); Standish McCleary (Histology and Pathology); Alexius McGlannan (Physiological Chemistry and demonstrator of Physiology); J. Hall Pleasants (Clinical Medicine); Melvin Rosenthal (Genito-urinary Surgery and Dermatology).

Demonstrators

Charles B. Canby (Pathology); Otto C. Glaser (Embryology); L. H. Hirshberg (Bacteriology and assistant in Neurology); H. C. Knapp (Clinical Laboratory); John Mason Knox, Jr. (Pathology and Physical Diagnosis); Glenn M. Litsinger (Obstetrics); G. W. Mitchell (Diseases of Nose, Throat, Chest and Osteology); W. W. Requardt (Surgery); C. W. G. Rhorer (Pathology and resident pathologist).

Assistant Demonstrator/Assistants

Albert F. Conrey (Gynecology); S. G. Davis (Anatomy); Samuel Rutler Grimes (Anatomy); W. Edward Magruder (Diseases of Children); L. J. Rosenthal (Diseases of Stomach); A. Samuels (Genito-urinary Surgery and demonstrator of Chemistry); Otto Schaeffer (Eye and Ear Diseases).

Tables B.1 and B.2   Daily Order of Lectures — First and Second Years[2]

Hour	Monday	Tuesday	Wednesday	Thursday	Friday	Saturday
9	Materia Medica	Chemistry	Materia Medica	Chemistry	Materia Medica	
10	Chemical and Histological	Osteology	Chemical and Histological	Osteology	Chemical and Histological	Osteology
11	Laboratories	Anatomy	Laboratories	Anatomy	Laboratories	Anatomy
12	Osteology	Physiology	Osteology	Physiology	Osteology	Physiology
1		Histology		Histology		
2						
3	Dissecting	Dissecting	Dissecting	Dissecting	Dissecting	Dissecting

Hour	Monday	Tuesday	Wednesday	Thursday	Friday	Saturday
9		Chemical Laboratory		Chemical Laboratory		
10	Pharmacology		Pharmacology		Pharmacology	Osteology
11	Bacteriological Laboratory	Anatomy	Bacteriological Laboratory	Anatomy	Physiological Laboratory	Anatomy
12		Physiology		Physiology		Physiology
1	Physiological Chemistry		Pathology and Med. Juris.			
2			Pathological Laboratory		Pathological Laboratory	
3	Dissecting	Dissecting	Dissecting	Dissecting	Dissecting	Dissecting

Table B.3 Daily Order of Lectures — Third Year[2]

Hour	Monday	Tuesday	Wednesday	Thursday	Friday	Saturday
9	Clinical Laboratory	Obstetrics	Clinical Laboratory	Clinical Laboratory	Obstetrics	Obstetrics
10	Surgery	Surgery	Surgery	Gynecology	Surgery	Surgery
11	Medicine	Clinical Medicine	Surgical Anatomy	Medicine	Operative Surgery	Medicine
12	Diseases of Nervous System	Pediatrics	Genito Urinary	Therapeutics	Diseases of Eye	Pharmacy Mental Diseases
1	Physical Diagnosis	Dermatology	Diseases of Ear	Diseases of Eye	Gynecology	
2					Diseases of Stomach	
3	Clinical Laboratory	Clinical Laboratory	Clinical Laboratory	Clinical Laboratory	Clinical Laboratory	

Table B.4 Daily Order of Lectures — Fourth Year[2]

	Hour	Monday	Tuesday	Wednesday	Thursday	Friday	Saturday
	9	Hospital Work		Hygiene, etc.	Hospital Work		Hospital Work
	10	Surgery	Surgery	Surgery	Gynecology	Surgery	Surgery
	11	Medicine	Clinical Medicine	Surgical Anatomy	Medicine	Operative Surgery	Medicine
Surgical Section	12	In Wards	In Wards	In Wards	In Wards	In Wards	In Wards
	1	Genito Urinary & Dermatology	Diseases Eye & Ear	Gynecology	Orthopedic Surgery	General Surgery	General Surgery
Medical Section	12	In Wards	In Wards	In Wards	In Wards	In Wards	In Wards
	1	Diseases of Stomach	Pediatrics	Medical Elective	Laryngology	Dis. Nervous System	Medicine
Dispensary Section	12						
	1	Dispensary	Dispensary	Dispensary	Dispensary	Dispensary	Dispensary
	3	Demonstration at Maternité		Obstetrics	Med. & Surg. Clinic	Obstetrics	

Table B.5 Student Registration, Samuel T. Darling, 1899–1903[3]

Course	Years	Name	Address	Ledger page
First Course	1899–1900	Samuel T. Darling	28 Brook St., Pawtucket, R.I.	153
Second Course	1900–1901	Samuel T. Darling	(no address given)	164
Third Course	1901–1902	Samuel T. Darling	College of P.& S.	181
Fourth Course	1902–1903	Samuel T. Darling	College of P.& S.	195

Table B.6   Student Grades, Samuel T. Darling, 1899–1903

Session	Year	Subject	Grade	Average
1899 – 1900[4]	First	Physiology	100	98.4
		Inorganic Chemistry	100	
		Materia Medica	100	
		Histology	93	
		Osteology	99	
1900 – 1901[5]	Second	Anatomy	98	99.0
		Physiology	100	
		Chemistry/ Bacteriology	100	
		Pathology/Med. Jurisprudence	100	
		Pharmacy	100	
		Hygiene	96	
1901 – 1902[6]	Third	Eye and Ear	100	93.90
		Principles and Practice of Medicine	80	
		Gynecology	91	
		Therapeutics	100	
		Surgical Anatomy	95	
		Physical Diagnosis	97	
		Surgery	94	
		Obstetrics	88	
		Nervous Diseases	90	
		Dermatology	98	
		Clinical Laboratory	100	
1902 – 1903[7]	Fourth	Medicine	100	93.83
		Surgery	100	
		Obstetrics	91	
		Gynecology	82	
		Operative Surgery	99	
		Mental Diseases	91	

Yearly averages for Samuel T. Darling:

		First year (1899-1900):	98.40	
		Second year (1900 – 1901):	99.0	
		Third year (1901 – 1902):	93.90	
		Fourth year (1902 – 1903):	93.83	
		Four-year average:		96.27

First Gold Medal awarded to Samuel T. Darling at 31st Annual Commencement Exercises on April 30, 1903, for obtaining the highest grade in his class at final examination.

Appendix C
Proceedings of the Canal Zone Medical Association

The medical staff of the isthmian hospitals organized the Canal Zone Medical Association and began its regular meetings in 1906.[1] Gorgas, who became president of the American Medical Association (A.M.A.) in 1908, at once helped to arrange for affiliation of the isthmian medical association to the national organization.[1] In the fall of 1909, an application was submitted to the A.M.A. for acceptance of the Canal Zone Medical Association as one of its constituent associations.[2] Following a recommendation of the General Secretary and endorsement by the appropriate committee, the House of Delegates approved recognition of the Canal Zone Medical Association as one of its component bodies at the sixty-first annual session of the A.M.A. in St. Louis on June 6, 1910.[2,3] At the time, it was the only medical association outside the United States permitting membership or fellowship in the A.M.A..[1] Darling became chairman of the Executive Committee and remained in that capacity for several years.[4] According to Herbert Clark, a colleague in Panama, Darling was the "guiding spirit" in the early organization of the Canal Zone Medical Association and was elected its president in 1908.[5,6]

Publication of the *Proceedings of the Canal Zone Medical Association* began in 1908.[7] The first volume consisted of 194 pages and was printed at the Isthmian Canal Commission Press in Mount Hope, Canal Zone. It contained twenty-three original reports by fifteen different authors.[7] The first article published in the *Proceedings* was a thirty-eight page compendium by Darling on the spirochetal relapsing fever of Panama.[8] If this was to become the standard by which subsequent reports were to be measured, the order was indeed a tall one. The article began with a historical review of the disease, followed by details from thirty-one cases of relapsing fever diagnosed in Canal Zone hospitals during a three-year period. The remaining twenty-six pages described the laboratory investigations made by Darling on inoculated white rats and mice to determine the morphological characteristics of the spirochete, animal reactions to inoculation, immune responses, prevention by vaccination, and treatment response to a number of dyes and quinine. Darling concluded that the relapsing fever of Panama was distinct from that observed in Africa, Europe, and Asia; that it was caused by a spirochete probably belonging to an already described group; that inoculation in macaque monkeys and white mice resulted in a recurring infection; that morphological variations of the spirochete made microscopic identification uncertain; that the mechanism of defense was by phagocytosis of the hepatic endothelium; and that the natural mode of infection was probably by means of an intermediary host such as a suctorial insect (mosquito) or acarid (tick).[8] Darling's presentation was an auspicious beginning for the fledgling journal and assured that the world of tropical medicine would follow with interest future issues.

Other original articles published by Darling in the first volume of the *Proceedings* dealt with rabies, varieties of anopheline mosquitoes, sarcosporidiosis, filariasis and elephantiasis. He also reported the pathological findings on a case of arterio-venous aneurysm of the aortic arch and on a case of anesthetic leprosy.

Darling contributed thirty-nine original articles, seven pathological and laboratory reports, and participated in twenty-nine discussions of other articles as recorded in the first five volumes of the *Proceedings*. This scientific output exceeded by far that of any other member of the association and comprised almost a quarter of the total pages of the *Proceedings* (283 out of 1,197 pages) during the five-year period 1908 to 1912.

Darling's participation at the meetings of the Canal Zone Medical Association and scientific contributions to the *Proceedings* slowed down after 1912. From 1913 to 1915, he contributed to the *Proceedings* only eight original articles and one pathological report, and participated in nine discussions. His last scientific study to appear in the *Proceedings* was entitled, "A note on typhus fever," published in 1914.[9] His last recorded discussion followed a paper presented by Herbert Clark on "Preliminary notes on neoplasms found in inhabitants of Panama Canal Zone," at the 105th meeting of the association on January 16, 1915, and his last entry was a question he posed during the discussion of a paper presented at the 106th meeting of the association dated February 20, 1915.[10,11] A decreased scholarly output toward the end of Darling's tenure in Panama may have been due in part to a six-month absence between October 1913 and April 1914, when he accompanied Gorgas to investigate increased deaths from pneumonia reported among workers in the Rand Mines of South Africa.[12] Darling also sensed, along with other employees, that construction of the canal was nearing completion and that their days on the isthmus were numbered.[13]

Publication of the *Proceedings* spanned a period of twenty years (1908 to 1927). The Canal Zone journal appeared in the form of yearly volumes in 1908 and 1909, followed by two-part yearly volumes from 1910 to 1920. The printing of the journal was discontinued between the years 1921 and 1926, and the *Proceedings* for those years were published as volume 14 in 1927.[14] The last volume of the *Proceedings* was for the year 1927 and consisted of only sixty-seven pages.[15] In 1912, the Medical Association of the Canal Zone changed its name to the Medical Association of the Isthmian Canal Zone and, accordingly, the journal became known as the *Proceedings of the Medical Association of the Isthmian Canal Zone*. An index to the name, year, and number of pages for each published volume of the *Proceedings* is shown in the following table.

Judging from both the quantity and quality of his contributions, it is safe to say that Darling was the driving force behind both the Canal Zone Medical Association and the *Proceedings of the Canal Zone Medical Association.*

Table C.7 Proceedings of the Canal Zone Medical Association, Volume Index, 1908–1927

Volume	Part	Date	Name	Pages
I		1908	Proceedings of the Canal Zone Medical Association	194
II		April 1909 to March 1910	Proceedings of the Canal Zone Medical Association	184
III	1	April to September 1910	Proceedings of the Canal Zone Medical Association	150
III*	2	October 1910 to March 1911	Proceedings of the Canal Zone Medical Association	114
IV	1	April to September 1911	Proceedings of the Canal Zone Medical Association	238
IV	II	October 1911 to March 1912	Proceedings of the Canal Zone Medical Association	152
V	1	April to September 1912	Proceedings of the Canal Zone Medical Association	165
V	2	October 1912 to March 1913	Proceedings of the Medical Association of the Isthmian Canal Zone	139
VI	1	April to September 1913	Proceedings of the Medical Association of the Isthmian Canal Zone	122
VI	2	October 1913 to March 1914	Proceedings of the Medical Association of the Isthmian Canal Zone	66
VII	1	April to September 1914	Proceedings of the Medical Association of the Isthmian Canal Zone	163
VII	2	October 1914 to March 1915	Proceedings of the Medical Association of the Isthmian Canal Zone	129
VIII	1/2	April to December 1915	Proceedings of the Medical Association of the Isthmian Canal Zone	169
IX	1	January to June 1916	Proceedings of the Medical Association of the Isthmian Canal Zone	190
IX	2	July to December 1916	Proceedings of the Medical Association of the Isthmian Canal Zone	133
X	1	January to June 1917	Proceedings of the Medical Association of the Isthmian Canal Zone	149
X	2	July to December 1917	Proceedings of the Medical Association of the Isthmian Canal Zone	174
XI	1	January to June 1918	Proceedings of the Medical Association of the Isthmian Canal Zone	118
XI	2	July to December 1918	Proceedings of the Medical Association of the Isthmian Canal Zone	73
XII	1/2	January to December 1919	Proceedings of the Medical Association of the Isthmian Canal Zone	54
XIII	1/2	January to December 1920	Proceedings of the Medical Association of	

		the Isthmian Canal Zone	139
XIV	1921 – 1926	Proceedings of the Medical Association of the Isthmian Canal Zone	133
XV	1927	Proceedings of the Medical Association of the Isthmian Canal Zone	67

*This is the first volume in the series assigned a part number (2); subsequent volumes IV to XIII consisted of two parts (given in either Roman or Arabic numerals, as shown above). Volumes I, XIV, and XV were assigned only years (no parts). The *Proceedings of the Canal Zone Medical Association* changed its name to *Proceedings of the Medical Association of the Isthmian Canal Zone* starting with volume V part 2 (October 1912 to March 1913).

Appendix D
Personnel and Staff, Board of Health Laboratories

The Board of Health Laboratories were created by a resolution of the Isthmian Canal Commission on June 14, 1905, for the purpose of supporting the broad responsibilities of the Board of Health.[1] The latter included the sanitation of the cities of Panama and Colon, laboratory services needed by the Commission hospitals, and research studies that would help to alleviate the burden of tropical diseases on the workforce involved in the construction of the canal.

Darling was appointed chief of the Board of Health Laboratories on October 5, 1906, and remained in that capacity for seven years and eight months until his resignation effective May 23, 1915.[2] The initial laboratory staff consisted of George V. Ridley, pathologist; R. W. Nauss, interne (chemistry); Paul M. Carpenter and Harry O'Connor, laboratory assistants.[1] A statement of the organization of the Board of Health Laboratory in 1908 gave the following personnel and respective annual salaries: S. T. Darling, chief of the laboratory ($4,000); Thomas R. Brown, bacteriologist ($3,000); Ralph W. Nauss, chemist ($3,000); James O. Meadows, physiologist ($2,700); Charles A. Herson, nurse ($720); Luis Ernst, laboratory assistant ($720 plus subsistence); James N. Keneally, laboratory assistant ($540 plus subsistence); Hutton Williams, laboratory assistant ($1,200 plus subsistence); and Ray A. Yunker, embalmer ($1,200).[3] Other personnel listed as "Silver Force" (in contrast to "Gold Force," as United States employees were designated) were: one morgue janitor ($480); two attendants ($300 each); and one messenger ($126).[3]

Running expenses for the Board of Health Laboratory for the months of July, August, September, and October 1908 (including payroll, material, steam, and light costs) were, respectively, $1,673.14, $1,686.66, $1,051.49, and $1,101.23.[3] These figures projected to an annual cost for operating Darling's laboratory well below $20,000. As comparison, annual salary costs for the Quarantine Division personnel exceeded $25,000, even though the United States Public Health and Marine Hospital Service paid more than half of the salaries for two of the quarantine officers, J. C. Perry and C. C. Pierce.[4] A permanent staff was established in

1909, with the following personnel listed, in addition to Darling: Lewis B. Bates, bacteriologist and serologist; Herbert C. Clark, pathologist; James E. Jacob, chemist; John R. Downes, water analyst; and Luis Ernst, assistant to Jacob and Downes.[1]

Among notables who worked with Darling at the Board of Health Laboratories were Arthur I. Kendall, who became professor of bacteriology at Northwestern University, and George H. Whipple, who became dean of the Rochester University School of Medicine and shared the Nobel Prize in Physiology or Medicine in 1934 for his work on treatment of pernicious anemia. Other colleagues and personnel of the Board of Health Laboratories during the period 1906 to 1936 are listed below.[1] Conspicuously absent from this list is Alleyne, Darling's first assistant in the morgue. Alleyne was a native Jamaican and, therefore, hired as a non-skilled worker on the "silver roll." Alleyne remained as an employee of the Board of Health Laboratories for forty years and reputedly participated in more than 15,000 autopsies at Gorgas Hospital.[5]

Chiefs of the Board of Health Laboratories

Arthur B. Herrick (1904–1906)
Samuel T. Darling (1906–1915) (First official chief)
Maj. Frederick F. Russell (1915–1917)
Maj. Oscar Teague (1917–1918)
Capt. William L. McFarland (1918–1919)
Lewis B. Bates (1919–to date) (1936)

Pathologists

Arthur B. Herrick (1904–1905)
Samuel T. Darling (1905–1906)
George Whipple (1907–1908)
Francis P. McCarthy (1908–1909)
Herbert C. Clark (1909–1922)
Ray S. Nelson (1917–1919)
William S.[*sic*] McFarland (1917–1919)
L. W. Gorton (1917–1919)
Capt. Virgil N. Cornell (1922–1926)
Maj. P. E. McNabb (19126–1928)
Maj. R. O. Dart (1928–1932)
Capt. E. Decoursey (1932–1934)
Maj. H. W. Mahon (1934–to date) (1936)

Bacteriologists

Arthur I. Kendall (1904–1906)
Thomas R. Brown (1907–1908)
Lewis B. Bates (1909–1918)
John N. Force (1918–1919)
Capt. J. H. St. John (1919–1922)
Capt. W. C. Cox (1922–1925)
Capt. S. D. Avery (1925–1928)

Capt. G. C. H. Franklin (1928–1931)
Capt. M. R. Reiber (1931–1934)
Capt. K. R. Lundeberg (1934 to date)

Chemists

R. W. Nauss (unofficial status) (1906–1908)
J. E. Jacob (1908 to date)
Sarah Vance (1918–1919)

Entomologists

A. H. Jennings
James Zetek (?–1919)
L. H. Dunn (1920–?)

Undertakers

Dunn
Ray E. Yunkers [sic]
William Hull
Alexander Mackenzie
G. F. Bohan

Appendix E
Discovery and Pathology of Histoplasmosis [1,2]

Darling received both graduate and post-graduate training in pathology in Baltimore. As a medical student, he assisted Nathaniel G. Keirle, professor of pathology and medical examiner of the City of Baltimore, at post-mortem examinations.[3] After graduation from the College of Physicians and Surgeons of Baltimore in 1903, Darling was appointed resident pathologist at Baltimore City Hospital and instructor in histology and pathology at his alma mater.[3] He also gained considerable experience in bacteriology working with Keirle at the Pasteur Rabies Institute in Baltimore, and as instructor in bacteriology at the Women's Medical College in Baltimore.[3,4]

These abilities were promptly recognized by his superiors in Panama, and within five months after his arrival, Darling was promoted from interne to pathologist and, a year later, to the post of chief of the Board of Health Laboratories.[5] In this latter capacity, he performed most of the autopsies done in the Canal Zone and considered this as a most important part of his work. During his nine-year tenure at Ancon Hospital, Darling performed more than four-thousand autopsies, aided by his able Jamaican assistant (Darling considered the term *deaner* as demeaning), Alleyne.[6]

Sir Ronald Ross visited Panama in 1904 and suggested that kala-azar (also called Oriental sore and visceral leishmaniasis) may be found in tropical America if properly sought among cases of splenomegaly (spleen enlargement).[7] Darling continued the search by examining microscopically smears from spleen, liver, and "rib-marrow" for the presence of Leishman-Donovan bodies — the name given by Ross to the causative parasite. As a result of this practice, on December 7, 1905, Darling found a new micro-organism in the post-mortem examination of a 27-year-old Martiniquan who died of a disease resembling kala-azar.[1] Within eight months, he encountered the same micro-organism in two additional autopsies and renewed acquaintances with his "old friend."[1] Meticulous attention to detail and remarkable powers of observation were evident in his description of the pathological findings in the three cases, published in the *Archives of Internal Medicine* in 1908.[1] The autopsy findings in the three cases of histoplasmosis are reproduced with permission below:

CASE 1.
Autopsy (No. 252). — The patient died December 6, [1905] 11:30 p.m. The autopsy was made on December 7, 8:30 a.m.

Macroscopic and Microscopic Examination. — Body of [N]egro, moderately emaciated; length 5 feet, 8 3/4 inches; inter-nipple distance, 7 3/16 inches; rigor mortis was plus. The odor on opening the thorax was suggestive of pulmonary tuberculosis. The right and left pleura were free. There were numerous red blotches (ecchymoses) beneath the visceral pleura of both lungs, 8 mm. in diameter. Many small nodules could be felt under the visceral pleura. The lungs on section were found studded with pale gray hyaline miliary tubercles from 2 to 3 mm. in diameter. The lungs were heavier and more voluminous than normal. The tubercles were not as closely packed or as numerous as is often found in miliary tuberculosis, and the general color of the lungs was bright red. The peribronchial lymph nodes contained a few small recently caseated tubercles. The nodes were enlarged and pigmented. The heart was small and normal. The liver was enlarged and pale, and there was slight atrophic cirrhosis. The spleen was enlarged to three times the normal size; the pulp was very firm. The Malphigian bodies were distinct. Here and there were a number of small yellow nodules resembling tubercles. In the kidneys there were a few depressions in a cortex diminished to 8 mm. in depth. The pancreas and bladder were normal, and the rib bone marrow normal and dry. Examination of the brain showed the pia-arachnoid slightly edematous and more generally adherent to the cortex than normal. The calvarium was very thick. Several specimens of *Tricocephalus dispar* were found in the cecum. There were a few small superficial circular ulcers from 2 to 4 mm. in diameter in the cecum and ileum. The mesenteric lymph nodes and those at hilum of the spleen were enlarged and pale.

Bacteriological Examination. — Spleen smears were negative for malarial parasites or pigment. Oval and round bodies were free in the plasma. In the rib bone marrow smears, there were traces of intracellular malarial pigment. A number of bodies similar to those in the spleen were seen. In lung smears tubercle bacilli were absent. There were myriads of intracellular and extracellular bodies similar to those found in the spleen and marrow. A moist coverslip preparation from the intestinal ulcers showed motile amebas.

Anatomic Diagnosis. — Acute miliary tuberculosis, pulmonary type. Tuberculous adenitis, peribronchial. Chronic interstitial splenitis. Atrophic cirrhosis. Chronic interstitial nephritis, slight. Lymphadenitis, mesenteric. Chronic leptomeningitis. Edema of pia-arachnoid. Ulcerative enterocolitis. Amebiasis. General infection by protozoon.

The micro-organism was not discovered in smears until late in the day, after the anatomical diagnosis had been made.

Appearance of the Parasite in Smears. — Lungs: This specimen was stained by carbolfuchsin and Gabbet's methylene blue, overstained with polychrome methylene blue, and differentiated with eosin. The polychrome blue was prepared as follows:

Methylene blue, pure medic, Grübb	1 gm.
Sodium carbonate, pure	.5 gm.
Distilled water	100 gm.

This was placed in the thermostat one week, and kept at room temperature for six months. The excess of blue was removed by washing the smear alternately with alcoholic solution of eosin (0.5 per cent. in 60 per cent. ethyl alcohol) one second and distilled water a few seconds, until the internal structure of the parasite showed plainly. The parasite was oviform or round and was surrounded by a clear, refractile, non-staining rim, in thickness about one-sixth the diameter of the parasite. This refractile rim was present in all smears, whether previously treated with acid blue or not. The structure was not homogenous, but consisted of faintly staining substance and a deeply staining one; a clear space or spaces; and chromatin granules. The chromatin granules were generally single; sometimes two or more were counted. One large parasite appeared to have six such dots of chromatin. The granules were often situated in a clear non-staining zone at one side of the darker staining substance; at other times they were situated on the margin or within this substance, and also frequently appeared in the clear refractile capsule. The chromatin granules were generally dot-shaped, very rarely elongated. Occasionally two chromatin dots placed together simulated a rod form.

The clear space or spaces resembled vacuoles; at times they resembled the clear non-staining spaces seen in filaria embryos and trypanosomes. The staining substance almost entirely filled the capsule or refractile rim of the parasite. The circular contour of the staining substance was at times broken on one side by the clear non-staining zone. This zone varied in shape, size, and in its relation to the staining substance, being circular, oval, or irregular in form; being three-fourths the size of the entire parasite, or at times barely perceptible on account of its minuteness; being centrally located or eccentric; and being single or multiple — two or three.

In size the parasites were one to four microns through their greatest diameter; commonly this diameter was three microns.

The parasite appeared to divide by fission into two equal or unequal elements. One parasite appeared to be dividing into four equal elements. Several parasites with chromatin dots scattered throughout their substances appeared as presegmenting bodies, ready to divide into five or six elements. Generally a smaller parasite might be seen close beside a larger one, as though separating from it; the smaller one being about one micron in diameter.

Although oval or round in outline, the staining substance, together with the clear, non-staining zone and chromatin granules, gave a varying picture, depending on the point of view. Forms suggesting the appearance of familiar objects, such as the eye, a shield, a conch shell, a bullet, or a shuttle, were seen. The resemblance of the deeply staining substance in certain parasites to a mammalian embryo in "fetal attitude" was very striking.

In the lung smears the parasite was apparently always intracellular and the cells contained from ten to one hundred or more parasites. The appearance of free parasites was probably due to the squeezing and breaking up of infected epithelial cells by pressure in making the smear. One unbroken alveolar epithelial cell occupied one-third the diameter of the field (1/12 oil im[mersion]. No.1 oe. B.& L.). Parasites had invaded the cell nucleus as well as the cytoplasm, and it was estimated that this cell contained more than three hundred.

Spleen and rib marrow smears showed fewer parasites, two or three to a field, and they appeared now and then to have been invaded. Each parasite had a definite refractile rim, as in the lung smears, and its internal structure could be well made out. Red blood corpuscles were never invaded.

Three flagellated forms were seen in a lung smear. The distal extremity of one of the flagella contained a rod of chromatin placed at right angles to the flagellum, simulating the relation of centrosome to chromatin filament in *Trypanosoma [l]ewisi*. The flagella were single, short and thick, without chromatin filaments, and were enclosed by the refractile capsule, continuous with that of the body of the parasite.

Examination of Sections . — Sections were fixed in Zenker's solution and stained by eosin and hematoxylin, Van Giesen's method, and polychrome-methylene blue.

Lung: The alveolar capillaries were tortuous and engorged with red blood corpuscles. In places the walls were broken down, stretched, or greatly distended. No leucocytes were seen within the capillaries. The epithelial cells of the alveolar walls was desquamating or completely shed. The alveoli were seen to be filled with red blood corpuscles, serum, and large swollen alveolar epithelial cells containing many parasites.

Polymorphonuclear leucoytes were rarely observed in the alveolar contents; a few mononuclear elements were noted. There were no tubercles. The pseudo-tuberculous areas were made up of alveoli with broken, distorted, or collapsed walls, containing many alveolar epithelial cells, distended by parasites. Small vessels or capillaries were seen to pass through the pseudo-tubercles, but there were no evidences of the hemorrhages seen in other alveoli. Within these areas there were enormous numbers of parasites generally contained within epithelial cells — rarely free. The nuclei of invaded cells stained well, though often more faintly than normal. The cytoplasm of badly infected cells was wanting, and there were numerous distended epithelial cells devoid of cytoplasm and parasites. The infected cells had a distinctly staining rim of cytoplasm, even when their nucleus and cytoplasm was gone.

Liver: There were numerous faintly staining areas ranging in size from that of a single liver cell to those one-third the size of a lobule in which the liver cells and endothelial cells of the portal capillaries were completely transformed by invading parasites. In the larger areas the cytoplasm and nuclei of the invaded cells had disappeared and did not stain. There was a mass of débris, embedded in which were myriads of parasites. In places the liver cells were normal; in others they had suffered cloudy change. In these latter localities there appeared to be a stasis of blood in the portal capillaries due to occlusion of capillaries by enormously distended endothelial cells filled with parasites.

There was a distinct primary invasion of liver cells in places, although oftener it seemed that many liver cells became invaded after they had had their nutrition cut off by the infected overlying endothelial cells.

Around the portal space the connective tissue was increased in amount and there was a recent round cell infiltration. The bile ducts and their epithelium were normal.

Spleen: The splenic spaces were greatly engorged with red blood corpuscles. The connective tissue was moderately increased, its cells were swollen, cloudy, and at times contained parasites. There was cloudy swelling of mononuclear cells in small areas here and there, and many of these cells contained parasites. There were also numerous free parasites.

Lymph Node From Hilum of Spleen. — The cortical follicles and medullary cords of the dense lymphoid tissue were, with the exceptions noted below, normal. The capsule and reticulum throughout the node were the seat of degenerative changes. The reticulum of the loose lymphoid tissue enclosed many large mononuclear cells containing parasites. The margins of these areas showed beginning degenerative changes; many fragmented nuclei were seen, as well as mononuclear cells distended by parasites.

Peribronchial Lymph Node. — This node contained several old fibrocaseous tubercles and one giant cell. The reticulum and capsule of the node were greatly thickened in places. A lymph vessel beneath the capsule contained mononuclear cells infected by parasites.

Case 2.
Autopsy (No. 306). — This was made Jan. 30, 1906, 8 a.m., four hours after death.

Negro from Martinique aged 29. The body was 5 feet 7 inches in length and much emaciated. Rigor mortis was plus. Pleura free — negative. Peribronchial lymph nodes enlarged. Pericardium, negative. Omentum contracted. No peritonitis noted. Lungs: The upper part of the lower lobes showed patches of bronchopneumonia. The upper lobes were negative. Heart: Small, flabby. Right heart considerably dilated. Valves negative; muscles light in color. Liver: Normal in size; color reddish brown. Adrenals: negative. Kidneys: Somewhat enlarged. Their capsules stripped with ease and both were much congested. Spleen: Five times its normal size, firm. There was an increase in its fibrous stroma. Its pulp was deep brown in color and smears contained aestivo-autumnal malarial parasites. Intestinal tract: The stomach contained considerable quantity of coffee-ground material and the mucosa, while very pale, showed no indications of hemorrhage. The intestines contained round worms, whip-worms and New World uncinaria worms.

Anatomic Diagnosis. — Bronchopneumonia; acute parenchymatous nephritis; uncinariasis; ascariasis; trichocephaliasis; malarial fever, e. a.

Smears from the spleen, bone marrow, liver and lymph nodes examined the following day showed numerous micro-organisms similar to those seen in Case 1.

Histopathology. — Kidney : The convoluted tubules were generally distended. The nuclei of the epithelial cells were swollen and did not stain deeply. Here and there a nucleus was missing. The lumen contained coagulated albumin and an occasional desquamated epithelial cell. Some of the straight tubules contained hyaline casts. The epithelium of the convoluted tubules were widely separated by a cellular exudation or proliferation. The cells making up this exudate or proliferate had eosin-staining protoplasm and most of them had deeply staining nuclei, eccentrically placed. Minute hemorrhages were also noted in these interstitial places. The cells of the glomeruli and of Bowman's capsule were swollen and their nuclei were swollen and pale. A few convoluted tubules showed colloid degeneration. The vessels appeared normal. Heart and pancreas: Negative. Spleen: The splenic spaces were distended by red blood cells. Numerous mono-phagocytes were dotted with parasites. The Malphigian bodies showed some disappearance of their lymphoid elements. Liver: There was a slight round-cell proliferation, around the portal spaces and in small foci here and there. The columns of the liver cells everywhere appeared flattened and attenuated, but the capillaries were not engorged. There appeared to have been a diffuse disappearance of liver cells. There were some very small areas about the size of a dozen liver cells in which there was an almost complete disappearance of liver cells; the space being occupied by endothelial cells containing malarial pigment and occasionally parasites. Throughout the section there was such much malarial pigment enclosed within endothelial cells lining the capillaries. Many of these endothelial cells were distended by parasites (*Histoplasma capsulatum*) as well as pigment. From this section the earliest lesion was apparently that in the endothelial cell. The areas of round-cell proliferation — apart from those around the portal spaces — were frequently associated on one side by the small areas of necrosis containing parasites. Some of these areas of necrosis extended outward from the portal space; others were in the intermediate zone; while others could not be oriented on account of their obscuration of the lobule outline. One of these small areas, where the liver cells had disappeared, contained a typical giant cell with a mural arrangement of its nuclei on one side. The giant cell was in the intermediate zone of a lobule. The giant cell was not a part of a tubercle, and around it were no round cells, epithelial cells, or nuclear fragmentation. The structures in the portal spaces were normal. In this instance the infection was a mixed one of the malarial parasite and *Histoplasma capsulatum*. Adrenal: Negative. Lung: The capillaries were tortuous and engorged with red blood cells. The alveoli contained red blood cells and polymorphonuclear leucocytes in about equal numbers, also a few desquamated alveolar epithelial cells. No parasites were seen. Lymph node: The spaces of the lymphoid tissue contained numerous large mononuclear phagocytes — some with double nuclei — many of which had engulfed red blood cells. There were no areas of necrosis, the changes being hyperplasia of large and small lymphoid cells. No parasites were seen in the section.

CASE 3.
Autopsy (No. 572). — Aug. 11, 1906, eighteen hours after death.

Body of a male Chinese, aged 55. Hair cropped short. Moderate pitting of feet, legs, thighs, lower abdomen and left side of face, which latter was congested. Rigor mortis was absent. There were three or four raised recent broad papules 8 mm. in diameter, on the left arm, outer aspect. External genitalia normal. Scrotum not edematous. Sub-cutaneous tissue slightly edematous. Muscles of chest, abdomen and legs very pale. Sartorius muscles a dull gray color. The knee joints normal. Lungs: Voluminous and the pleura free. Right and left upper lobes and middle lobe contained a few raised hyaline dense areas resembling tubercles. They were from 2 to 6 mm. in diameter and were often irregular in contour and elongate. They were always surrounded by a raised hemorrhagic zone about 4 mm. in thickness. The peribronchial lymph nodes were slightly enlarged, pigmented black, and contained no tubercles. Pericardium normal, containing about 30 c.c. clear fluid. Heart: Rather small and flaccid; valves normal; musculature dull brown color. Liver: Enlarged, capsule smooth. Organ presented a unique appearance, due to a grayish yellow arborescence. The limbs of the arborescence were 4 mm. in diameter and apparently followed portal radicals. Their centers were gray, their peripheries rather yellow. The areas contained only four or six limbs, but were scattered thickly throughout the entire organ, save in one portion of the liver near the falciform ligament about 16 e.e. elongate anteroposteriorly. There was much fatty infiltration of the parenchyma. The gall bladder was normal. The portal lymph nodes were enlarged, pale, yellow, slightly edematous and friable. Spleen: Enlarged, long and relative narrow; its pulp was firm, and tense. Kidneys and Adrenals: Negative. The peritoneal surface of the sigmoid flexure, descending colon and perirectal peritoneum near Poupart's ligament was intensely pigmented black in spots. Aorta: Normal. Testes: Normal. The colon contained about twenty-four small 6 mm. round pigmented areas of hyperplasia and ulceration. Small Intestines: The entire ileum and lower two-thirds of the jejunum contained altogether about 50 circumscribed areas of hyperplasia infiltration, necrosis, ulceration and hemorrhage. There were several stages to the process. 1. A pigmented raised area five to six mm. without ulceration. 2. The same with much infiltration of periphery. 3. Necrosis. 4. Recent ulceration with fresh blood clotted on the surface of the ulcer (8 mm.). 5. A puckered, pigmented scar 8 mm. in diameter. The mesenteric lymph nodes were not appreciably enlarged. The postperitoneal lymph nodes were enlarged and were similar to the portal nodes. The upper jejunum, duodenum, stomach and esophagus were normal. The calvarium was thin and the cranium markedly brachycephalic in type. Brain: Pale, normal. Accessory sinuses; normal. Smears from liver, intestinal ulcers and spleen contained many histoplasma bodies.

Cause of death. — Protozoon infection — histoplasmosis.

Histopathology. — Kidney: There was some edema. The epithelium of the convoluted tubercle was swollen and in places desquamated and cloudy. Most of the nuclei failed to take the stain. Many of the tubules contained granular débris, desquamated epithelium and occasionally a hyaline cast. There was a slight increase in the intertubular connective tissue and in Bowman's capsule. The space between the glomerulus and Bowman's capsule frequently contained a large amount of coagulated albumin.

Liver: The section showed extensive destruction of the parenchyma by coagulative necrosis having a reticulated character; and the replacement of these areas of necrosis to connective tissue, old and newly formed. The cells of the latter showed an extensive invasion by the micro-organism; many of the cells contained thirty or forty parasites. The process was so extensive that a zonal arrangement could not be positively made out. The older and more extensive areas of necrosis and replacement appeared to be in the portal spaces, where the areas of connective tissue were frequently broader than a liver lobule. The areas of coagulative necrosis varied in size from two or three liver cells up to one-half the diameter of a lobule. These areas of necrosis were scattered everywhere; sometimes isolated, at other times on the margin of a large area, which had apparently undergone necrosis and been replaced by connective tissue. There did not appear to be a shrinkage in this substitutive fibrosis, and there was apparently no distortion of the liver lobule. The areas of necrosis always contained parasites; some parasites appeared to be free, others were enclosed in large vesicular cells, resembling endothelial cells. The heaviest invasion by parasites was in the connective tissue cells, which had replaced the areas of necroses, and these areas corresponded to the hyaline opalescence noted at autopsy. The connective tissue of the capsule of the liver was thickened and frequently communicated with the infected underlying areas of necroses, but the capsule showed no invasion by parasites. The hepatic vein occasionally was surrounded by connected [*sic*] tissue which had been invaded by parasites. The epithelium of the bile ducts showed no appreciable proliferation and its epithelium was not invaded by parasites.

Ulcer, Ileum: The peritoneum and muscle wall were normal. The mucous membrane was pushed away from the muscle wall by an oval mass of large round and oval cells, most of which had a large amount of eosin-staining cytoplasm, which was more or less replaced by micro-organisms. The periphery of this granuloma, nearest the lumen of the intestine, was denuded of mucous membrane, almost to the depth of the muscularis mucosa. Under the higher power there was seen to be an extraordinary invasion of certain cells in the granuloma by the micro-organism. The nucleus of the invaded cell was either eccentric, or pushed to one side and the micro-organism was closely packed in a clear achromatic space. This achromatic space had no definite membrane and was surrounded by eosin-staining cytoplasm of the cell. Some of the invaded cells did not show this achromatic space, but merely showed a mass of micro-organisms embedded in the cytoplasm of the cell. In this section the blood vessels were not involved, but the lymph spaces everywhere showed an invasion of their lining endothelium by parasites. While most of the micro-organisms were intracellular there was quite a large number apparently free. The epithelium of the tubular glands was everywhere from an invasion by micro-organisms, yet the interglandular connective tissue stroma and the basement membrane were crowded with parasites. The denuded surface of the ulcer was rich in infected cells and there were detached cells and parasites lying free on the surface. The morphology of these free parasites on the surface was the same as those embedded in tissue. Flagella apparently were not present. The cells making up the granuloma were generally large, with small and deeply staining, or large and vesicular nuclei; most of them had a large amount of eosin-staining cytoplasm, while others had a slight affinity for hematoxylin. This section showed a more intense invasion by parasites than that of any other tissue. Epithelial cells, blood vessels and smooth muscles were not invaded. In this tissue the micro-organisms had spread along the lymph spaces. A peribronchial lymph node showed several large areas in which the lymphoid tissue of the node has been replaced by dense fibrous tissue, in the periphery of which there was a good deal of black pigment. Here and there where the lymphoid tissue still remained there were large cells, sometimes appearing to be a part of the reticulum, at other times endothelial cells bulging out into the lymph spaces, packed with parasites.

Spleen: The splenic spaces were greatly distended by red blood cells and there was a very striking absence of leucocytes in the splenic spaces. The reticulum did not appear to be increased in amount by the proliferation of its elements, but there was an extensive invasion of large cells in the reticulum by parasites; on the whole, however, the most extensive invasion was that of cells making up the reticulum of the organ. There as an almost complete disappearance of the lymphoid cells of the Malphigian bodies, the reticulum of which was thickened and fibrous.

Lung: Section of granuloma 2.5 mm. in diameter. The pulmonary alveoli surrounding the granuloma were full of red blood cells. The granuloma consisted of a reticulum conveying small blood vessels. The reticulum was not alveolated but consisted of whorls and strands of loose, connective tissue, small blood vessels, and what appeared to be the remains of alveoli, filled with very large cells containing micro-organisms. In places there were alveoli partly collapsed, containing very large cells with single or double nuclei; these cells showed an enormous invasion by parasites. The alveoli also contained red blood cells and desquamated epithelial cells, containing both parasites and pigment (dust cells).

Darling named the novel micro-organism *Histoplasma capsulatum*, a descriptive term encompassing its morphological characteristics: "plasmodia"-like organisms seen in "histiocytes" and surrounded by a "capsule."[8,9] However, Darling erroneously classified *Histoplasma capsulatum* as a protozoon, based on his observations of a few flagellated forms in a lung smear in Case 1, which resembled the Leishman-Donovan bodies typically found in kala-azar.[1] This misperception was strengthened by the respected opinion of Ross, who reviewed Darling's histologic preparations and agreed with his interpretation.[10] Attempts at cultivation of the micro-organism failed and innumerable microscopic examinations of water pellicles (as found in kala-azar), animals (including calves, iguanas, raccoons, monkeys, rats, mice, snakes, and marsupials), and various insects, also failed to disclose *Histoplasma capsulatum*.[11] With a measure of scientific caution, Darling remarked that "it will be necessary to cultivate the micro-organism from splenic pulp from a patient during life in order to determine its morphology in the flagellated stage."[12]

In 1912, da Rocha-Lima studied Darling's material and concluded that the tinctorial properties and budding forms were more consistent with yeast forms and that Darling's observations of flagellated forms were probably spurious.[13] Classification of *Histoplasma capsulatum* and its subsequent cultivation as a yeast, as well as characterization of histoplasmosis as a mycosis or fungal infection, probably would have pleased Darling. As a scientific investigator, Darling strived for the truth and respected scientific facts.

Appendix F
Visitors and Workers, Field Station for Studies in Malaria, Leessburg, Georgia

The following list was given by Darling in a report to the International Health Board on the activities of the Field Station for Studies in Malaria for the year 1924.[1]

Dr. Charles A. Bailey; Mr. M. M. Balfour; Dr. M. E. Barnes; Dr. George Bevier; Dr. S. B. Bieker, Alabama State Board of Health; Dr. C. B. Blaisdell; Dr. R. W. Bradshaw; Mr. R. B. Broughman, Florida State Board of Health; Dr. Émile Brumpt, University of Paris; Mr. T. L. Coggeshell, University of Indiana; Dr. R. K. Collins; Miss Adah Corpening, Virginia State Board of Health; Dr. J. H. L. Cumpston, Australia; Dr. K. Drensky, of Bulgaria; Dr. E. C. Faust, Peking Medical College; Dr. John A. Ferrell; Dr. R. G. Hamilton, South Carolina State Board of Health; Mr. Wm. Hoffman; Dr. R. N. Holland, Florida State Board; Dr. A. L. Hoops, Straits Settlements; Dr. Ross Hopkins, Missouri State Board of Health; Dr. W. P. Jacocks; Mr. Dr. J. H. Janney; Dr. Peter de Jarnette, Georgia State Board of Health; H. A. Johnson; Dr. C. A. Kane, Virginia State Board of Health; Dr. Vernon L. Kellogg; Dr. John F. Kendrik; Dr. C. H. Kinaman, Florida State Board of Health; Dr. F. E. Kitchens, Tennessee State Board; Dr. R. Kudo, University of Illinois; Dr. Chas. N. Leach; Mr. Thos. LeBlanc, U.S.P.H.S; Dr. Gustavo de Lessa, Brazil; Mr. F. F. Longley; Dr. Thorvald Madsen, Denmark; Dr. Leroy Maeder; Dr. J. R. Mahone, Texas State Board; Miss Marion Maitland, University of Toronto; Dr. Martin, Alabama; Dr. Henry Meleney, Peking Medical College; Dr. F. T. Milam; Dr. P. H. Muse, Tennessee State Board of Health; Dr. W. N. Newcomb; Dr. W. H. Nicholls, Tennessee; Dr. Massimo Pantaleoni, Italy; Dr. George Payne; Dr. V. G. Presson; Dr. Carl Puckett, Oklahoma State Board of Health; Dr. H. C. Ricks, Oklahoma State Board; Dr. F. F. Russell; Dr. W. A. Sawyer; Mr. T. F. Sellers, Georgia State Board of Health; Dr. W. G. Smillie; Mr. Jack Soundground, Johns Hopkins University; Mr. E. S. Talbot, Florida State Board; Dr. H. A. Taylor; Dr. R. M. Taylor; Dr. Wu Lien The, China; Dr. and Mrs. E. Walch, Holland and Java; Mr. J. S. Wise, South Carolina State Board; Dr. S. W. Welch, Alabama; Dr. David B. Wilson.

Appendix G
Obituaries and Condolences

OBITUARIES, SAMUEL T. DARLING

American Journal of Public Health
Association News. S. T. Darling, M.D., 1872–1925 Norman V. Lothian, D.P.H.,
1889–1925. 1925; 15: 714.

American Journal of Tropical Medicine
Samuel Taylor Darling 1872–1925. 1925; 5 (No. 5): 319–21.

British Medical Journal
Obituary. 1925; 1 (May 30): 1024.
Samuel Taylor Darling, M.D. 1925; 1 (June 13): p. 1111.

Bulletin de la Société de Pathologie Exotique
Nécrologie. Samuel Darling (Séance du 10 juin 1925). 1925; 18 (No. 6): 31–2.

International Health Board Bulletin
Samuel Taylor Darling 1872–1925. 1925; 6 (No. 1 July): 1–25.

Journal of the American Medical Association
Deaths. Samuel Taylor Darling. Vol 84 (No. 22) May 30, 1925. p. 1681.

Journal of Parasitology
Obituary. Samuel Taylor Darling 1872–1925. 1926; 12 (No. 3 March): 17–18.
The Helminthological Society of Washington (88th Meeting held on September
19, 1925). 1926; 12: 110.

Lancet
Obituary. Samuel Taylor Darling. 1925; 1 (June 30): 1320–1.

Science
Hegner R.W.: Samuel Taylor Darling 1872–1925. 1925 (New Series); 62 (No.
1593 July 10): 23–24.

Section on Preventive and Industrial Medicine and Public Health of the American Medical Association. Resolution on the Death of Dr. Darling.
International Health Board Annual Report 1925.

Transactions of the Royal Society of Tropical Medicine & Hygiene
Obituary. Dr. Samuel Taylor Darling. 1925; 19 (No. 3): 186–7.

The New York Times
Dr. Darling killed in Syrian car wreck. May 23, 1925.

CONDOLENCES

These messages are arranged chronologically, as received and filed at the International Health Board offices, Rockefeller Foundation, between May and July, 1925.

May 1925[1]

1. Henry Carr, Ralph K. Collins, The Laboratory Staff, Leesburg, Georgia, to Mrs. Darling, May 22, 1925: "The tremendous shock of the news of Dr. Darling's fatal accident has just come to us. We are grieved beyond words for [he] has always been to us the essence of good and our guiding hand in what feeble efforts we could make to carry out the important work he initiated and so faithfully sponsored here in Georgia."

2. R. R. Forrester, Leesburg, Georgia, to Mrs. Darling, May 22, 1925: "Condolences from the Mayor and Council of City."

3. Selskar M. Gunn, Director International Health Board, Paris, to Frederick F. Russell, May 22, 1925: "Sir Eric Drummond notified Vincent and Hackett; I have cabled you and telegraphed Hackett. This is a terrible thing and a very serious loss to the IHB and to malaria control work in the world."

4. John A. Ferrell to Mrs. Darling (Telegram), May 22, 1925: "Deepest sympathy for you and children in your distressing loss."

5. George E. Vincent/F. F. Russell to Mrs. Darling, May 22, 1925: "Our deepest sympathy goes to you. Doctor Darling's death is a tragedy keenly felt by all of us. As a friend and as a distinguished man of science his loss is irreparable."

6. Marshall C. Balfour to John A. Ferrell, May 23, 1925.

7. Eric C. Drummond, Société des Nations, Geneva, to Mr. Vincent, Esq., Chairman of I. H. B., May 23, 1925.

8. Abercrombie to Rockefeller Foundation, May 23, 1925: "I am grieved over Doctor Darling's death. Science and public health in particular has lost a valuable man."

9. Kligler, Haifa, to Russell, n.d.*: "Tragic death Darling his visit great[ly] stimulus have deeply felt irreplaceable."

10. Ernest Whitehead, Leesburg (Telegram), May 24, 1925.

11. M. E. Barnes, P. F. Russell, Singapore, to Mrs. Darling, May 25, 1925: "Please accept our . . . sympathy."

12. High Commissioner, Jerusalem, to I. H. B., n.d.: "Please convey to his relatives sincere sympathy of Palestine Government and myself."

13. E. Walch, Amsterdam, to Russell, May 26, 1925: "You know what he has been to us: a faithful guide and a dear friend, in every sense of the world. How we admired him when he was talking of his ideals!"
14. Clayton Lary [?*] to Russell, May 26, 1925.
15. T. H. D. Griffits [?], Epidemiologist, Public Health Service, Montgomery, Alabama, May 26, 1925.
16. Prof. Dr. W. Schüffner and J. J. van Loghem, Tropical Institute, Amsterdam, to Russell, May 27, 1925.
17. Henry Beewkes [?] to F. F. Russell, May 27, 1925.
18. Dr. Stingily [?], Jackson Infirmary, Miss., to Russell, May 29, 1925.

June 1–15, 1925[2]

19. S. P. James, Ministry of Health, Whitehall, to Russell, June 1, 1925: "Condolences left with Professor Hechtday [?sp] at accident. Knew Darling since 1912 in Canal Zone."
20. George K. Strade, Rio de Janeiro, Conselho Sanitario Internacional, to F. F. Russell, June 5, 1925.
21. Mark F. Boyd, Rio de Janeiro, June 6, 1925.
22. Lambert, São Paulo, to Mrs. Darling, June 8, 1925.
23. Souza to I. H. B., n.d.
24. Dias to Rockefeller Foundation, n.d.: "Professors and medical faculty condolences."
25. Dr. Edward Escomel, Peru, n.d.
26. Dr. Émil Brumpt to Russell, June 11, 1925.
27. Prof. Donato Ottolenghi, Bologna, June 13, 1925.

June 16–30, 1925[3]

28. Herbert C. Clark, Tela Railroad Co., Honduras, June 22, 1925.
29. Madsen, Health Commission, League of Nations, to Russell, June 23, 1925.
30. Lewis B. Bates, Ancon, Canal Zone, to C. C. W., June 27, 1925.

July 1925[4]

31. J. Juan Lonkhuijzcn, Chief Medical Services, Netherland East Indies, n.d.
32. Societa de Biologia et Hygiene to F. F. Russell, n.d.
33. Dr. Bastiandelli, International Congress Malaria in Rome, July 14, 1925.

*n.d. (no date given); [?] spelling/handwriting not clear.

Appendix H
Societies, Honors, and Commemoratives

APPENDIX H.1 — **Membership in Societies and Honors** [1-3]

American College of Physicians (fellow)
American Helminthological Society
American Medical Association
American Society of Museum Curators
American Society of Tropical Medicine (president in 1924)
Canal Zone Medical Association (president in 1908 and chairman of Executive Committee)
Helminthological Society
Sociedad de Medicina e Cirugia de São Paulo, Brazil
Société de Pathologie Exotique
Society of the Chagres (Canal Zone)
Society of Parasitologists (vice-president 1925)

Honorary Doctor of Science (Sc.D.) conferred by the University of Maryland in 1923.
Honorary Fellowship in the Royal Society of Tropical Medicine and Hygiene (this honor at the time had been given to only two other Americans: William Gorgas and Theobald Smith).

Commemoratives

"Samuel Taylor Darling 1872–1925." *International Health Board Bulletin* 1925; 6: 1–35.
"A Memorial Meeting for Dr. Samuel Taylor Darling." *International Health Board Bulletin* 1926; 6: 247–263.
League of Nations established a Darling Memorial Prize and Medal to be awarded periodically to outstanding contributors for achievements in the field of malaria (see Appendix H.2).
Gorgas (Ancon) Hospital Medical Library named "Samuel Taylor Darling Memorial Library" in 1972 (see Appendix H.3).

Liberty ship named in his honor: S.S. *Samuel T. Darling* (see Appendix H.4).
Three species named in his honor (see Appendixes H.5–H.7):

> *Anopheles darlingi*
> *Besnoitia darlingi*
> *Diplomys darlingi*

APPENDIX H.2 — Darling Medal and Prize, League of Nations and World Health Organization

A fund was established by the League of Nations to honor the memory of Samuel Taylor Darling following the tragic motor car accident near Beirut that took his life on April 1925.[1] Contributions to the Darling Memorial Fund were sought from friends and colleagues. On July 26, 1926, The International Health Board of the Rockefeller Foundation transmitted to Dr. Ludwik Rajchman, medical director of the Health Section of the Secretariat of the League of Nations, the sum of $1,086.77, "representing the contributions to the Darling Memorial Prize Fund of fourteen officers of the Rockefeller Foundation and its boards, forty-five members of the Board's field staff, and the following friends of Dr. Darling outside the staff: Dr. Lewis B. Bates, chief of laboratories, Board of Health Laboratories, Ancon, Canal Zone; Judge Frank Feuille; Dr. Herbert C. Clark; Dr. W. E. Deeks; Dr. Roland C. Connor, of the United Fruit Company; and Dr. R. W. Hegner, of the Johns Hopkins School of Hygiene and Public Health."[1]

At the Sixth Session of the Health Committee of the League of Nations, held from April 26 to May 1, 1926, the following details were given about the Darling Memorial Prize:

> It is probable that the total contributions to the Darling Memorial Prize will be somewhere in the neighborhood of 11,000 Swiss francs. Such a sum would be sufficient for the biennial award of a medal in bronze and a prize approximating 1,000 Swiss francs.
>
> The medal might suitably be 2 1/4 inches in diameter, bearing on one side the protrait and name of Dr. Darling — with the years of birth and death — and around the margin, "The Darling Prize: Prix Darling"; and on the reverse, around the margin, "League of Nations-Health Organization," in French and English, and in the center, "For distinguished Malaria Research," and the name of the prize-winner and the year of the award.[1]

As a result, the Darling Foundation was created on November 1, 1929, through private subscription by the League of Nations and a starting capital of 10,076 Swiss francs.[2,3] The purpose of the foundation was to award the Darling prize, consisting of a bronze medal and a fixed sum of 1,000 Swiss francs, to an outstanding contributor for achievements in the pathology, etiology, epidemiology, therapy, prophylaxis or control of malaria.[3,4]

The administration of the Darling award was transferred from the League of Nations to the United Nations in June 1947, and again in September 1948, to the World Health Organization (WHO).[3] According to the present governance of the foundation, the fixed sum consists of 2,500 CHF to be awarded, along with the medal, at a special ceremony during the World Health assembly.[4]

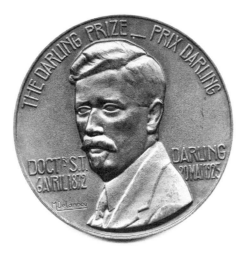

Darling Prize Medal. Reproduced with permission, courtesy of Professor H. M. Gilles, Liverpool School of Tropical Medicine, Liverpool, United Kingdom.

The administrator of the foundation ascertains every six months from the trustee of the foundation funds when the interest accumulated is sufficient for the award (after deducting the cost of striking the medal) and invites member states and associate members of the organization, members of the WHO Expert Committee on Malaria, to nominate within six months the name of any person who qualifies for the award. The Expert Committee on Malaria evaluates the candidates and recommends to the Darling Foundation Committee its selection and this, in turn, to the Executive Board, who designates the recipient(s) of the prize.[4]

To date, 28 persons from 12 countries have been honored as recipients of the Darling Medal and Prize.[4]

Table H.8 Darling Medal and Prize Recipients (1932–1999)[4]

Year	Recipient	Country
1932	Col. S. P. James	United Kingdom
1936	Prof. N. H. Swellengrebel	Netherlands
1951	Prof. H. E. Shortt	United Kingdom
1951	Dr. P. C. C. Garnham	United Kingdom
1954	Dr. G. Robert Coatney	USA
1954	Prof. George Macdonald	United Kingdom
1957	Dr. P. F. Russell	USA

1959	Dr. E. J. Pampana	Italy
1960	Sir Gordon Covell	United Kingdom
1960	Dr. Arnoldo Gabaldón	Venezuela
1963	Dr. Martin D. Young	USA
1964	Col. M. K. Afridi	Pakistan
1966	Prof. M. Ciuca	Romania
1966	Prof. P. G. Sergiev	USSR
1968	Dr. G. Giglioli	Italy
1968	Dr. Jaswant Singh	India
1971	Prof. L. J. Bruce-Chwatt	United Kingdom
1971	Prof. A. Corradetti	Italy
1974	Dr. I. A. McGregor	United Kingdom
1974	Dr. Amar Prasad Ray	India
1980	Dr. M. A. Farid	Egypt
	Dr. W. Trager	USA
1986	Prof. R. H. Black	Australia
1986	Prof. D. F. Clyde	USA
1990	Prof. H. M. Gilles	United Kingdom
1990	Dr. S. Pattanayak	India
1999	Dr. Agostinho Cruz Marques	Brazil
1999	Dr. Vinod Prakash Sharma	India

APPENDIX H.3 — Samuel T. Darling Collection, Johns Hopkins School of Hygiene and Public Health, Baltimore, Maryland

A memorial meeting was held on January 17, 1926, at the Johns Hopkins School of Hygiene and Public Health honoring Darling.[1] Mrs. Darling took the opportunity to contribute her husband's two-hundred books and several thousand pamphlets and periodicals to the library of the Johns Hopkins School of Hygiene and Public Health.[2] This collection was set up initially as the "Samuel Taylor Darling Library."[3] Upon the retirement of Dr. W. W. Cort, a memorial library was set up in his name and the Darling collection was incorporated into it.[4] Dr. Gerald Baum searched in 1956 and found only a handful of books and pamphlets, including a 1912 edition of *Trypanosomes et trypanosomiasis* (signed by A. Laveran to his colleague S. Darling), plus reprints of Darling's work inscribed with his name and initials.[4] These apparently were removed with the renovation of the reading room and a search for them in 1987 failed to identify any of the original items.[5]

Samuel Taylor Darling Memorial Library
Gorgas Hospital, Canal Zone

The Gorgas Hospital medical library was dedicated as the "Samuel Taylor Darling Memorial Library" in a ceremony convened at 10:30 a.m., on October 27, 1972, in Ancon, Canal Zone.[6] A bronze plaque was unveiled, with the inscription:

SAMUEL TAYLOR DARLING
MEMORIAL LIBRARY
IN RECOGNITION OF HIS CONTRIBUTIONS
TO MEDICAL KNOWLEDGE
CHIEF OF LABORATORIES — ANCON HOSPITAL 1905–1915
PHYSICIAN, PATHOLOGIST AND PARASITOLOGIST
1872–1925

The ceremony was attended by two of Darling's close relatives: a sister, Ruth Darling Mannhardt, and a son, Dashwood Peyton Darling. Others attending the ceremony were Governor David S. Parker; Dr. William A. Boyson, Canal Zone Health Director; Dr. Robert W. Irvin, Jr., Gorgas Hospital Director; and guests from the Canal Zone and Panama.[6]

This act was the culmination of dogged efforts by the Gorgas Hospital medical librarian, Mrs. Virginia Ewing Stich, who was dedicated to preserving Darling's memory. The library contained several exhibits of Darling's contributions to tropical medicine, as well as a model of Ancon Hospital which Darling had commissioned for the Panama Canal Sanitary Exhibit at the 1915 San Francisco Panama-Pacific International Exposition to commemorate the completion of the Panama Canal. The model represented the old section "C" building erected by the French in 1881 and repaired by the Americans in 1907, and formerly known as the Nurses' Quarters. The building was located at the site where the Middle American Research Unit was later built.[7]

Due to the termination of services by the Gorgas Army Community Hospital in Ancon on October 1, 1997, and transfer of the hospital buildings to the Panama government jurisdiction, the Samuel Taylor Darling Memorial Library was transferred to Fort Sam Houston, Texas, for safeguarding of its valuable collection of documents and books.[8,9]

APPENDIX H.4 — Darling's Liberty Ship: S.S. *Samuel T. Darling*

The United States Maritime Commission authorized in 1941 the construction of Liberty ships to meet the demand for readily available means to transport troops, ammunition and war materiel during World War II.[1] The British idea, proposed before the United States entered the war, was conceived to replace as rapidly as possible the losses of the British Navy from torpedo attacks by German submarines.[2] These losses were staggering: during the first twelve months of the war, British shipping losses amounted to 385 ships or ten per cent of the total available at the start of the war.[2] The Germans were sinking ships three times as fast as British and Commonwealth yards could replace them.[3] It made sense to both Roosevelt and Churchill to utilize the American shipyards and abundant available manpower for mutual benefit. According to Admiral Land, when Roosevelt first saw the profile plans for the ship, he commented that, although she could carry a good load and would serve well, she wasn't much to look at — a real "ugly duckling."[4] This sobriquet became the ship's famous nickname.

The ships were built according to a standardized, mass-produced design provided and supervised initially by Cyril Thompson, head of the British

Shipbuilding Mission to the United States, and also known as the "Father of the Liberty ship."[5,6] The cost of building a Liberty vessel was a little less than $2 million.[7] The 250,00 component parts were pre-fabricated in 250-ton sections and welded together in about seventy days into a ship 441 feet long and 56 feet wide.[8] The result was a vessel powered by a three-cylinder, reciprocating steam engine capable of producing 2,500 horsepower and 11 knots.[8] One Liberty ship could carry 9,000 tons of cargo, including airplanes, tanks and locomotives, or 2,840 jeeps, 440 tanks or 230 million rounds of rifle ammunition.[8] A crew usually consisted of about 44 seamen and 12 to 25 Naval Armed Guard personnel.[8] A total of 2,571 Liberty ships were built and about 200 of these were lost during the war.[8] Because of their endowed ability to rapidly move troops and military cargo, these ships became an indispensable part of naval operations and were credited as "the ships that won the war."[9] The cost in human lives lost, however, was substantial: an estimated 8,300 U.S. Merchant Marine seamen died as a result of enemy action in World War II.[10]

Liberty ships were named after prominent deceased Americans, starting with Patrick Henry and the signers of the Declaration of Independence.[11] Any group that raised $2 million in War Bonds could suggest a name for a Liberty ship.[8] On November 1, 1943, Mrs. Samuel T. Darling wrote to Mr. Harry F. Byrd, senator from Virginia, suggesting that a Liberty ship be named for her late husband.[12] Senator Byrd forwarded this request to Admiral E. S. Land, chairman of the United States Maritime Commission, and on November 9, 1943, Admiral Land informed Senator Byrd that the Ship Naming Committee would be glad to assign the suggested name to one of the southern yards in the near future.[13] Mrs. Ernest du Pont, Jr., (Darling's daughter, Virginia) had the honor of sponsoring the ship.[14]

The S.S. *Samuel T. Darling* (type of vessel: EC2–S-C1; MC Hull No. 2433) was built at the Southeastern Shipbuilding Corporation in Savannah, Georgia.[15] Her keel was laid on November 26, 1943 and fifty-three days later she was launched on January 18, 1944.[15] According to the *Savannah Morning News*, Mrs. Ernest du Pont, Jr., " . . . smashed a beribboned bottle of champagne across the bow in traditional style."[16] Mrs. Samuel T. Darling was unable to attend due to a fractured ankle.[17] However, Dashwood Peyton Darling, Dr. Darling's son and an executive at W. R. Grace (Grace Line, Inc.), attended the ceremony in her place.[17] The vessel was allocated to the Grace Line on December 11, 1943, and delivered on January 31, 1944.[18]

APPENDIX H.5 — Darling's Mosquito: *Anopheles darlingi*

The original description of the mosquito *Anopheles darlingi* was made by Francis M. Root in 1926.[1] Root was a faculty member and in charge of the Department of Medical Entomology at the Johns Hopkins School of Hygiene and Public Health.[2,3] He was responsible for directing and organizing the work in medical entomology from the time the school was established there until his death.

Although Root's main object of interest was the dragon fly, he was involved in important studies about mosquitoes in Puerto Rico, West Indies, Central America, Venezuela, and Brazil.[2,3] In 1924 he published the results of an investigation of the mosquitoes in Lee County, Georgia, suggesting that he and

Darling probably collaborated in this area of mutual interest.[4] It is not surprising, therefore, that in 1926 Root honored the memory of his recently lost colleague by naming a new species of mosquitoes from Brazil as *Anopheles darlingi*.[1] A more detailed description of the larval and adult female forms of *Anopheles darlingi* was given by W. H. W. Komp, Senior Medical Entomologist of the U.S. Public Health Service, in *The Anopheline Mosquitoes of the Caribbean Region*.[5]

The importance of *Anopheles darlingi* in the transmission of malaria in regions of South America, such as Brazil and Peru, had been recognized since the 1930s. By the 1950s this species of mosquito was regarded as the most efficient indigenous malaria vector in north and northeastern Brazil.[6] Although reported to be eradicated in 1968, *Anopheles darlingi* reemerged in the 1990s and malaria incidence increased significantly since the 1970s in the Belem region of Brazil.[7] Deforestation was blamed for this phenomenon and it was estimated that for every one per cent in deforestation, the number of *Anopheles darlingi* was increased by eight per cent. The dominance of this species in deforested regions of the Amazon basin was explained by the fact that it thrives in open, sunlit ponds.[7,8]

Low-cost and effective vector repellents have been developed by Samuel Darling (Samuel Taylor Darling's grandson) in attempts to reduce the burden of malaria in regions of Central and South America.[9] A repellent derived from plant sources has proved to be highly effective (>98 per cent protection up to five hours after application) and affordable ($.07 cost per day for adults) against various malaria vectors, including *Anopheles darlingi*.[9] These studies are the result of a collaboration between the Puerta del Cielo Foundation and the London School of Hygiene and Tropical Medicine.[9]

Anopheles darlingi has emerged as a dominant species in malaria transmission in Brazil, Peru and Chile. Its name serves to remind us, almost a century later, of the seminal and lasting contributions Darling made in the field of malariology.

APPENDIX H.6 — *Besnoitia darlingi*

Darling reported in 1908, in the *Proceedings of the Canal Zone Medical Association*, and again the following year in the *Archives of Internal Medicine*, a case of a 20-year-old Barbadian who had fever, headache, and stiffness of the muscles and joints.[1,2] A muscle biopsy obtained from the right arm was found to have "hundreds of little oval vesicular bodies having a round nucleus at one end."[1,2] A second biopsy done ten days later showed "older amoebiform sporozoa" and a smaller number of parasites which appeared "elongated, sickle-shaped and nucleated, with eosin staining cytoplasm."[1,2] A third biopsy taken after the patient had recovered clinically failed to show any parasites.

Darling classified the parasite he found as belonging to the group *Sarcosporidia*, based on similarities with previously described cases.[3,4] However, important morphological differences led him to investigate the possibility that the parasite in question could undergo morphological changes when harbored by an unusual host. To test this concept, Darling devised experimental studies by feeding guinea pigs with rat muscle infected with *Sarcocystis muris*.[5,6] The results appeared to confirm his hypothesis, as he later found in two of the guinea pigs parasites similar to those he had seen in the Barbadian. Darling concluded that the parasite he had found represented an aberrant form of sarcosporidium developing in the muscle of an unusual host.[5,6]

Darling's interest in the morphological variation of this parasite was rekindled when he found it again occurring naturally in an opossum caught at the dairy of Ancon Hospital.[6] He decided this time to conduct inoculation experiments and injected a saline suspension of the parasite into the muscles of the hind legs of two guinea pigs. After waiting for a period of sixty days, he found in one of the guinea pigs a few small intramuscular sarcosporidia which corresponded in morphology to the ones found by him previously in the Barbadian patient and naturally in the opossum.[6] Darling designated this parasite as *Sarcocystis* sp. opossum.[6]

Darling's original contribution was recognized by Émil Brumpt, of the Faculty of Medicine in Paris and professor of the Faculty of Medicine in São Paulo, Brazil, who named the parasite *Sarcosporidia darlingi* in the second edition of his authoritative *Précis de Parasitologie* published in 1913.[7] Along with fifteen other species of the genus *Sarcocystis*, Brumpt described the new species as: "Discovered by Darling in Panama in an opossum (*Didelphis*). It is found within striated muscles, cardiac fibers, smooth muscles, connective tissue of various organs. The parasitic cysts may reach 1.5 to 2 mm. The sporozoites measure 8 to 12 m by 2 to 4 m."[7] Nevertheless, the exact classification of this parasite remained in doubt and others thought that it could belong to the genus *Toxoplasma*.[8]

Mandour, of the London School of Hygiene and Tropical Medicine, compared the morphology of various species of *Sarcocystis* found in marsupials in South America.[9] He studied the descriptions, drawings and photomicrographs given by Darling and, based on the structure of the cyst wall (particularly the absence of the characteristic spines), concluded that the parasite Darling had described probably belonged to the genus *Besnoitia* rather than to *Sarcocystis*.[9]

Previous confusion about the taxonomy of this organism can be partly explained by the limited resolution of the monocular microscope that Darling used in his work. Perhaps one should be more impressed by what Darling was able to see than what he missed in his detailed descriptions of *Besnoitia darlingi*. Correct classification of these parasites may require not only accurate descriptions of their morphology, but knowledge about their distribution in muscle and other tissues of each animal studied, as well as elucidation of their complete life cycle. Almost seventy years after Darling's initial description, Smith and Frenkel established that cats served as definitive hosts and opossums as intermediate hosts for *Besnoitia darlingi*.[10,11] More recently, Dubey and his colleagues applied modern techniques such as cell culture propagation, ultrastructural examinations, and nuclear ribosomal DNA studies to differentiate among different species of *Toxoplasma*, *Sarcosporidia* and *Besnoitia*, substantiating the complexity of these coccidian parasites and the difficulties encountered in their correct classification.[12]

APPENDIX H.7 — Darling's Spiny Rat: *Diplomys darlingi*

This species of arboreal rat was first obtained by Darling at Ancon, Panama.[1] No member of the genus had previously been collected on the Panama mainland, although an insular form described as *Loncheres labilis* Bangs had been discovered on San Miguel Island in the Bay of Panama. The new species was named after

Darling by Goldman.[1] Although ascribed initially to the genus *Isothrix*, Darling's spiny rat was subsequently assigned to the genus *Diplomys*.[2] The spiny rats of the genus *Diplomys* are distinguishable from those of the other genera occurring in Panama by the short and conspicuously tufted ears and the blackish hairs projecting about half an inch beyond the margins. The face is marked by narrow vertical stripes at the posterior base of the whiskers. The dorsal pledge is bristly, but softer than in *Hoplomys* and *Proechimys*.[2]

The *Diplomys labilis* is known locally (San Miguel Island) as *ratón marinero* (marine rat).

During ecological studies of vesicular stomatitis virus in Panama, a team from the Middle America Research Unit (MARU), National Institute of Allergy and Infectious Diseases, National Institutes of Health, collected seventy-four specimens of *Diplomys darlingi* among more than a thousand arboreal and terrestrial mammals obtained from El Aguacate, a small, isolated rural community in central Panama.[3] All specimens were collected from tree holes, usually at some distance above the ground, and in trees located near streams. This arboreal rat is strictly nocturnal and in captivity demonstrated aggressive behavior and a high-pitched whine when disturbed. Weight varied between 55 and 492 g. Minimum gestation was estimated at fifty-five days and the young were relatively well developed at birth. Few specimens of *Diplomys darlingi* have been collected due to its arboreal and nocturnal habits.[3]

Notes

Darling's Quotation (page ii)

Darling to Florence Read (assistant secretary), November 4, 1922, folder 151, series 305L, Record Group (RG) 1.1, Rockefeller Foundation (RF), Rockefeller Archive Center (RAC), Sleepy Hollow, New York.

Preface

1. "Construction Days. Ancon Hospital. 1904–1914." *The Panama Canal Review* (Diamond Jubilee Supplement), November 1, 1957, pp. 7–11.
2. Secretary of the Isthmian Canal Commission to Darling, February 8, 1905, Personnel Bureau Files, Panama Canal Company (PCC), Ancon, Canal Zone.
3. Campbell to Stich, June 11, 1968, Virginia E. Stich personal correspondence, Samuel T. Darling Memorial Library (STDL), Gorgas Hospital, Ancon, Canal Zone.
4. "Gorgas Library Dedicated in Honor of Dr. Darling." *The Panama Canal Spillway,* November 17, 1972.
5. Baum GL. *Samuel Taylor Darling.* Cincinnati: Private edition, 1958.
6. Takos to Stich, January 28, 1957, Virginia E. Stich personal correspondence. (STDL)
7. Chaves-Carballo E. Samuel T. Darling and human sarcosporidiosis or toxoplasmosis in Panama. *Journal of the American Medical Association* 1970; 211: 1687–1689.
8. Chaves-Carballo E. Samuel T. Darling: Studies on malaria and the Panama Canal. *Bulletin of the History of Medicine* 1980; 54: 95–100.
9. Chaves-Carballo E. Ancon Hospital: An American hospital during the construction of the Panama Canal, 1904–1914. *Military Medicine* 1999; 164: 725–730.
10. Chaves Carballo E. Las contribuciones de Samuel Darling para la salubridad de Panamá durante la construcción del canal y una bibliografía completa de su obra científica [The contributions of Samuel Darling to the sanitation of Panama during the construction of the canal and a complete bibliography of his scientific works]. *Revista Cultural La Lotería* (Panama) 2001; (No. 436, May/June): 89–107.

11. Chaves Carballo E. El hospital de Ancón durante la construcción del canal [Ancon Hospital during the construction of the canal]. *Revista Cultural La Lotería* (Panama) 2001; (No. 437, July/August): 62–77.
12. Balfour AC. Some British and American pioneers in tropical medicine and hygiene. *Transactions of the Royal Society of Tropical Medicine and Hygiene* 1925; 19: 189–231.

Chronology

1. Baum, Gerald L. *Samuel Taylor Darling.* Cincinnati: Private edition, 1958.
2. "Darling, Samuel Taylor, Movements." S. T. Darling File, Secretary's Office, Record Group 15, Rockefeller Foundation (RF), Rockefeller Archives Center (RAC), Sleepy Hollow, New York.

Prologue: Aboard the *Cristobal*

1. Collins JO. "The Year 1914 in Canal History." *Society of the Chagres Year Book 1914.* Balboa Heights, Canal Zone: John O. Collins, Publisher, 1914, pp. 77–79.
2. "Steamship 'Cristobal' Makes Test Trip Between Entrance Channels." *Canal Record*, Vol. VII, No. 50 (August 5, 1914), p. 493.
3. "Official Trip of the 'Ancon.'" *Canal Record*, August 19, 1914, Vol VII, No. 52, p. 521.
4. The estimated combined cost of the French and American efforts to construct the Panama Canal is based on the following figures: French expenditures (1881–1889) $287 million (Mack, G. *The Land Divided: A History of the Panama Canal and Other Isthmian Canal Projects.* New York: Alfred A. Knopf, 1944, p. 355); American expenditures: $333 million ["Classified Expenditures – The Panama Canal," *Canal Record*, vol VIII, No. 6 (September 30, 1914), p. 54], including $7 million for canal fortifications; added to these totals are $40 million paid to the French for equipment and buildings and $10 million paid to Panama, for a total of $383 million. The combined total for French ($287 million) and American ($383) expenditures is $670 million. This sum is multiplied by 19.5 [Consumer Price Index average in 2005 (195.3) and in 1914 (10.0), from Bureau of Labor Statistics, U.S. Department of Labor] to convert to $13.1 billion in present day dollars.
5. The estimated losses in human lives are derived from Gorgas' review of French hospital records showing 22,189 deaths (Gorgas WC. Sanitation in Panama. *J Am Med Assoc* 1912; 58: 908) and during the American construction period of 6,630 men (Gorgas WC. *Sanitation in Panama.* New York: D. Appleton and Company, 1915, p. 283), for a combined total of 28,819 deaths. This is surely an underestimate since many sick employees died outside hospitals and were unaccounted for.
6. The length of the Panama Canal is about forty miles from shore-line to shore-line and about fifty miles from deep-water in the Atlantic Ocean to deep-water in the Pacific Ocean (Bishop JB. *The Panama Gateway.* New York: Charles Scribner's Sons, 1913, pp. 351–354). The latter figure of fifty miles (eighty kilometers) is commonly used as the official length of the canal. The narrowest part of the isthmus is approximately 35 miles wide.

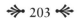

7. Acosta J. *Natural and Moral History of the Indies.* (Edited by Jane E. Mangan and translated by James M. López-Morillas.) Durham, North Carolina: Duke University Press, 2002, p. 124.

8. Gorgas WC. *Sanitation in Panama.* New York: D. Appleton and Company, 1915, p. 227.

9. Chaves-Carballo E. Carlos Finlay and yellow fever: Triumph over adversity. *Military Medicine* 2005: 187: 881–885.

10. Reed W, Carroll J, Agramonte A. The etiology of yellow fever: An additional note. *Journal of the American Medical Association* 1901; 36: 431–440. Reprinted in *Military Medicine* 2001; 166 (Suppl 1): 44–53.

11. Mack G. *The Land Divided. A History of the Panama Canal and other Isthmian Canal Projects.* New York: Octagon Books, 1974, p. 355.

12. Chamberlain WP. *Twenty-five Years of American Medical Activity on the Isthmus of Panama: A Triumph of Preventive Medicine.* Mt. Hope, Canal Zone: Panama Canal Press, 1929, p. 8.

13. Simmons JS. *Malaria in Panama.* Baltimore: The Johns Hopkins Press, 1939, p. 67.

14. "Gorgas Hospital Autopsies and Pathology Reports, 1900–1970's." Otis Historical Archives, National Museum of Health and Medicine, Armed Forces Institute of Pathology, Walter Reed Army Medical Center, Washington, D.C. (OHA)

15. Clark HC. A chart presenting the incidence of the more common causes of death on the Panama Canal Zone as found at autopsy during the years 1904 to 1916, inclusive. *Proceedings of the Medical Association of the Isthmian Canal Zone* 1917; X (Part 2): 20–23.

16. Chaves-Carballo E. Samuel T. Darling: Studies on malaria and the Panama Canal. *Bulletin of the History of Medicine* 1980; 54: 95–100.

17. Darling ST. *Studies in Relation to Malaria.* Mt. Hope, Canal Zone: Panama Canal Press, 1910. Also published by the U.S. Government Printing Office in 1910.

18. Baum GL. *Samuel Taylor Darling,* Cincinnati: Private edition, 1958, p. 14.

19. Murphy to Darling, February 1, 1905, Personnel Bureau Files, Panama Canal Company, Ancon, Canal Zone. (PCC)

20. Daniel TM, Baum GL. *Drama and Discovery. The Story of Histoplasmosis.* (Contributions in Medical Studies, No. 48) Westport, Connecticut: Greenwood Press, 2002, pp. 21–24.

21. Darling ST. Protozoön general infection producing pseudo-tubercles in lungs and local necrosis in liver, spleen, and lymph nodes. *Journal of the American Medical Association* 1906; 46: 1283–1285.

22. "Message of Congratulations from the Secretary of War." *Canal Record,* Vol. VII, No. 52 (August 19, 1914), p. 521.

23. "Executive Order to Create a Committee to Formally and Officially Open the Panama Canal." *Canal Record,* Vol. VII, No. 41 (June 3, 1914), p. 399.

24. MCullough D. *The Path Between the Seas. The Creation of the Panama Canal 1870–1914.* New York: Simon & Schuster, 1977, p. 608.

25. "No Gratuity Pay for Time off Account of Trip Through Canal." *Canal Record,* Vol. VII, No. 51 (August 12, 1914), p. 518.

26. Darling to Florence Read (assistant secretary), November 4, 1922, folder

151, series 305L, Record Group (RG) 1.1, Rockefeller Foundation (RF), Rockefeller Archive Center (RAC), Sleepy Hollow, New York.

1 Scottish Ancestry

1. Baum GL. *Samuel Taylor Darling.* Cincinnati: Private edition, 1958, p. 5.
2. Mannhardt, Ruth Darling. Interview with the author on September 12, 1987, in Cromwell, Connecticut.
3. Peabody JB. *The Founding Fathers: John Adams. A Biography in His Own Words.* (Vol. 1) New York: Newsweek, 1973, p. 65.
4. Ferling J. *John Adams. A Life.* New York: Henry Holt and Co., 1992, pp. 9–11.
5. Sprague WC. *The President John Adams and President John Quincy Birthplaces, Quincy, Massachusetts.* Quincy: Quincy Historical Society, 1959 (reprinted 1964), p. 14.
6. Edwards WC, Coates FA. *Third Centennial Celebration of the Incorporation of the Ancient Town of Braintree 1640–1940.* Quincy: First Parish Church, 1940, (no pagination given).
7. Daniel TL, Baum GL. *Drama and Discovery. The Story of Histoplasmosis.* (Contributions in Medical Studies, No. 48) Westport, Connecticut: Greenwood Press, 2002, pp. 24–25.
8. College of Physicians and Surgeons, Baltimore, Maryland. *Annual Announcement and Catalogue 1899–1900. 28th Annual Session.* Baltimore: The Sun Book and Job Printing Office, 1899. Historical/Special Collections of the Health Sciences and Human Services Library, University of Maryland, Baltimore. (UMHL)

2 New Century

1. The Cocksure Era. *1900–1910.* This Fabulous Century Series. (Vol. 1) Brown E. (ed.). New York: Time-Life Books, 1969, p. 29.
2. *The 1902 Edition of The Sears, Roebuck Catalogue.* (Facsimile) New York: Bounty Books, Crown Publishers, 1969, p. 2.
3. *Sears Catalogue,* p. 165.
4. *Sears Catalogue,* p. 203.
5. *Sears Catalogue,* p. 276.
6. *Sears Catalogue,* p. 339.
7. *Sears Catalogue,* p. 367.
8. *Sears Catalogue,* p. 321.
9. *Sears Catalogue,* p. 260.
10. *Sears Catalogue,* p. 245.
11. *Sears Catalogue,* pp. 440–468.
12. *Sears Catalogue,* p. 446.
13. Pringle HF. *Theodore Roosevelt. A Biography.* New York: Harcourt, Brace and Company, 1931, pp. 428–429.
14. Lord W. The Wright Brothers' Incredible Flying Machine. In *The 1900s.* Immell MH (ed.). San Diego: Greenwood Press, 2000, pp. 165–177.
15. The Automobiling Fad. *1900–1910.* This Fabulous Century Series. (Vol. 1) Brown E (ed.). New York: Time-Life Books, 1969, p. 228.

16. Holbrook SH. Henry Ford and his Motorcar for the Masses. In *The 1900s*. Immell MH (ed.). San Diego: Greenwood Press, 2000, pp. 178–184.
17. Woog A. *The 1900s*. Through the Decades. A Cultural History of the United States. San Diego: Lucent Books, Inc., 1999, p. 83.
18. The American Colossus. *1900–1910*. This Fabulous Century Series. (Vol. 1) Brown E. (ed.). New York: Time-Life Books, 1969, pp. 61–62.

3 College of Physicians and Surgeons of Baltimore

1. College of Physicians and Surgeons, Baltimore, Maryland: *Annual Announcement and Catalogue. 1899–1900. 28th Annual Session*. Baltimore: The Sun Book and Job Printing Office, 1899. Historical/Special Collections of the Health Sciences and Human Services Library, University of Maryland, Baltimore. (UMHL)
2. Freidenwald E. Student Days at the College of Physicians and Surgeons. A Memorial Meeting for Dr. Samuel Taylor Darling. *International Health Board Bulletin* 1926; 6: 247–250.
3. Baum GL. *Samuel Taylor Darling*. Cincinnati: Private edition, 1958, pp. 6, 14.
4. College of Physicians and Surgeons of Baltimore, Matriculation records and class lists 1882–1912. Historical /Special Collections of the Health Sciences and Human Services Library, University of Maryland, Baltimore, p. 153. (UMHL)
5. Merck & Co. *Merck's 1899 Manual of Materia Medica*. (Facsimile of 1899 edition.) New York, 1999.
6. *The Pharmacopoeia of the United States*. 7th decennial revision (1890). Philadelphia: J. B. Lippincott Co., 1893.
7. American Pharmaceutical Association. *The National Formulary of Unofficial Preparations*. (3rd ed.) Baltimore, Maryland, 1906.
8. Flexner A. *Medical Education in the United States and Canada. A Report to the Carnegie Foundation for the Advancement of Teaching*. Boston: D. B. Updyke, The Merrymount Press, 1910, pp. 235–236.
9. Bernheim BM. *The Story of The Johns Hopkins*. New York: McGraw-Hill Book Co., Inc., 1948.
10. Cordell EF. *Historical Sketch of the University of Maryland School of Medicine (1807–1890)*. Baltimore: Press of Isaac Friedenwald, 1891, p. 158.
11. College, Matriculation records, p. 181. (UMHL)
12. *College of Physicians and Surgeons of Baltimore 1905–6*. (Annual announcement and catalogue; no date, place, or publisher given.) (UMHL)
13. Abrahams HJ. *The Extinct Medical Schools of Baltimore, Maryland*. Baltimore: Maryland Historical Society, 1969, pp. 71–72.
14. Abrahams, *Extinct Medical Schools*, p. 37.
15. College of Physicians and Surgeons, Baltimore, MD. *Annual Announcement and Catalogue. 1900–1901. 29th Annual Session*. Baltimore: The Sun Printing Office, 1900. (UMHL)
16. Cullen TS. *Early Medicine in Maryland*. (Address of the President of the Medical and Chirurgical Faculty of Maryland, delivered at the Faculty Building, 1211 Cathedral St., April 26, 1927.) 1927, 15 pp.

17. Ballard MA. *A University is Born.* (Appendix VII. College of Physicians and Surgeons of Baltimore.) Old Hundred Union, West Virginia, 1965, pp. 270–280.

18. Cordell EF. *The Medical Annals of Maryland (1799–1899).* Baltimore: Williams & Wilkins Co., 1903, pp. 464–465.

19. College of Physicians and Surgeons of Baltimore. *31st Annual Announcement. Session of 1902–1903.* Baltimore, 1902. (UMHL)

20. "Dr. N. G. Keirle Dead." The *Baltimore Sun*, n.d. (newspaper clipping). (UMHL)

21. College of Physicians and Surgeons of Baltimore: *31st Annual Commencement. Thursday, April Thirtieth, 1903.* (No place or publisher given.)

22. College of Physicians and Surgeons of Baltimore. *32nd Annual Announcement. Session of 1903–1904.* (No place, date, or publisher given.) (UMHL)

23. College of Physicians and Surgeons of Baltimore. (Annual Announcement.) Baltimore: Press of Guggenheim, Weil & Co., 1904. (UMHL)

24. Chaves-Carballo E. Samuel T. Darling: Studies on malaria and the Panama Canal. *Bulletin of the History of Medicine* 1980; 54: 95–100.

25. Fleming D. *William H. Welch and the Rise of Modern Medicine.* Baltimore: The Johns Hopkins University Press, 1987.

26. Flexner S, Flexner JT. *William Henry Welch and the Heroic Age of American Medicine.* New York: Dover Publications, Inc., 1941.

27. Ludmerer KM. *Learning to Heal. The Development of American Medical Education.* New York: Basic Books, Inc., Publishers, 1985, pp. 57–63.

28. Fleming, *Welch*, p. 20.

29. Fleming, *Welch*, p. 28.

30. Fleming, *Welch*, pp. 33–34.

31. Fleming, *Welch*, p. 56.

32. Fleming, *Welch*, p. 59.

33. Fleming, *Welch*, p. 67.

34. Fleming, *Welch*, p. 34.

35. "Twenty-four blocks burned in heart of Baltimore." The *Baltimore Sun*, February 8, 1904 (extra edition), front page.

36. College of Physicians and Surgeons of Baltimore: *Yearbook 1907.* (UMHL)

37. The *Baltimore Sun*, February 13, 1905.

38. Abbott HL. *Problems of the Panama Canal; including climatology of the isthmus, physics and hydraulics of the river Chagres cut at the continental divide, and discussion of plans for the waterway, with history from 1870 to date.* New York: Macmillan, 1907, p. 77.

39. Abbott, *Problems*, p. 98.

40. "Panama bill passed." The *Baltimore Sun*, February 17, 1905.

4   Isthmian Explorations

1. Marco Polo. *The Travels (Description of the World).* Köln, Germany: Könemann, 1996, p. 239.

2. Mack G. *The Land Divided. A History of the Panama Canal and other Isthmian Canal Projects.* New York: Octagon Books, 1974, pp. 3–17.

3. Morison SE. *Admiral of the Ocean Sea. A Life of Christopher Columbus.* Boston: Little Brown and Co., 1942, pp. 586–589.

4. Morison, *Admiral*, pp. 596–601.

5. Morison, *Admiral*, p. 580.

6. Voltes P. *Colon.* Barcelona: Salvat Editores, 1986, pp. 137–142.

7. Winsor J. *Christopher Columbus and How He Received and Imparted the Spirit of Discovery.* Boston: Houghton, Mifflin and Co., 1891.

8. Mack, *Land Divided*, pp. 18–26.

9. Bishop JB. *The Panama Gateway.* New York: Charles Scribner's Sons, 1913, pp. 27–29.

10. Mack, *Land Divided*, pp. 27–39.

11. Mack, *Land Divided*, pp. 40–47.

12. Acosta J de. *Natural and Moral History of the Indies.* (Edited by Jane E. Mangam and translated by Frances M. López-Morillas.) Durham, North Carolina: Duke University Press, 2002, p. 124.

13. Gorgas WC. *Sanitation in Panama*, New York: D. Appleton and Company, 1915, p.135.

14. Mack, *Land Divided*, pp. 71–77.

15. Otis FN. *Illustrated History of the Panama Railroad; together with a Traveler's Guide and Business Man's Hand-book for the Panama Railroad and its Connections with Europe, the United States, the North and South Atlantic and Pacific Coasts, China, Australia, and Japan, by Sail and Steam.* (2nd ed.) New York: Harper & Brothers, Publishers, 1862, pp. 31–36.

16. Castillero EJ. *Historia de Panama [History of Panama].* (10th ed.) Panama: (no publisher given), 1989, pp. 34–35.

17. "Panama. Tropical journeyings by Oran." *Harper's New Monthly Magazine.* Vol 19, No. 112 (September 1859), pp. 433–454.

18. Bishop, *Panama Gateway*, pp. 14–17.

19. Collins JO. *The Panama Guide.* Mount Hope, Canal Zone: I.C.C. Press, 1912, pp. 107–108.

20. Anderson CLG. *Old Panama and Castilla del Oro.* New York: North River Press, 1944, p.183.

21. Bishop, *Panama Gateway*, p. 7.

22. Castillero, *Historia*, p. 27.

23. Thomas H. *Rivers of Gold. The Rise of the Spanish Empire, from Columbus to Magellan.* New York: Random House Trade Paperbacks, 2005, p. 336.

24. Wood P. *The Spanish Main.* Alexandria, Virginia: Time-Life Books Inc., 1979, p 21

25. Mack, *Land Divided*, p. 69.

26. Réclus A. *Panama et Darien. Voyages d'Exploration [Panama and Darien. Voyages of Exploration].* Paris: Librairie Hachette et Cie., 1881.

27. Beatty C. *De Lesseps of Suez. The Man and his Times.* New York: Harper & Brothers, 1956.

28. Mack, *Land Divided*, pp. 287–297.

29. Mack, *Land Divided*, pp. 303–304.

30. "First Stroke of the Pick at Panama." (Reproduced from *Bulletin du Canal Interocéanique*, February 1, 1880.) *Canal Record*, Vol. I, No. 48 (July 29, 1908), p. 383.

31. Mcullough D. *The Path Between the Seas. The Creation of the Panama Canal 1870–1914*. New York: Simon and Schuster, 1977, p. 172.
32. Mack, *Land Divided*, p. 346.
33. Mack, *Land Divided*, pp. 480, 489.
34. Mack, *Land Divided*, p. 355.
35. Chamberlain WP. *Twenty-Five Years of American Medical Activity on the Isthmus of Panama: A Triumph of Preventive Medicine*. Mt. Hope, Canal Zone: Panama Canal Press, 1929, p. 8.

5 Lure of Panama

1. Richards A. "Retrospect of the Panama Canal. My Five Years in the Canal Zone." May, 1964, Personal Papers, Library of Congress, Washington, D.C. (LOC)
2. Medical News. *Journal of the American Medical Association*. December 17, 1904.
3. The *Panama-American*, February 5, 1905.
4. Isthmian Canal Commission. *Manual of Information Concerning Employments for Service on the Isthmus of Panama*. (Revised November 15, 1910.) Washington, D.C.: Government Printing Office, 1910, p. 27.
5. Secretary of the Isthmian Canal Commission to Welch, January 27, 1905, Personnel Bureau Files, Panama Canal Company, Ancon, Canal Zone. (PCC)
6. Welch to Murphy, February 1, 1905, Personnel Bureau Files, Panama Canal Company, Ancon, Canal Zone. (PCC)
7. Murphy to Darling, February 8, 1905, Personnel Bureau Files, Panama Canal Company, Ancon, Canal Zone. (PCC)
8. Darling to Murphy, February 12, 1905. Personnel Bureau Files, Panama Canal Company, Ancon, Canal Zone. (PCC)
9. Isthmian Canal Commission, *Manual,* p. 26.
10. The *Panama-American*, February 9, 1905.
11. Baum GL. *Samuel Taylor Darling*. Cincinnati: Private edition, 1958, pp. 8, 10.
12. Daniel TM, Baum GL. *Drama and Discovery. The Story of Histoplasmosis*. Westport, Connecticut: Greenwood Press, 2002, p. 26.
13. Meeting for Dr. Samuel Taylor Darling. *International Health Board Bulletin* 1926; 6: 250–257, p. 250.
14. Carter HR. A note on the interval between infecting and secondary cases of yellow fever from the records of the yellow fever at Orwood and Taylor, Mississippi in 1898. *New Orleans Medical and Surgical Journal* 1900; 52: 617–636. Reprinted in part in *Military Medicine* 2001; 166 (Suppl 1); 12–16.
15. Finlay CJ. El mosquito considerado hipotéticamente como agente transmisor de la fiebre amarilla [The mosquito hypothetically considered as the agent of transmission of yellow fever]. Read before the Royal Academy of Medical, Physical and Natural Sciences of Havana, session of August 14, 1881, Havana, Cuba. Translated by J. C. Finlay in *Finlay Obras Completas* (Vol. 1) pp. 263–276, Havana: Academia de Ciencias de Cuba, 1965. Reproduced in abridged form in *Military Medicine* 2001; 166 (Supplement 1): 6–10.
16. Reed W, Carroll J, Agramonte A, Lazear JW. The etiology of yellow fever –

a preliminary note. *Philadelphia Medical Journal* Oct 27, 1900. Reprinted in part in *Military Medicine* 2001; 166 (Suppl 1): 29–37.

17. Gorgas WC. *Sanitation in Panama*. New York: D. Appleton and Co., 1915, pp. 238–239.
18. Le Prince JA, Orenstein AJ. *Mosquito Control in Panama. The Eradication of Malaria and Yellow Fever in Cuba and Panama*. New York: G. P. Putnam's Sons, 1916.
19. "Panama Railroad Company. Time Table No. 19. Taking Effect April 1st, 1907." *Canal Record*, Vol. I, No. 3, (September 18, 1907), p. 23.
20. The *Baltimore Sun*, Monday, February 13, 1905.
21. Abbott HL. *Problems of the Panama Canal; including climatology of the isthmus, physics and hydraulics of the river Chagres cut at the continental divide, and discussion of plans for the waterway, with history from 1890 to date*. New York: Macmillan, 1907.
22. Otis FN. *Illustrated History of the Panama Railroad*. (2nd ed.) New York: Harper & Brothers, Publishers, 1862, pp. 75, 86–127.
23. Collins JO. *The Panama Canal Guide*. Mount Hope, Canal Zone: I.C.C. Press, 1912, p. 27.
24. Collins, *Guide*, p. 36.
25. "Early Days on the Isthmus." From an address by W. C. Haskins, of the Department of Material and Supplies, before his fellow-citizens, at Oelwein, Iowa, in July last. *Canal Record*, Vol. I, No. 2 (September 11, 1907), p. 15.
26. Scott WR. *The Americans in Panama*. New York: The Statler Publishing Company, p. 206.
27. Gorgas MD, Hendrick BJ. *William Crawford Gorgas. His Life and His Work*. Philadelphia, Lea & Febiger, 1924, pp. 155–157.
28. "Commission Hospital Service. Ancon Hospital. I." *Canal Record*, Vol. 1 No. 48 (July 29, 1908), p. 381.
29. Gorgas, *Sanitation*, pp. 228–229.

6 Ancon Hospital

1. Roosevelt T. *Message of the President of the United States Communicated to the Two Houses of Congress at the Beginning of the First Session of the Fifty-ninth Congress*. Washington, D.C.: Government Printing Office, 1905, p. 54.
2. Roosevelt to Taft, May 9, 1904, quoted by Martin, Thomas W. *Doctor William Crawford Gorgas of Alabama and the Panama Canal*. New York: The Newcomen Society of England, 1947, p. 21.
3. Gorgas WC. *Sanitation in Panama*. New York: D. Appleton and Company, 1915, p. 146.
4. Gorgas, *Sanitation*, p. 72.
5. "Solving the Mystery of Yellow Fever. The 1900 U.S. Army Yellow Fever Board." Pierce JR, Writer JV (eds.). *Military Medicine* 2001; 166 (Supplement 1): 1–82.
6. Isthmian Canal Commission. *The First Annual Report of the Isthmian Canal Commission*. Washington, D.C.: Government Printing Office, 1905, p. 49.
7. Gorgas, *Sanitation*, p. 224.
8. Réclus A. *Paname et Darien. Voyages of Exploration [Panama and Darien. Voyages of Exploration]*. Paris: Librairie Hachette et Cie., 1881, p. 26.

9. Boyland GH. The De Lesseps canal and its relation to hygiene. *The Practitioner* 1880; 1: 317–334.

10. Shiffert HO. The sanitary conditions and the diseases common to the isthmus of Panama. *Sanitarian* 1904; 52: 120–124.

11. Chaves-Carballo E. Carlos J. Finlay and yellow fever: Triumph over adversity. *Military Medicine* 2005; 170: 881–885.

12. Turney JJR. Panama or isthmus fever. *Boston Medical and Surgical Journal* 1851; 45: 361–364, p. 361.

13. Leigh JG. Sanitation and the Panama Canal. II. The solution of certain climatic and hygienic problems. *Lancet* 1905; 1 (June 10): 1597–1601, p. 1597.

14. "French Days. L'Hôpital Central du Panama 1882–1904." *The Panama Canal Review* (Diamond Jubilee Supplement), November 1, 1957, pp. 2–6.

15. Minton R, Muller S, Cohen G. Fifty years of American medicine on the isthmus of Panama. *American Journal of Tropical Medicine and Hygiene* 1954; 3: 951–963, p. 951.

16. Leigh JG. Sanitation and the Panama Canal. *Lancet* 1905; 1: 1726–1730, p. 1727.

17. Gorgas WC. Sanitation at Panama. *Journal of the American Medical Association* 1912; 58: 907–909, p. 908.

18. Ziperman HH. A medical history of the Panama Canal. *Surgery, Gynecology and Obstetrics* 1973; 137: 104–114.

19. Governor to Sister Marie Brezard, November 21, 1904, file 71–A-18, box 385, Record Group (RG) 185, Department of Sanitation, Commission Hospital Service, Ancon Hospital Records of the Panama Canal Commission. Second Isthmian Canal Commission. General Correspondence, 1905–1914. National Archives, College Park, Maryland. (NA II)

20. Sister Marie Brezard to Secretary of State Taft (translated from French), December 5, 1904, file 71–A-18, box 385, RG 185. (NA II)

21. Chaves-Carballo E. Ancon Hospital: An American hospital during the construction of the Panama Canal (1904–1914). *Military Medicine* 1999; 164: 725–730.

22. Gorgas WC. *Sanitation in Panama.* New York: D. Appleton and Company, 1915, pp. 219–223.

23. "Construction Days. Ancon Hospital 1904–1914." *The Panama Canal Review* (Diamond Jubilee Supplement), November 1, 1957, pp. 7–11.

24. "Commission Hospital Service. Ancon Hospital I." *Canal Record*, Vol. I, No. 48 (July 29, 1908), pp. 381–382.

25. "The Transformation. Ancon Into Gorgas 1914–1941." *The Panama Canal Review* (Diamond Jubilee Supplement), November 1, 1957, pp. 12–13.

26. "Commission Hospital Service. Ancon Hospital." (Typed manuscript, 9 pp.) File 71–A-18, box 385, Record Group (RG) 185. (NAII)

27. Gorgas WC. Sanitation at Panama. *Journal of the American Medical Association* 1912; 58: 907–909, p. 908.

28. Gorgas, *Sanitation*, p. 283.

29. Gorgas, *Sanitation*, p. 148.

30. Gorgas MD, Hendrick BJ. *William Crawford Gorgas. His Life and Work.* Philadelphia: Lea & Febiger, 1924, p. 222.

31. Martin TW. *Doctor William Crawford Gorgas of Alabama and the Panama Canal.* New York: The Newcomen Society of England (American Branch), 1947, pp. 23–24.
32. Gorgas, *Sanitation*, pp. 151–152.
33. Gillett MC. *The Army Medical Department 1865–1917.* Washington, D.C.: Center of Military History, United States Army, 1995, p. 266.
34. "The Sanitary Problem in Panama." *Journal of the American Medical Association* 1905; 45: 1065–1066.
35. Reed CAL. Isthmian Sanitation. The Panama Canal Mismanagement. Report to the Government by Dr. Charles A. L. Reed, Showing How the Commission Makes Efficient Sanitation Impossible. *Journal of the American Medical Association* 1905; 44: 812–818.
36. Gorgas, *Sanitation*, pp.154–155.
37. Gorgas MD, *Gorgas*, p. 201.
38. Mack G. *The Land Divided. A History of the Panama Canal and other Isthmian Canal Projects.* New York: Octagon Books, 1974, p. 155.
39. Gorgas MD, *Gorgas*, p. 187.
40. Carter HR. Notes on the sanitation of yellow fever and malaria, from isthmian experience. *Medical Record* (N.Y.) 1909; 76: 56–59, p. 58.
41. Simmons JS. *Malaria in Panama.* (The American Journal of Hygiene Monographic Series No. 13.) Baltimore: The Johns Hopkins Press, 1939, p. 121.
42. Rocco F. *Quinine. Malaria and the Quest for a Cure that Changed the World.* London: HarperCollins*Publishers* (Perennial), 2004, pp. 78–80.
43. Bishop JB. *The Panama Gateway.* New York: Charles Scribner's Sons, 1913, pp. 249–257.
44. Gorgas WC. The sanitary organization of the isthmian canal as it bears upon antimalarial work. *Military Surgeon* 1909; 24: 261–267.
45. Darling ST. *Studies in Relation to Malaria.* Mt. Hope, Canal Zone: Panama Canal Press, 1910, p. 22.
46. Le Prince JA, Orenstein AJ. *Mosquito Control in Panama. The Eradication of Malaria and Yellow Fever in Cuba and Panama.* New York: G. P. Putnam's Sons, 1916.

7 Board of Health Laboratories

1. Personnel Bureau Files, Panama Canal Company, Ancon, Canal Zone. (PCC)
2. Chaves-Carballo E. Samuel T. Darling: Studies on malaria and the Panama Canal. *Bulletin of the History of Medicine* 1980; 54: 95–100.
3. Gorgas WC. *Report of the Chief Sanitary Officer of the Canal Zone.* February 20, 1905. Washington, D.C.: U.S. Government Printing Office, 1905, pp. 8–9.
4. Clark HC. "Laboratory Development on the Isthmus of Panama. January 11, 1936." (Typed manuscript, 8 pp.) Otis Historical Archives, National Museum of Health and Medicine, Armed Forces Institute of Pathology, Walter Reed Army Medical Center, Washington, D.C. (OHA)
5. Kean BH. *M.D. One Doctor's Adventures Among the Famous and the Infamous from the Jungles of Panama to a Park Avenue Practice.* New York: Ballantine Books, 1990, pp. 81, 295.

6. "Commission Hospital Service. Ancon Hospital." (Typed manuscript, 9 pp.) File 71–A-18, box 385, Record Group 185, Records of the Panama Canal, Second Isthmian Canal Commission, General Correspondence (1905–1914), National Archives II, College Park, Maryland. (NA II)

7. Russell FF. Darling's Work in Panama and in the United States. *International Health Board Bulletin* 1926; 6: 250–257.

8. Gorgas WC. *Sanitation in Panama.* New York: D. Appleton and Company, 1915, pp. 238–239.

9. Watson M. *Rural Sanitation in the Tropics: Being Notes and Observations in the Malay Archipelago, Panama and Other Lands.* New York: E. P. Dutton & Co., 1915, p. 225.

10. Mears JE. The Triumph of American Medicine in the Construction of the Panama Canal. *Medical Record* (N.Y.) 1911: 80: 409–417.

11. Gorgas WC. *Annual Report of the Department of Sanitation of the Isthmian Canal Commission for the Year 1907.* Washington, D.C.: U.S. Government Printing Office, 1908.

12. Baum GL. *Samuel Taylor Darling.* Cincinnati: Private edition, 1958, p. 6.

13. Clark HC. Samuel Taylor Darling. *International Board of Health Bulletin* 1925; 6: 10–11.

14. Baum, *Darling*, p. 10.

15. Darling ST. The morphology of the parasite (*Histoplasma capsulatum*) and the lesions of histoplasmosis, a fatal disease of tropical America. *Journal of Experimental Medicine* 1909; 11: 515–531, pp. 515–516.

16. Darling ST. Histoplasmosis: A fatal infectious disease resembling kala-azar found among natives of tropical America. *Archives of Internal Medicine* 1908; 2:107–123, pp. 110–117.

17. Darling ST. Notes on histoplasmosis — A fatal disorder met with in tropical America. *Maryland Medical Journal* 1907; 50: 125–129.

18. Lopez JF, Grocott RG. Demonstration of *Histoplasma capuslatum* in peripheral blood by the use of methamphetamine-silver nitrate stain (Grocott's). *American Journal of Clinical Pathology* 1968; 50: 692–694.

19. Gorgas WC. *Annual Report of the Department of Sanitation of the Isthmian Canal Commission for the Year 1907.* Washington, D.C.: U.S. Government Printing Office, 1908, p. 7.

20. Gorgas WC. *Annual Reports of the Department of Sanitation of the Isthmian Canal Commission for the Years 1906–1913.* Washington, D.C.: U.S. Government Printing Office, 1907–1914.

21. Gorgas WC. Malaria in the tropics. *Journal of the American Medical Association* 1906; 46: 1416–1417.

22. "Gorgas Hospital Autopsies and Pathology Reports, 1900–1970's." Otis Historical Archives, National Museum of Health and Medicine, Armed Forces Institute of Pathology, Walter Reed Army Medical Center, Washington, D.C. (OHA)

23. Thayer WS. *Lectures on the Malarial Fevers.* New York: D. Appleton and Company, 1897, pp. 84–86.

24. Darling ST. *Studies in Relation to Malaria.* Laboratory of the Board of Health, Department of Sanitation, Isthmian Canal Commission. Washington, D.C.: U.S. Government Printing Office, 1910, pp. 12–17.

25. Darling, *Malaria*, pp. 26–27.
26. Darling, *Malaria*, pp. 22–24.
27. Simmons JS. *Malaria in Panama*. Baltimore: The Johns Hopkins Press, 1939, p. 103.
28. Darling, *Malaria*, pp. 29–31.
29. Darling ST. A mosquito larvacide[*sic*]-disinfectant and the methods of its standardization. *American Journal of Public Health* 1912; 2: 89–92.
30. King WG. Applied hygiene in the tropics. Darling's larvicide. *Tropical Disease Bulletin* 1914; 4: 199–200.
31. Darling, *Malaria*, pp. 31–33.
32. Darling, *Malaria*, pp. 33–35.
33. Montgomery DW. Impressions of the Panama Canal. *American Medicine* (Complete Series) 1912; 7: 147,150,152.
34. Russell PF. Darling's work in Panama and in the United States. *International Health Board Bulletin* 1925; 6: 250–257.
35. Darling ST. The examination of stools for cysts of *Entamoeba tetragena*. *American Journal of Tropical Medicine and Hygiene* 1912; 15: 257–259.
36. Darling ST. The rectal inoculation of kittens as an aid in determining the identity of pathogenic entamoeba. *Southern Medical Journal* 1912; 6: 509–511.
37. Darling ST. Observations on the cysts of *Entamoeba tetragena*. *Archives of Internal Medicine* 1913; 11: 1–14.
38. Darling ST. Budding and other forms in trophozoites of *Entamoeba tetragena* simulating the "spore cyst" forms attributed to "*Entamoeba histolytica*." *Archives of Internal Medicine* 1913; 11: 495–506.
39. Craig CF. In discussion, Darling ST. The identification of the pathogenic entamoeba of Panama. *Transactions of the 15th International Congress of Hygiene and Demography*, Sept. 23–28, 1912. Washington, D.C.: U.S. Government Printing Office, 1913, pp. 166–167.
40. Darling, *Transactions*, 1912, p. 168.
41. Craig CF. The identity of *Entamoeba histolytica* and *Entamoeba tetragena*: A preliminary note. *Journal of the American Medical Association* 1913; 60: 1353–1354.
42. Darling ST. Murrina, a trypanosomal disease of equines in Panama. *Journal of Infectious Diseases* 1911; 8: 467–485.
43. Darling ST. Sarcosporidiosis: with report of a case in man. *Archives of Internal Medicine* 1909; 3: 183–192.
44. Darling ST. Experimental sarcosporidiosis in the guinea pig and its relation to a case of sarcosporidiosis in man. *Journal of Experimental Medicine* 1910; 12: 19–28.
45. Darling ST. Sarcosporidiosis in the opossum and its experimental production in the guinea pig by the intramuscular injection of sporozoites. *Bulletin Société de Pathologie Exotique* 1910; 3: 513–518.
46. Kean BH, Grocott RG. Sarcosporidiosis or toxoplasmosis in man and guinea pig. *American Journal of Pathology* 1945; 21: 467–483.
47. Chaves-Carballo E. Samuel T. Darling and human sarcosporidiosis or toxoplasmosis in Panama. *Journal of the American Medical Association* 1970; 211: 1687–1689.
48. Splendore A. Sur un nouveau protozoaire parasite du lapin: Deuxiéme note

preliminaire. *Bulletin Société de Pathologie Exotique* 1909; 2: 462–465.

49. Wolf A, Cowen D, Paige BH. Toxoplasmic encephalomyelitis: III. New case of granulomatous encephalomyelitis due to protozoon. *American Journal of Pathology* 1929; 15: 657–694.

50. Darling ST. Oriental sore. *Journal of Cutaneous Diseases* 1911; 26: 617–627.

51. Darling ST. Two cases of anaphylactic serum disease over six years after primary injection of horse serum (Yersin's antipest serum). *Proceedings of the Canal Zone Medical Association* 1912; 5 (Part I): 37–45.

52. "Report on La Chorrera and Chame with Regard to Infant Mortality and Smallpox dated September 1, 1910, to the Secretary of Fomento, Panama." File 37–F-101, Box 252, Record Group 185, Records of the Panama Canal, Second Isthmian Canal Commission, General Correspondence, 1905–1914, National Archives, College Park, Maryland. (NA II)

53. Darling to Chief Sanitary Officer, October 31, 1910, file 37–F-101, Box 252, RG 185. (NA II)

54. Gorgas WC. Sanitary conditions as encountered in Cuba and Panama, and what is being done to render the Canal Zone healthy. *Medical Record* (N.Y.) 1905; 67: 161–163.

55. Gorgas WC. Recommendations as to sanitation concerning employees of the mines on the Rand made to the Transvaal Chamber of Mines. *Journal of the American Medical Association* 1914; 62: 1855–1865.

56. Gorgas, *Sanitation*, p. 238.

57. Balfour A. *War Against Tropical Disease*. London: Baillier, Tindall and Co., 1920, p. 67.

58. Chamberlain WP. *Twenty-five years of American medical activity on the isthmus of Panama 1904–1929: A triumph of preventive medicine*. Mount Hope, Canal Zone: Panama Canal Press, 1929, p. 9.

8   Rand Mines, South Africa

1. Baum GL. *Samuel Taylor Darling*. Cincinnati: Private edition, 1958, p. 14.

2. Darling ST. South Africa. *Proceedings of the Medical Association of the Isthmian Canal Zone* 1914; 7: 7–15, p. 7.

3. Gorgas MD, Hendrick BJ. *William Crawford Gorgas*. Philadelphia: Lea & Febiger, 1924, pp. 264–268.

4. Gorgas, *Gorgas*, pp. 277–279.

5. Gorgas, *Gorgas*, pp. 280–282.

6. Darling, *Proceedings*, p. 14.

7. Darling, *Proceedings*, pp. 8–9.

8. Gorgas WC. Recommendations as to sanitation concerning employees of the mines on the Rand made to the Transvaal Chamber of Mines. *Journal of the American Medical Association (JAMA)* 1914; 62: 1855–1865, p. 1855.

9. Gorgas, *JAMA*, p. 1859.

10. Gorgas, *JAMA*, p. 1861.

11. Darling, *Proceedings*, p. 11.

12. Gorgas, *JAMA*, p. 1863.

13. Gorgas, *JAMA*, p. 1865.

14. Gorgas, *Gorgas*, pp. 285–289.

9   Uncinariasis Commission to the Far East

1. Ferrell to Darling, January 7, 1915, folder 232, box 15, series 1.2 (Correspondence, Projects), Record Group (RG) 5 (International Health Board), Rockefeller Foundation Archives (RF), Rockefeller Archive Center, Sleepy Hollow, New York. (RAC)
2. Farley J. *To Cast Out Disease. A History of the International Health Division of the Rockefeller Foundation (1913–1951).* Oxford: Oxford University Press, 2004, p. 4.
3. Stapleton DH. "The Rockefeller (University) Effect: A Phenomenon in Biomedical Science." In *Creating a Tradition of Biomedical Research. Contributions to the History of the Rockefeller University.* Stapleton DH (ed.), New York: The Rockefeller University Press, 2004, pp. 5–15. <http://archive.rockefeller.edu/faqs>, accessed February 23, 2005.
4. Farley, *Cast*, p. 3.
5. Farley, *Cast*, p. 5.
6. Fosdick RB. *The Story of the Rockefeller Foundation.* New York: Harper & Brothers, Publishers, 1952, p. 10.
7. Ettling J. *The Germ of Laziness. Rockefeller Philanthropy and Public Health in the New South.* Cambridge, Massachusetts: Harvard University Press, 1981, p. 107
8. Ettling, *Germ*, p. 110.
9. Ettling, *Germ,* p. 11.
10. Fosdick, *Story*, p. 38.
11. Ettling, *Germ*, p. 138.
12. Ettling, *Germ*, p. 164.
13. Ettling, *Germ*, p. 178.
14. Ettling, *Germ*, p. 186.
15. Fosdick, *Story*, p. 24.
16. Fosdick, *Story*, p. 34.
17. Gorgas to Ferrell, December 12, 1914, folder 232, box 15, series 1.2, RG 5, RF, RAC.
18. Simon Flexner to Ferrell, December 1, 1914, folder 232, box 15, series 1.2, RG 5, RF, RAC.
19. Darling to Ferrell, January 7, 191[5], folder 232, box 15, series 1.2, RG 5, RF, RAC.
20. Darling ST, Barber MA, Hacker HP. *Hookworm and Malaria Research in Malaya, Java, and the Fiji Islands. Report of the Uncinariasis Commission to the Orient 1915–1917.* (Rockefeller Foundation International Health Board Publication No. 9), New York, 1920, p. 15.
21. Darling ST. *Some phases of hookworm treatment questions, treatment in malarial communities and suggestions for a campaign.* (15 pp.) Series 2 (Reports Special), RG 5, RF, RAC.
22. Darling to Intercom (Western Union Cablegram), January 19, 1915, folder 232, box 15, series 1.2, RG 5, RF, RAC.
23. "Itemized list of contents of cases comprising shipments of medical equipment from the Rockefeller Foundation, International Health Commission, for Dr. Darling, destination Singapore, manifested at New York on the

Adriatic, sailing April 21 for Liverpool, England," folder 232, box 15, series 1.2, RG 5, RF, RAC.

24. Darling to Rose, May 4, 1915, folder 232, box 15, series 1.2, RG 5, RF, RAC.

25. Meyer to Darling, June 8, 1915, folder 232, box 15, series 1.2, RG 5, RF, RAC.

26. Darling to Rose, August 27, 1915, folder 232, box 15, series 1.2, RG 5, RF, RAC.

27. Darling to Rose, September 1, 1915, folder 232, box 15, series 1.2, RG 5, RF, RAC.

28. Darling to Heiser, October 4, 1915, folder 232, box 15, series 1.2, RG 5, RF, RAC.

29. Darling to Kirk, February 16, 1915, folder 232, box 15, series 1.2, RG 5, RF, RAC.

30. Kirk to Darling, February 17, 1916, folder 232, box 15, series 1.2, RG 5, RF, RAC.

31. Brown ER. *Rockefeller Medicine Men. Medicine & Capitalism in America.* Berkeley: University of California Press, 1979, p. 128.

32. Darling to Rose, July 6, 1916a, folder 232, box 15, series 1.2, RG 5, RF, RAC.

33. Darling, *Hookworm*, p. 3.

34. Darling to Rose, July 6, 1916b, folder 232, box 15, series 1.2, RG 5, RF, RAC.

35. Darling to Heiser, July 6, 1916, folder 232, box 15, series 1.2, RG 5, RF, RAC.

36. Darling to Heiser, August 20, 1916, folder 35, box 18, series 1.2, RG 5, RF, RAC.

37. Darling to Rose, July 29, 1916, folder 232, box 15, series 1.2, RG 5, RF, RAC.

38. Darling ST. "Comparative helminthology as an aid in the solution of ethnological problems." (Presidential address read, in part, by Dr. V.G. Heiser at the twenty-first annual meeting of the American Society of Tropical Medicine, May 5 and 6, 1925, Washington, D.C.). *American Journal of Tropical Medicine* 1925; 5: 323–337.

39. Darling to Rose, November 15, 1916, folder 232, box 15, series 1.2, RG 5, RF, RAC.

40. Darling to Heiser, December 12, 1916, folder 232, box 15, series 1.2, RG 5, RF, RAC.

41. Darling to Rose, January 20, 1917, folder 794, box 53, series 1.2, RG 5, RF, RAC.

42. Darling to Rose, April 6, 1917, folder 794, box 53, series 1.2, RG 5, RF, RAC.

43. Darling to Rose, May 18, 1917, folder 794, box 53, series 1.2, RG 5, RF, RAC.

44. Darling to Rose and Heiser, July 11, 1917, folder 794, box 53, series 1.2, RG 5, RF, RAC.

45. Darling, *Hookworm*, p. 21.

46. Darling to Rose, August 10, 1918, folder 906, box 62, series 1.2, RG 5, RF, RAC.

47. Darling, *Hookworm*, 191 pp.
48. Darling to Williamson, August 7, 1922, series 2, Reports Special, RG 5, RF, RAC.
49. Darling, *Hookworm*, p. 16.
50. Darling, *Hookworm*, p. 25.
51. Darling, *Hookworm*, p. 27.
52. Darling, *Hookworm*, p. 28.
53. Darling, *Hookworm*, p. 31.
54. Darling to Director General, International Health Board, December 11, 1916. *Report of an investigation in Java to determine the extent and character of hookworm infection among the native.* (13 pp.) Series 2, Reports Special, RG 5, RF, RAC.
55. Smillie WG. Dr. Darling's Hookworms Studies. *International Health Board Bulletin* 1925; 6: 26–30.
56. Barnes ME. Samuel Taylor Darling. *International Health Board Bulletin* 1925; 6: 20–23.
57. Gorgas to Rose, March 24, 1917, folder 627, box 40, series 1.1, RG 5, RF, RAC.
58. Rose to Gorgas, March 26, 1917, folder 627, box 40, series 1.1, RG 5, RF, RAC.
59. Mrs. ST Darling to Rockefeller Foundation, August 16, 1917, folder 794, box 53, series 1.2, RG 5, RF, RAC.
60. Darling to Rose, September 18, 1917, folder 794, box 53, series 1.2, RG 5, RF, RAC.

10   Institute of Hygiene, São Paulo, Brazil

1. Fosdick RB. *The Story of the Rockefeller Foundation.* New York: Harper & Brothers, Publishers, 1952, p 41.
2. Fosdick, *Rockefeller*, p. 42.
3. Flexner S, Flexner JT. *William Henry Welch and the Heroic Age of American Medicine.* New York: Dover Publications, Inc., 1941, p. 364.
4. Fleming D. *William H. Welch and the Rise of Moderm Medicine.* Baltimore: The Johns Hopkins University Press, 1954, pp. 182–184.
5. "International Health Board minutes," October 23, 1917, folder 151, series 305 L, Record Group (RG) 1.1, Rockefeller Foundation Archives (RF), Rockefeller Archive Center (RAC), Sleepy Hollow, New York.
6. Rose to Darling, September 20, 1917, folder 151, series 305 L, RG 1.1, RF, RAC.
7. Darling to Lund, November 2, 1917, folder 794, series 1.2, RG 5, RF, RAC.
8. Darling to Rose, January 23, 1918, folder 151, series 305 L, RG 1.1, RF, RAC.
9. "Plan of Co-operation between Dr. L. W. Hackett, Director for Brazil, and Dr. S. T. Darling, Professor of Hygiene and Director of Hygienic Laboratories in the Medical School of São Paulo," November 17, 1917, folder 151, series 305 L, RG 1.1, RF, RAC.
10. Vieira de Carvalho to Pearce and Rose, February 14, 1918, folder 151, series 305 L, RG 1.1, RF, RAC.

11. Darling to Meyer, March 16, 1918, folder 151, series 305 L, RG 1.1, RF, RAC.
12. Darling to Rose, June 25, 1918, folder 151, series 305 L, RG 1.1, RF, RAC.
13. Darling to Rose, March 1, 1919, folder 151, series 305 L, RG 1.1, RF, RAC.
14. Baum GL. *Samuel Taylor Darling.* Cincinnati: Private edition, 1958, pp. 18, 20.
15. Darling to Pearce, June 26, 1918, folder 151, series 305 L, RG 1.1, RF, RAC.
16. Smillie to Rose, October 15, 1918, folder 151, series 305 L, RG 1.1, RF, RAC.
17. Darling to Rose, November 13, 1918, folder 151, series 305 L, RG 1.1, RF, RAC.
18. "Darling, S. T. Reports 1918," folder 154, series 305 L, RG 1.1, RF, RAC.
19. Smillie to Rose, November 14, 1918, folder 151, series 305 L, RG 1.1, RF, RAC.
20. Darling to Rose, January 17, 1919, folder 151, series 305 L, RG 1.1, RF, RAC.
21. "Memorandum on Brazil" by R. M. Pearce (copy), 1919, folder 151, series 305 L, RG 1.1, RF, RAC.
22. Rose to Pearce, February 24, 1919, folder 151, series 305 L, RG 1.1, RF, RAC.
23. Pearce to Rose, April 6, 1919, folder 151, series 305 L, RG 1.1, RF, RAC.
24. Darling to Rose, February 28, 1919, folder 151, series 305 L, RG 1.1, RF, RAC.
25. Darling to Rose, May 16, 1919, folder 151, series 305 L, RG 1.1, RF, RAC.
26. Darling to Rose, June 26, 1919, folder 151, series 305 L, RG 1.1, RF, RAC.
27. Darling to Rose, July 10, 1919, folder 151, series 305 L, RG 1.1, RF, RAC.
28. Darling ST, Reports 1919, folder 154, series 305 L, RG 1.1, RF, RAC.
29. "Preliminary Report of Field Research on Hookworm Infection and Treatment for 1920 of the Institute of Hygiene," Darling to Rose, May 24, 1920, Reports Special, series 2, RG 5, RF, RAC.
30. Darling ST, Smillie WG. *Studies on Hookworm Infection in Brazil. First Paper.* (Monographs of the Rockefeller Institute for Medical Research No. 14, February 1, 1921.) New York: The Rockefeller Institute for Medical Research, 1921.
31. Smillie WG. *Studies on Hookworm Infection in Brazil 1918–1920. Second Paper.* (Monographs of The Rockefeller Institute for Medical Research No. 17, May 12, 1922.) New York: The Rockefeller Institute for Medical Research, 1922.
32. Darling to Rose, folder151, series 305L, RG 1.1, RF, RAC.
33. Souza to Rose, December 30, 1920, folder 154, series 305 L, RG 1.1, RF, RAC.
34. "Terms of the agreement between the Government of the State of São Paulo, Brazil and the International Health Board, New York City for the organization of a Department of Hygiene to be annexed to the Facultade de Medicina of São Paulo" (copy and translation), February 9, 1918, folder 151, series 305 L, RG 1.1, RF, RAC.
35. Fosdick, *Rockefeller*, p. 34.

36. Souza to Soper, November 18, 1941 (author's translation from Portuguese), folder 154, series 305 L, RG 1.1, RF, RAC.
37. Rose to Campos, December 20, 1920, folder 151, series 305 L, RG 1.1, RF, RAC.
38. Farley J. *To Cast Out Disease. A History of the International Health Division of the Rockefeller Foundation (1913–1951)*. Oxford: Oxford University Press, 2004, p. 206.
39. Smillie to Rose, August 31, 1921, folder 152, box 18, series 305 L, RG 1.1, RF, RAC.
40. Farley, *Cast Out*, p. 207.
41. Souza to Russell, October 30, 1923, folder 152, box 18, series 305 L, RG 1.1, RF, RAC.
42. Farley, *Cast Out*, p. 209.

11 Darling's Paralysis

1. Baum GL. *Samuel Taylor Darling*. Cincinnati: Private edition, 1958, pp. 8, 10.
2. Darling to Rose, August 19, 1920, folder 151, series 305L, Record Group (RG) 1.1, Rockefeller Foundation (RF), Rockefeller Foundation (RF), Rockefeller Archive Center (RAC), Sleepy Hollow, New York.
3. Mrs. Darling to Rose, November 22, 1920, folder 151, series 305L, RG 1.1, RF, RAC.
4. Mrs. Darling to Edyth Miller (librarian), December 23, 1920, folder 151, series 305L, RG 1.1, RF, RAC.
5. Mrs. Darling to Rose, December 27, 1920, folder 151, series 305L, RG 1.1, RF, RAC.
6. Rose to de Campos, December 20, 1920, folder 151, series 305L, RG 1.1, RF, RAC.
7. Rose to Mrs. Darling, December 29, 1920, folder 151, series 305L, RG 1.1, RF, RAC.
8. Darling to Miller, February 3, 1921, folder 151, series 305L, RG 1.1, RF, RAC.
9. Darling to Miller, February 22, 1921, folder 151, series 305L, RG 1.1, RF, RAC.
10. Miller to Darling, February 25, 1921, folder 151, series 305L, RG 1.1, RF, RAC.
11. Darling to Rose, March 14, 1921, folder 151, series 305L, RG 1.1, RF, RAC.
12. Darling to Ruth Ann Mannhardt, March 25, 1921, folder 151, series 305L, RG 1.1, RF, RAC.
13. Darling to Rose, July 2, 1921, S. T. Darling file, Secretary's Office, RG 15, RF, RAC.
14. Darling to Rose, July 11, 1921, folder 151, series 305L, RG 1.1, RF, RAC.
15. Darling to Rolling Dean, October 11, 1921, folder 151, series 305L, RG 1.1, RF, RAC.
16. Darling to Miller, October 19, 1921, folder 151, series 305L, RG 1.1, RF, RAC.
17. Darling to Ruth Ann Mannhardt, October 26, 1921, Ruth Ann Mannhardt personal correspondence.

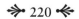

18. Hegner RW. "At the School of Hygiene and Public Health." A Memorial Meeting for Dr. Samuel Taylor Darling. *International Health Board Bulletin* 1926; 6: 261–263.
19. Samuel Darling (Samuel T. Darling's grandson), personal correspondence with the author.
20. Darling ST. The tertian characters of quotidian aestivo-autumnal fever. *American Journal of Tropical Medicine* 1921; 1: 397–408.
21. Darling to Miller, February 24, 1922, folder 151, series 305L, RG 1.1, RF, RAC.
22. Darling to Rose, June 26, 1922, folder 151, series 305L, RG 1.1, RF, RAC.
23. Darling to Rose, July 3, 1922, folder 151, series 305L, RG 1.1, RF, RAC.
24. Darling to Miller, August 1, 1922, folder 151, series 305L, RG 1.1, RF, RAC.
25. Darling to Ruth Ann Mannhardt, November 26, 1922, Ruth Ann Mannhardt personal correspondence.
26. Darling to Miller, November 4, 1922, folder 151, series 305L, RG 1.1, RF, RAC.

12   Station for Field Studies in Malaria, Leesburg, Georgia

1. Ferrell to Darling, January 13, 1923, folder 959, box 68, series 1.1, Record Group (RG) 5, Rockefeller Foundation Archives (RF), Rockefeller Archive Center (RAC), Sleepy Hollow, New York.
2. Darling to Deane, March 21, 1923, folder 960, box 68, series 1.1, RG 5, RF, RAC.
3. Darling to Read, March 28, 1923, folder 960, box 68, series 1.1, RG 5, RF, RAC.
4. Darling to Ferrell, March 28, 1923, folder 960, box 68, series 1.1, RG 5, RF, RAC.
5. Darling to Ferrell, March 30, 1923, folder 960, box 68, series 1.1, RG 5, RF, RAC.
6. Darling to Russell, April 3, 1923, folder 961, box 68, series 1.1, RG 5, RF, RAC.
7. Darling to Miller, no date, folder 961, box 68, series 1.1, RG 5, RF, RAC.
8. Darling to Russell, April 16, 1923, folder 961, box 68, series 1.1, RG 5, RF, RAC.
9. Kirk to Darling, April 19, 1923, folder 961, box 68, series 1.1, RG 5, RF, RAC.
10. Russell to Darling, April 13, 1923, folder 961, box 68, series 1.1, RG 5, RF, RAC.
11. Darling to Russell, April 18, 1923, folder 961, box 68, series 1.1, RG 5, RF, RAC.
12. Darling to Russell, May 22, 1923, folder 962, box 68, series 1.1, RG 5, RF, RAC.
13. Darling to Ferrell, June 4, 1923, folder 962, box 68, series 1.1, RG 5, RF, RAC.
14. Darling to Ferrell, July 11, 1923, folder 963, box 68, series 1.1, RG 5, RF, RAC.
15. Darling to Russell, May 16, 1924, folder 1095, box 77, series 1.1, RG 5, RF, RAC.

16. Darling to Ruth Ann Mannhardt, September 17, 1924, Personal correspondence.
17. Darling to Russell, May 23, 1924, folder 1095, box 77, series 1.1, RG 5, RF, RAC.
18. Darling to Ferrell, September 20, 1923, folder 964, box 68, series 1.1, RG 5, RF, RAC.
19. Darling to Ferrell, October 30, 1923, folder 965, box 68, series 1.1, RG 5, RF, RAC.
20. Darling to Ferrell, December 11, 1923, folder 966, box 68, series 1.1, RG 5, RF, RAC.
21. Darling to Ferrell, December 12, 1923, folder 966, box 68, series 1.1, RG 5, RF, RAC.
22. Darling to Ferrell, June 23, 1923, folder 962, box 68, series 1.1, RG 5, RF, RAC.
23. Darling to Williamson, June 10, 1924, folder 1096, box 77, series 1.1, RG 5, RF, RAC.
24. Darling to Ferrell, February 24, 1925a , folder 1269, box 89, series 1.1, RG 5, RF, RAC.
25. Darling to Ferrell, February 24, 1925b, folder 1269, box 89, series 1.1, RG 5, RF, RAC.
26. Russell to Darling, January 22, 1925, folder 959, box 68, series 1.1, RG 5, RF, RAC.
27. Darling to Russell, January 22, 1925, folder 959, box 68, series 1.1, RG 5, RF, RAC.
28. Darling to Russell, March 13, 1923, folder 960, box 68, series 1.1, RG 5, RF, RAC.
29. Darling to Russell, March 13, 1923b, folder 960, box 68, series 1.1, RG 5, RF, RAC.
30. Darling to Russell, March 30, 1923, folder 460, box 68, series 1.1, RG 5, RF, RAC.
31. Darling to Russell, April 9, 1923, folder 961, box 68, series 1.1, RG 5, RF, RAC.
32. Darling to Russell, June 16, 1923, folder 962, box 68, series 1.1, RG 5, RF, RAC.
33. Darling to Russell, September 18, 1923, folder 964, box 68, series 1.1, RG 5, RF, RAC.
34. Darling to Russell, September 27, 1923, folder 964, box 68, series 1.1, RG 5, RF, RAC.
35. Darling to Russell, December 10, 1923, folder 966, box 68, series 1.1, RG 5, RF, RAC.
36. Darling to Russell, December 10, 1923, folder 966, box 68, series 1.1, RG 5, RF, RAC.
37. Darling to Russell, December 11, 1923, folder 966, box 68, series 1.1, RG 5, RF, RAC.
38. Darling to Williamson, January 3, 1924, folder 1091, box 77, series 1.1, RG 5, RF, RAC.
39. Darling to Russell, February 12, 1924, folder 1092, box 77, series 1.1, RG 5, RF, RAC.

40. Darling to Russell, May 5, 1924, folder 1095, box 77, series 1.1, RG 5, RF, RAC.
41. Darling to Russell, February 13, 1924, folder 1092, box 77, series 1.1, RG 5, RF, RAC.
42. Darling to Russell, February 12, 1924, folder 1092, box 77, series 1.1, RG 5, RF, RAC.
43. Darling to Russell, August 28, 1924, folder 1098, box 77, series 1.1, RG 5, RF, RAC.
44. Darling to Russell, December 23, 1924, folder 1102, box 77, series 1.1, RG 5, RF, RAC.
45. Carter HR. "Comments on Post-mortem Examination of Yellow Fever Cases." From Carter to Read, January 14, 1925, series 2 Reports Special, RG 5, RF, RAC.
46. Darling to Russell, September 25, 1924, folder 1099, box 77, series 1.1, RG 5, RF, RAC.
47. Darling to Russell, February 21, 1924, folder 1092, box 77, series 1.1 RG 5, RF, RAC.
48. Darling to Dean, August 8, 1924, folder 1098, box 77, series 1.1, RG 5, RF, RAC.
49. Darling to Russell, April 23, 1924, folder 1094, box 77, series 1.1, RG 5, RF, RAC.
50. Lambert to Russell, May 2, 1924, folder 1096, box 77, series 1.1, RG 5, RF, RAC.
51. Darling to Read, June 2, 1924, folder 1096, box 77, series 1.1, RG 5, RF, RAC.
52. Darling to Russell, October 1, 1924, folder 1100, box 77, series 1.1, RG 5, RF, RAC.
53. Reye RDK, Morgan G, Baral L. Encephalopathy and fatty degeneration of the viscera: A disease entity in childhood. *Lancet* 1963; 2: 749–752.
54. Darling to Abercrombie, January 15, 1924, folder 1091, box 77, series 1.1, RF, RG 5, RAC.
55. Darling to Ferrell, January 29, 1924, folder 1091, box 77, series 1.1, RG 5, RF, RAC.
56. Darling to Ferrell, June 12, 1924, folder 1096, box 77, series 1.1, RG 5, RF, RAC.
57. "Extracts with some Additions from Journal of Dr. S. T. Darling, Leesburg, Georgia," October 1924, series 2 Reports Special, RG 5, RF, RAC.
58. Darling to Russell, July 1, 1924, folder 1097, box 77, series 1.1, RG 5, RF, RAC.
59. Fricks to Darling, January 31, 1924, folder 1091, box 77, series 1.1, RG 5, RF, RAC.
60. Darling to Ferrell, July 18, 1924, folder 1097, box 77, series 1.1, RG 5, RF, RAC.
61. Darling to Read, July 18, 1924, folder 1097, box 77, series 1.1, RG 5, RF, RAC.
62. Darling to Ruth Ann Mannhardt, September 17, 1924, Personal correspondence.
63. Baum GL. *Samuel Taylor Darling.* Cincinnati: Private edition, 1958, p. 21.

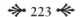

64. Darling to Ferrell, October 29, 1924, folder 1100, box 77, series 1.1, RG 5, RF, RAC.
65. Ferrell to Darling, October 8, 1924, folder 1100, box 77, series 1.1, RG 5, RF, RAC.
66. Russell to Darling, October 21, 1924, folder 1100, box 77, series 1.1, RG 5, RF, RAC.
67. Darling to Ferrell, October 29, 1924, folder 1100, box 77, series 1.1, RG 5, RF, RAC.
68. Ferrell to Darling, December 9, 1924, folder 1102, box 77, series 1.1, RG 5, RF, RAC.
69. Darling to Ferrell, December 13, 1924, folder 1102, box 77, series 1.1, RG 5, RF, RAC.

13 Malaria Commission, League of Nations

1. The *Baltimore Sun*, March 26, 1925.
2. Harned to Darling, March 5, 1925, folder 1270, box 89, series 1.1, Record Group (RG) 5, Rockefeller Foundation Archives (RF), Rockefeller Archive Center (RAC), Sleepy Hollow, New York.
3. Read to Ferrell, March 5, 1925 and Russell to Gunn, March 19, 1925, folder 1270, box 89, series 1.1, RG 5, RF, RAC.
4. Darling to Ferrell, March 6, 1925, folder 1270, box 89, series 1.1, RG 5, RF, RAC.
5. Harned to Darling, March 19, 1925, folder 1270, box 89, series 1.1, RG 5, RF, RAC.
6. Read to Mrs. Darling, March 23, 1925, folder 1270, box 89, series 1.1, RG 5, RF, RAC.
7. Read to Ferrell, March 5, 1925, folder 1270, box 89, series 1,1, RG 5, RF, Series 1.1, RAC.
8. Hackett, Lewis B. Samuel Taylor Darling 1872–1925. *International Health Board Bulletin* 1925; 6: 1–35, pp. 14–18.
9. Darling to Read, April 15, 1925, folder 1270, box 89, series 1.1, RG 5, RF, RAC.

14 Death Near Beirut

1. Drummond to Vincent (telegram from Geneva), May 22, 1925, folder 1271, box 89, series 1.1, Record Group (RG) 5, Rockefeller Foundation (RF) , Rockefeller Archive Center (RAC), Sleepy Hollow, New York.
2. Carley to Russell, June 8, 1925, folder 1272, box 89, series 1.1, RG 5, RF, RAC.
3. "The disaster at Beitmery," (translation from French) *La Syrie*, May 23, 1925, folder 1272, box 89, series 1.1, RG 5, RF, RAC.
4. Russell to Mrs. Darling, May 22, 1925, folder 1271, box 89, series 1.1, RG 5, RF, RAC.
5. "Dr. Darling killed in Syrian car wreck," *The New York Times*, May 23, 1925, and "Three killed when auto leaps cliff," The *New York Herald* (Paris edition), May 27, 1925 (photocopies of newspaper clippings), folder 1271, box 89, series 1.1, RG 5, RF, RAC.

6. Drummond to Vincent, May 23, 1925, folder 1272, box 89, series 1.1, RG 5, RF, RAC.

7. Kligler to Heiser, May 26, 1925, folder 1272, box 89, series 1.1, RG 5, RF, RAC.

8. P. F. Russell to F. F. Russell, June 5, 1925, folder 1272, box 89, series 1.1, RG 5, RF, RAC.

9. Russell to Mrs. Darling, December 21, 1925, folder 1276, box 89, series 1.1, RG 5, RF, RAC.

10. Mrs. Darling to Read, June 20, 1925, folder 1272, box 89, series 1.1, RG 5, RF, RAC.

11. Dandy to International Health Board, June 25, 1925, folder 1272, box 89, series 1.1, RG 5, RF, RAC.

12. Dandy to Russell, June 29, 1925, folder 1272, box 89, series 1.1, RG 5, RF, RAC.

13. Harned to Glassford, June 17, 1925, folder 1273, box 89, series 1.1, RG 5, RF, RAC.

14. Russell to Mrs. Darling, December 21, 1925, folder 1276, box 89, series 1.1, RG 5, RF, RAC.

15. "Memorandum from Read," May 26, 1925, folder 1271, box 89, series 1.1, RG 5, RF, RAC.

16. Balfour, Andrew C. Some British and American pioneers in tropical medicine and hygiene. *Transactions of the Royal Society of Tropical Medicine and Hygiene* 1925; 19: 189–231, pp. 225–226.

Appendixes

A: Bibliography of Publications by Samuel T. Darling

1. A list of Darling's publications first appeared in 1925 (*International Health Board Bulletin* 1925; 6: 30–35) and consisted of 73 entries. A compilation of Darling's bibliography by W. W. Cort and published by Gerald L. Baum in 1958 (Baum GL. *Samuel Taylor Darling*. Cincinnati: Private edition, 1958, pp. 32–35) listed 102 total publications. An additional 102 citations are included in the present bibliography. The discrepancy consists, in part, by the inclusion of twenty-nine discussions following paper presentations, four papers presented at meetings, four letters to the editors, forty-eight abstracts (mostly appearing in *Tropical Diseases Bulletin*), and thirty-two articles published in more than one journal. The decision to include these publications was not made to inflate the total number of publications by Darling, but to make the bibliography as complete as possible.

B: Faculty, Class Schedules, Registration, and Grades, College of Physicians and Surgeons of Baltimore

1. College of Physicians and Surgeons of Baltimore. *31st Annual Commencement. Thursday, April Thirtieth, 1903.* (No place or publisher given.)

2. College of Physicians and Surgeons of Baltimore. *Annual Announcement and Catalogue 1900–1901. 29th Annual Session.* Baltimore: The Sun Printing

Office, 1900, pp. 23–26. Historical/Special Collections, Health Sciences and Human Services Library, University of Maryland, Baltimore, Maryland. (UMHL)

3. College of Physicians and Surgeons of Baltimore. Matriculation records and class lists 1882–1912. (UMHL)
4. Matriculation records, p. 22. (UMHL)
5. Matriculation records, p. 38. (UMHL)
6. Matriculation records, p. 58. (UMHL)
7. Matriculation records, p. 78. (UMHL)

C: Proceedings of the Canal Zone Medical Association

1. Clark HC. "Some historical notes, Medical Association of the Isthmian Canal Zone." (Typed mansucript, 2 pp.), Otis Historical Archives, National Museum of Health and Medicine, Armed Forces Institute of Pathology, Walter Reed Army Medical Center, Washington, D.C. (OHA)
2. "Application from the Medical Association of the Isthmian Canal Zone," First Meeting — Monday Morning, June 6, Official Minutes — House of Delegates, Proceedings of the Sixty-first Annual Session held at St. Louis, June 6–10, 1910, House of Delegates Proceedings, American Medical Association, 1910.
3. "Isthmian Canal Zone," American Medical Association — Organization and Administration, Digest of Official Actions, 1846–1958, American Medical Association, 1959, vol. 1, p. 24.
4. "Officers of the Canal Zone Medical Association for the corresponding period." *Proceedings of the Canal Zone Medical Association* 1909; 2: 3
5. Clark HC. Samuel Taylor Darling 1872–1925. *Bulletin of the International Health Board* 1925; 6: 10–11.
6. Bennett IE. *History of the Panama Canal. Its Construction and Builders.* Washington, D.C.: Historical Publishing Co., 1915, p. 468.
7. *Proceedings of the Canal Zone Medical Association* 1908; 1: 1–194.
8. Darling ST. The relapsing fever of Panama. *Proceedings of the Canal Zone Medical Association* 1908; 1: 3–38.
9. Darling ST. A note on typhus fever. *Proceedings of the Medical Association of the Isthmian Canal Zone* 1914; 7 (Part 1): 152–162.
10. Darling ST. Discussion following paper by Herbert C. Clark, "Preliminary notes on neoplasms found in inhabitants of Panama Canal Zone, with special reference to their occurrence in the negro and mestizo." *Proceedings of the Medical Association of the Isthmian Canal Zone* 1915; 7 (Part 2): 63–64.
11. Darling ST. Discussion following paper, *Proceedings of the Medical Association of the Isthmian Canal Zone* 1915; 7 (Part 2): 91.
12. Darling ST. South Africa. *Proceedings of the Medical Association of the Isthmian Canal Zone* 1914; 7 (Part 1): 7–15.
13. Baum GL. *Samuel Taylor Darling.* Cincinnati: Private edition, 1958, p. 14.
14. *Proceedings of the Medical Association of the Isthmian Canal Zone,* 1921–1926; 14: 1–133.
15. *Proceedings of the Medical Association of the Isthmian Canal Zone,* 1927; 15: 1–67.

D: Personnel and Staff, Board of Health Laboratories

1. Clark HC. "Laboratory Development on the Isthmus of Panama. Miscellaneous Records Assembled by Herbert C. Clark," 11 January 1936, Panama Canal Company, Ancon, Canal Zone. (PCC)
2. Baum GL. *Samuel Taylor Darling.* Cincinnati: Private edition, 1958, p. 10.
3. "Organization of the Board of Health Laboratory," Statement No. 7, file 70–A-11, Records Group 185, Records of the Panama Canal, Second Isthmian Canal Commission, General Correspondence, 1905–1914, National Archives II, College Park, Maryland. (NA II)
4. "Organization of the Quarantine Division," Statement No. 11, file 70–A-11, RG 185. (NA II)
5. Kean BH. *M.D. One Doctor's Adventures Among the Famous and the Infamous from the Jungles of Panama to a Park Avenue Practice.* New York: Ballantine Books, 1990, pp. 81, 295.

E: Discovery and Pathology of Histoplasmosis

1. Darling ST. Histoplasmosis: A fatal infectious disease resembling kala-azar found among natives of tropical America. *Archives of Internal Medicine* 1908; 2: 107–123, pp. 110–117. (Copyright© 1908, American Medical Association. All rights reserved.)
2. "Gorgas Hospital Autopsies and Pathology Reports, 1900–1970s," Otis Historical Archives, National Museum of Health and Medicine, Armed Forces Institute of Pathology, Walter Reed Army Medical Center, Washington, D.C. (OHA)
3. Baum GL. *Samuel Taylor Darling.* Cincinnati: Private edition, 1958, p. 6.
4. Chaves-Carballo E. Samuel T. Darling: Studies on malaria and the Panama Canal. *Bulletin of the History of Medicine* 1980; 54: 95–100, p. 97.
5. Baum, *Darling*, p. 10.
6. Kean BH. *M.D. One Doctor's Adventures Among the Famous and Infamous from the Jungles of Panama to a Park Avenue Practice.* New York: Ballantine Books, 1990, p. 81.
7. Darling ST. The morphology of the parasite (*Histoplasma capsulatum*) and the lesions of histoplasmosis, a fatal disease of tropical America. *Journal of Experimental Medicine* 1909; 11: 515–531, pp. 515–516.
8. Baum, *Darling*, p. 14.
9. Daniel TM, Baum GL. *Drama and Discovery. The Story of Histoplasmosis.* Westport, Connecticut: Greenwood Press, 2002, p. 22.
10. Darling ST. Notes on histoplasmosis — A fatal disorder met with in tropical America. *Maryland Medical Journal* 1907; 50: 125–129, p. 128.
11. Darling ST. Histoplasmosis. A fatal infectious disease resembling kala-azar found among natives of tropical America. *Archives of Internal Medicine* 1908; 2: 118–119.
12. Darling, *Archives*, p. 122.
13. Schwarz J, Baum GL. The history of histoplasmosis, 1906 to 1956. *New England Journal of Medicine* 1957; 256: 253–258.

F: Visitors and Workers, Station for Field Studies in Malaria, Leesburg, Georgia

1. "Brief summary of the outstanding features of the year's work in Field Studies in Malarial Control, Lee County, Georgia," pp. 24–25, Darling to F. F. Russell, General Director, International Health Board, December 31, 1924, Reports Special, series 2, Record Group (RG) 5, Rockefeller Foundation Archives (RF), Rockefeller Archives Center (RAC), Sleepy Hollow, New York.

G: Obituaries and Condolences

1. "Condolences," file 1271, box 89, series 1.1, Record Group (RG) 5, Rockefeller Foundation (RF), Rockefeller Archive Center (RAC), Sleepy Hollow, New York.
2. "Condolences," file 1272, box 89, series 1.1, RG 5, RF, RAC.
3. "Condolences," file 1273, box 89, series 1.1, RG 5, RF, RAC.
4. "Condolences," file 1274, box 89, series 1.1, RG 5, RF, RAC.

H: Societies, Honors, and Commemoratives

H.1: *Membership in Societies and Honors*

1. Baum GL. *Samuel Taylor Darling.* Cincinnati: Private edition, 1958, p. 25.
2. Samuel Taylor Darling 1872–1925. *Bulletin of the International Board of Health* 1925; 6: 1–35, pp. 5–6.
3. "Dr. Darling's Work in the Canal Zone Laboratory Raised to Important Position." The *Star & Herald* (Panama), January 6, 1915, (Part Two), p. 9.

H.2: *Darling Gold Medal and Prize*

1. "The Darling Memorial Prize Fund." *International Health Board Bulletin* 1926; 7: 160–162.
2. Baum GL. *Samuel Taylor Darling.* Cincinnati: Private edition, 1958, p. 25.
3. Baum, *Darling*, p. 32.
4. WHO Darling Foundation. <www.who.int.governance/awards/darling/winners> (accessed July 26, 2004).

H.3: *Samuel T. Darling Collection, Johns Hopkins School of Hygiene and Public Health, Baltimore, Maryland, and Samuel Taylor Darling Memorial Library, Gorgas Hospital, Ancon, Canal Zone*

1. A Memorial Meeting for Dr. Samuel Taylor Darling. *International Health Board Bulletin* 1926; 6: 247–263.
2. Baum GL. *Samuel Taylor Darling.* Cincinnati: Private edition, 1958, p. 22.
3. Samuel Taylor Darling (1872–1925). *International Health Board Bulletin* 1925; 6: 1–35.
4. Baum, *Darling*, p. 29.
5. Noel R. Rose, Johns Hopkins University School of Public Health and Hygiene, September 21, 1987, correspondence with the author.
6. "Gorgas Library Dedicated In Honor of Dr. Darling." *Panama Canal Spillway*, November 17, 1972, p. 3.

7. Samuel T. Darling Memorial Library, Gorgas Hospital, Ancon, Canal Zone, document dated April 12, 1960. (STDL)
8. *Panama Canal Spillway,* March 27, 1997.
9. Norma Sellers, Stimson Library, U.S. Army Medical Department (AMEDD) Center and School, Academy of Health Sciences, Fort Sam Houston, Texas, personal communication with the author.

H.4: *Darling's Liberty Ship: S.S.* Samuel T. Darling

1. Lane FC. *Ships for Victory. A History of Shipbuilding under the U.S. Maritime Commission in World War II.* Baltimore: Johns Hopkins Press, 1951.
2. Elphick P. *Liberty. The Ships that Won the War.* Annapolis, Maryland: Naval Institute Press, 2001, p. 13.
3. Elphick, *Liberty*, p. 14.
4. Elphick, *Liberty*, p. 18.
5. Elphick, *Liberty*, p. 30.
6. Elphick, *Liberty*, p. 35.
7. Elphick, *Liberty*, p. 85.
8. "Liberty Ships Built by the United States Maritime Commission in World War II," <www.usmn.org/libertyships/html> (accessed July 5, 2004).
9. Elphick, *Liberty*, p. 17.
10. Herbert B. *The Forgotten Heroes: The Heroic Story of the United States Merchant Marine,* New York: Forge, 2004, p. 79.
11. Elphick, *Liberty*, p. 102.
12. Mrs. S. T. Darling to Senator Harry F. Byrd, November 1, 1943, Mrs.Virginia Darling, Charlottesville, Virginia, personal correspondence with the author.
13. E. S. Land to Harry F. Byrd, November 9, 1943, Mrs. Virginia Darling, Charlottesville, Virginia, personal correspondence with the author.
14. "Wilmington Woman Will Sponsor Ship Named for Father," *Wilmington Morning News,* January 17, 1944.
15. "Liberty Ships, Master List of Names," <www.fiu.edu~thompsop/liberty/liberty_listS.html> (accessed July 5, 2004).
16. "Another Vessel Goes Down Ways. Southeastern Launches 38th, S.S. Samuel T. Darling," *Savannah Morning News,* January 19, 1944.
17. "Ship Bears Name of Dr. S.T. Darling," *Charlottesville Daily Progress,* January 1, 1944.
18. Lamark, War Shipping Administration, to D. P. Darling, December 11, 1943. Mrs. Virginia Darling, Charlottesville, Virginia, personal correspondence with the author.

H.5: *Darling's mosquito:* Anopheles darlingi

1. Root FM. Studies on Brazilian mosquitoes. I. The Anophelines of the Nyssorhyncous group. *American Journal of Hygiene* 1926; 6: 684–717.
2. Hegner R. Francis Metcalf Root. *Journal of Parasitology* 1935; 21: 67–69.
3. In Memoriam: Francis Metcalf Root (1889–1934). *Journal of Parasitology* 1933–1934; 20: 342–343.

4. Root FM. Notes on mosquitoes of Lee County, Georgia. *American Journal of Hygiene* 1924; 4: 449–455.

5. Komp WHW. *The anopheline mosquitoes of the Caribbean region.* (National Institutes of Health Bulletin No. 179), Washington, D.C.: U.S. Government Printing Office, 1942.

6. Foote RH, Cook DR. *Mosquitoes of Medical Importance.* (Agriculture Handbook No. 152, Agriculture Research Service), Washington, D.C.: U.S. Department of Agriculture, 1959, p. 118.

7. Povoa MM., Conn J, Schlichting CD, et al. Malaria vectors, epidemiology, and the re-emergence of *Anopheles darlingi* in Belem, Para, Brazil. *Journal of Medical Entomology* 2003; 40: 379–386.

8. <www.guardian.co.uk/life/dispatch> December 4, 2003 (accessed July 21, 2004).

9. Moore S, Darling S. "The development of a broad-spectrum, plant-based mosquito repellent for use in malaria endemic regions of the Americas." (Typed manuscript, 20 pp.) Samuel Darling, personal correspondence with author.

H.6: Besnoitia darlingi

1. Darling ST. Sarcosporidiosis with report of a case in man. *Proceedings of the Canal Zone Medical Association* 1908; 1: 141–152.

2. Darling ST. Sarcosporidiosis with report of a case in man. *Archives of Internal Medicine* 1909; 3: 183–192.

3. Baraban L, St. Remy G: Sur un cas de tubes sporospermiques observe chez l'homme. *Comptes Rendus Société Biologique* 1894; 10: 201–203.

4. Lindemann K. Über die hygienische bedeutung der gregarinen. *Staatsarzneikunde* 1868; 2: 326–352.

5. Darling ST. Experimental sarcosporidiosis in the guinea pig and its relation to a case of sarcosporidiosis in man. *Journal of Experimental Medicine* 1910; 12: 19–28.

6. Darling ST. Sarcosporidiosis in the opossum and its experimental production in the guinea pig by the intra-muscular injection of sporozoites. *Bulletin Société Pathologie Exotique* 1910; 3: 513–518.

7. Brumpt É. *Précis de Parasitologie.* (2nd ed.) Paris: Masson et Cie., 1913, p 109.

8. Chaves-Carballo E. Samuel T. Darling and human sarcosporidiosis or toxoplasmosis in Panama. *Journal of the American Medical Association* 1970; 59: 609–612.

9. Mandour AM. *Sarcocystis garnhami* n. sp. in the skeletal muscle of an opossum, *Didelphis marsupialis. Journal of Protozoology* 1965; 12: 606–609.

10. Smith DD, Frenkel JK. *Besnoitia darlingi* (Protozoa: Toxoplasmatinae): Cyclic transmission by cats. *Journal of Parasitology* 1977; 63: 1066–1071.

11. Smith DD, Frenkel JK. *Besnoitia darlingi* (Apicomplexa, Sarcocystidae, Toxoplasmatinae): Transmission between opossums and cats. *Journal of Protozoology* 1984; 31: 584–587.

12. Dubey JP, Lindsay DS, Rosenthal BM, et al. Establishment of *Besnoitia*

darlingi from opossums (*Didelphis virginiana*) in experimental intermediate and definitive hosts, propagation in cell culture, and description of ultra-structural and genetic characteristics. *International Journal of Parasitology* 2002; 32: 1053–1064.

H.7: *Darling's Spiny Rat:* **Diplomys darlingi**

1. Goldman EA. New mammals from Eastern Panama. *Smithsonian Miscellaneous Collections* 1912; 60: 12–13.
2. Goldman EA. Mammals of Panama. *Smithsonian Miscellaneous Collections* 1920; 69: 124–125.
3. Tesh RB. Observations on the natural history of *Diplomys darlingi*. *Journal of Mammalogy* 1970; 51: 197–199.

Bibliography

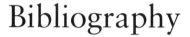

Abbreviations

LHL   Linda Hall Library of Science, Engineering and Technology, Kansas City, Missouri.

LOC   Library of Congress, Washington, D.C.

NA   National Archives, Washington, D.C.

NAII   National Archives II, College Park, Maryland.

NLM   National Library of Medicine, National Institutes of Health, Bethesda, Maryland.

OHA   Otis Historical Archives, National Museum of Health and Medicine, Armed Forces Institute of Pathology, Walter Reed Army Medical Center, Washington, D.C.

PCC   Panama Collection (The Panama Collection was transferred from the Canal Zone Library, Civil Affairs Bureau, Canal Zone Government, to the Technical Resources Center, Balboa, Panama, and was accessed by the author in January 1995.)

RAC   Rockefeller Archive Center, Rockefeller Foundation, Sleepy Hollow, New York.

STDL   Samuel T. Darling Memorial Library, Gorgas Hospital, Ancon, Panama. (Gorgas Army Community Hospital in Ancon closed its doors on October 1, 1997. Anticipating the reversion of the Panama Canal territories and facilities to the Republic of Panama on December 31, 1999, documents and books from the "Samuel T. Darling Memorial Library," were transferred to the Stimson Library, AMEDD (Army Medical Department) Center and School, Fort Sam Houston, Texas.)

UMHL   University of Maryland Health Sciences and Human Services Library, Historical and Special Collections, Baltimore, Maryland.

Manuscripts and Archives

B. Nichols, Panama Canal Notebooks (circa 1906–1920) (LHL)
Annual Reports of the Health Bureau (1883–1977) (NA II)
Henry R. Carter Papers (NLM)
Gorgas Collection (1903–1933) (OHA)

Gorgas Hospital Autopsies and Pathological Reports (1900–1970s) (OHA)
Gorgas Hospital Mortuary Records (1906–1999) (NA II)
Photographic Records of the Panama Canal (Still Pictures) (1887–1979) (NA)
Records of the International Health Board (RAC)
Records of the Isthmian Canal Commission (NAII)
Records of the Isthmian Historical Society (NAII)
Siler Collection (includes Ancon Hospital photographs) (1910–1929) (OHA)
Surgeon General's Office Records (1861–1970s) (OHA)
William Gorgas Papers (NLM)
Ziperman Collection (1957–1963) (OHA)

Newspapers and Periodicals

Baltimore Sun (LOC)
Bulletin du Canal Interocéanique (LH)
Canal Record (PCC)
La Estrella de Panamá (LOC)
La Lotería. Revista Cultural de Panamá
New York Herald Tribune (LOC)
Panama-American (LOC)
Panama Star & Herald (LOC)
Proceedings of the Canal Zone Medical Association (NAII)
Proceedings of the Medical Association of the Isthmian Canal Zone (NAII)
The New York Times (LOC)
The Panama Canal Review (PCC)
The Panama Canal Spillway (PCC)

Interviews and Correspondence

Dr. Gerald L. Baum, Tel-Aviv, Israel (2005)
Mrs. Nina Curran, Williamsburg, Virginia (2005)
Mr. Samuel Darling, Vancouver, Canada (2005)
Mrs. Virginia Darling, Charlottesville, Virginia (1981)
Mrs. Virginia Darling Lloyd, Charlottesville, Virginia (2005)
Mrs. Ruth Ann Mannhardt, Cromwell, Connecticut (1989)
Mrs. Virginia Ewing Stich, New Orleans, Louisiana

Bibliography

1. Abbott HL. *Problems of the Panama Canal; including climatology of the isthmus, physics and hydraulics of the river Chagres cut at the continental divide, and discussion of plans for the waterway, with history from 1870 to date.* New York: The MacMillan Company, 1907.
2. Abbott WJ. *Panama and the Canal in Picture and Prose.* London: Syndicate Publishing Company, 1913.
3. Abrahams HJ. *The Extinct Medical Schools of Baltimore, Maryland.* Baltimore: Maryland Historical Society, 1969.
4. Acosta J de. *Natural and Moral History of the Indies.* (Edited by Jane E. Mangan and translated by Frances M. López-Morillas.) Durham, North Carolina: Duke University Press, 2002.

5. Adams CF. *History of Braintree, Massachusetts.* Cambridge, Maryland: no publisher given, 1981.
6. American Geographical Society. Interoceanic Ship Canal Discussion. *Bulletin of the American Geographical Society.* New York: 1880. (Pamphlet)
7. *Ancon Hospital.* (Operated by the Health Department of the Panama Canal at Ancon, Canal Zone.) Mt. Hope, Canal Zone: The Panama Canal Press, 1923. (Pamphlet) PCC
8. Anderson CLG. *Old Panama and Castilla Del Oro.* New York: North River Press, 1938.
9. Anguizola G. *Philippe Bunau-Varilla. The Man Behind the Panama Canal.* Chicago: Nelson Hall, Inc., 1980.
10. Avery RE. *The Panama Canal and Golden Gate Exposition.* (No place or publisher given), 1915.
11. Bakenhus R, Knapp HS, Johnson ER. *The Panama Canal. Comprising its History and Construction, and its Relation to the Navy, International Law and Commerce.* New York: John Wiley & Sons, Inc., 1915.
12. Ballard MB. *A University is Born.* Old Hundred Union, West Virginia: (no publisher given), 1965.
13. Balfour A. *War Against Tropical Diseases.* London: Baillier, Tindall and Co., 1920.
14. Barber MA. *A Malariologist in Many Lands.* Lawrence, Kansas: University of Kansas Press, 1946.
15. Barry JM. *The Great Influenza. The Epic Story of the Deadliest Plague in History.* New York: Penguin Books, 2004.
16. Baum GL. *Samuel Taylor Darling.* Cincinnati: Private edition, 1958.
17. Baum GL. The history of histoplasmosis. In Sweany HC, ed. *Histoplasmosis.* Springfield, Illinois: Charles C Thomas, Publisher, 1960, pp. 14–39.
18. Beatty C. *De Lesseps of Suez. The Man and His Times.* New York: Harper & Brothers, 1956.
19. Bennett IE. *History of the Panama Canal. Its Construction and Builders.* Washington, D.C.: Historical Publishing Co., 1915.
20. Bernheim BM. *The Story of Johns Hopkins.* New York: McGraw-Hill Book Co., Inc, 1941.
21. Bishop F. *Panama Past and Present.* New York: The Century Co., 1913.
22. Bishop JB. *The Panama Gateway.* New York: Charles Scribner's Sons, 1913.
23. Bishop JB. *Uncle Sam's Panama Canal and World History.* New York: John Wanamaker for The World Syndicate Co., 1913.
24. Bishop J. *Goethals. Genius of the Panama Canal.* New York: Harper & Bothers, Publishers, 1930.
25. Bonner TN. *Iconoclast. Abraham Flexner and a Life in Learning.* Baltimore: Johns Hopkins University Press, 2002.
26. Bovallius C. *Viaje al Istmo 1881–1883 [Voyage to the Isthmus 1881–1883].* Translated from the Swedish by Abel Lombardo Vega, Panama: Ministerio de Educacion, 1972.
27. Boyson WA. *The Relationship of Disease and Sanitation to the Panama Canal Company.* (Typewritten manuscript, 7 pp.), Balboa Heights, Canal Zone, 1973. PCC

28. Braun M. *The Animal Parasites of Man. A Handbook for Students and Medical Men.* New York: William Wood and Company, 1907.

29. Breunle PC. *The Historical Development of the Management of the Health Care Delivery System in the Canal Zone.* (Thesis prepared for the Committee on Credentials in partial fulfillment for Fellowship to the American College of Hospital Administrators, 193 pp.), 1975. PCC

30. Brown ER. *Rockefeller Medicine Men: Medicine & Capitalism in America.* Berkeley: University of California Press, 1979.

31. Brumpt É. *Précis de Parasitologie.* (Collection de Précis Médicaux.) Paris: Masson & Cie., 1913.

32. Bunau-Varilla P. *Panama: The Creation, Destruction, and Resurrection.* London: Constable & Company, Ltd., 1913.

33. Cameron I. *The Impossible Dream. The Building of the Panama Canal.* New York: William Morrow and Company, Inc., 1972.

34. Capper A. *Panama Canal as Seen by a Kansan.* (No date or place of publication given) (Pamphlet).

35. Carles RD. *Old Panama.* (Panamá Vieja, translated by Patrick J. Smyth). Panama: La Estrella de Panamá, 1960 (Pamphlet).

36. Carles RD. *The Centennial City of Colon 1852 – 1952.* Panama: Imprenta Nacional, n.d. (Pamphlet).

37. Castillero EJ. *Historia de Panama [History of Panama].* 10th ed. Panama, 1989.

38. Castro Vega O. *Pedrarias Dávila. La Ira de Dios [Pedrarias Davila, The Wrath of God].* Costa Rica: Litografía e Imprenta LIL, 1996.

39. Chamberlain WP. *Twenty-five Years of American Medical Activity on the Isthmus of Panama 1904–1929: A triumph of preventive medicine.* Mount Hope, Canal Zone: Panama Canal Press, 1929.

40. Clark HC. "Some historical notes, Medical Association of the Isthmian Canal Zone," (typed manuscript, 2 pp.). OHA

41. Clark HC. "Laboratory Development on the Isthmus of Panama. Miscellaneous Records Assembled by Herbert C. Clark. 11 Jan. 1936." (Typed manuscript, 8 pp.; Appendix No. 3, 2 pp.; Plate I, 1 p.; Handwritten notes, 1 p.) OHA

42. Coates A. "En la Historia Geológica, Panamá ha Cambiado al Mundo [In Geological History, Panama has Changed the World]," In Hackedon-Moreno S (ed.) *Panamá: Puente Biológico, Las Charlas Smithsonian del Mes: 1996–1999 [Panama: Biological Bridge, Smithsonian Talks of the Month: 1996–1999].* Panama: Instituto Smithsonian de Investigaciones Tropicales, 2001, pp. 18–25.

43. College of Physicians and Surgeons of Baltimore. *Annual Announcement and Catalogue, 1899–1900, 28th Annual Session,* Baltimore: The Sun Book and Job Printing Office, 1899. UMHL

44. College of Physicians and Surgeons of Baltimore. *Annual Announcement and Catalogue, 1900–1901, 29th Annual Session.* Baltimore: The Sun Printing Office, 1900. UMHL

45. College of Physicians and Surgeons of Baltimore. *Annual Announcement and Catalogue, 1901–1902, 30th Annual Session.* Baltimore: The Sun Printing House, 1901. UMHL

46. College of Physicians and Surgeons of Baltimore. *31st Annual Announcement, Session of 1902–1903*. Baltimore (no publisher or date given). UMHL

47. College of Physicians and Surgeons of Baltimore. *31st Annual Commencement. Order of Exercises. Thursday, April Thirtieth, 1903*. Baltimore (no publisher or date given).

48. College of Physicians and Surgeons of Baltimore. *32nd Annual Announcement, Session of 1903–1904*. Baltimore (no publisher or date given). UMHL

49. *College of Physicians and Surgeons of Baltimore*. Baltimore: Free Press of Guggenheim, Weil & Co., 1904. UMHL

50. College of Physicians and Surgeons of Baltimore. *Yearbook 1907*. UMHL

51. Compagnie Nouvelle du Canal de Panama. *Short Notice Descriptive of the Exhibit of the Company*. (Pan-American Exposition, Buffalo, New York), 1901. (Pamphlet)

52. Companyo L. *Projet d'Organisation du Service de Santé de la Compagnie du Canal Interocéanique de Panama. Lettre a M. le Comte Ferdinand de Lesseps, President Fondateur et Directeur des Compagnies Universelles des Canaux Maritimes de Suez et Interocéanique de Panama [Project of Organization of the Health Service of the Panama Interoceanic Canal Company. Letter to M. the Count Ferdinad de Lesseps, President Founder of the Universal Companies of the Maritime Canals of Suez and Interoceanic of Panama]* . Paris: Librairie J. B. Baillere et Fils, 1880.

53. Cordell EF. *Historical Sketch of the University of Maryland, School of Medicine (1807–1890)*. Baltimore: Baltimore Press of Isaac Friedenwald, 1891.

54. Cordell EF. *The Medical Annals of Maryland. 1799–1899*. Baltimore: Williams & Wilkins Co., 1903.

55. Cornish V. *The Panama Canal and its Makers*. Boston: Little, Brown & Co., 1909.

56. Cueto M. *Missionaries of the Rockefeller Foundation & Latin America*. Bloomington: Indiana University Press, 1994.

57. Cullen TS. Early Medicine in Maryland. (Address of the President of the Medical and Chirurgical Faculty of Maryland, delivered at the Faculty Building, 1211 Cathedral St., Baltimore, April 26, 1927). UMHL

58. Daniel TM, Baum GL. *Drama and Discovery: The Story of Histoplasmosis*. (Contributions in Medical Studies, No. 48), Westport, Connecticut: Greenwood Press, 2002.

59. Dario Carles R. *Old Panama*. (*Panamá Vieja*, translated by Patrick J. Smyth). Panama: La Estrella de Panamá, 1960 (Pamphlet).

60. Darling ST. *Studies in Relation to Malaria*. Laboratory of the Board of Health, Department of Sanitation, Isthmian Canal Commission. Washington, D.C.: U.S. Government Printing Office, 1910.

61. Darling ST, Barber MA, Hackett HP. *Hookworm and Malaria Research in Malaya, Java, and the Fiji Islands. Report of the Uncinariasis Commission to the Orient 1915–1917*. (The Rockefeller Foundation International Board of Health, Publication No. 9), New York: Rockefeller Foundation, 1920.

62. Darling ST, Smillie WG. *Studies on Hookworm Infection in Brazil. First*

Paper. (Monographs of the Rockefeller Foundation Institute for Medical Research No. 14), New York: The Rockefeller Institute for Medical Research, 1921.

63. Desowitz RS. *The Malaria Capers. More Tales of Parasites and People, Research and Reality.* New York: W.W. Norton & Company, 1991.
64. Desowitz RS. *Tropical Diseases from 50,000 BC to 2500 AD.* London: Harper Collins Publishers, 1997.
65. Diamond Jubilee Supplement: Seventy Five Years of Medical Service. *The Panama Canal Review.* November 1, 1957.
66. *Dictionary of American Biography.* Vol. III (Cushman-Fraser), Johnson, Allen and Malone, Dumas (eds.). New York: Charles Scribner's Sons, 1959.
67. DuVal MP Jr. *And The Mountains Will Move. The Story of the Building of the Panama Canal.* Westport, Connecticut: Greenwood Press, 1975.
68. Easley SC. *From Atlantic to Pacific. 115 Years of Medicine on Ancon Hill.* (No date or place of publication given)
69. Edwards WC, Coates FA. *Third Centennial Celebration of the Incorporation of the Ancient Town of Braintree 1640–1940.* Quincy, Massachusetts: First Parish Church, 1940. (Pamphlet)
70. Elphick P. *Liberty. The Ships that Won the War.* Annapolis, Maryland: Naval Institute Press, 2001.
71. Enock CR. *The Panama Canal (Its Past, Present, and Future).* London: Collins' Clear-type Press, (no date given).
72. Ettling J. *The Germ of Laziness. Rockefeller Philanthropy and Public Health in the New South.* Cambridge, Massachusetts: Harvard University Press, 1981.
73. Falk IS. *A Survey of Health Services and Facilities in the Canal Zone, 1958.* PCC.
74. Farley J. *To Cast Out Disease. A History of the International Health Division of the Rockefeller Foundation (1913–1951).* Oxford: Oxford University Press, 2004.
75. Fast H. *Goethals and the Panama Canal.* New York: Julian Messner, Inc., 1942.
76. Ferling J. *John Adams. A Life.* New York: Henry Holt and Co., 1992.
77. Fleming D. *William H. Welch and the Rise of Modern Medicine.* Baltimore: The Johns Hopkins University Press, 1987.
78. Flexner A. *Medical Education in the United States and Canada. A Report to the Carnegie Foundation for the Advancement of Teaching.* Boston: D.B. Updyke, The Merrymout Press, 1910.
79. Flexner S, Flexner JT. *William Henry Welch and the Heroic Age of American Medicine.* New York: Dover Publications, Inc., 1941.
80. Foote RH, Cook DR. *Mosquitoes of Medical Importance.* (Agriculture Handbook No. 152, Agriculture Research Service), Washington, D.C.: U.S. Department of Agriculture, 1959.
81. Forbes L. *Panama the Isthmus and Canal.* Philadelphia: The John C. Winston Co., 1906.
82. Forbes L. *The Story of Panama and the Canal.* Philadelphia: The John C. Winston Co., 1906.
83. Forbes L. *Panama and the Canal Today.* (No place given): L.C. Page & Company, 1913.

84. Fosdick RB. *The Story of the Rockefeller Foundation.* New York: Harper & Brothers, Publishers, 1952.

85. Franck HA. *Zone Policeman 88.* New York: The Century Co., 1913.

86. Fraser J. *Panama and What It Means.* London: Cassell and Company, 1913.

87. Garrison OV. *Balboa: Conquistador. The Soul-Odyssey of Vasco Núñez, Discoverer of the Pacific.* New York: Lyle Stuart, Inc., 1971.

88. Gause FA, Carr CC. *The Story of Panama. The New Route to India.* New York: Silver, Burdett and Company, 1912.

89. Gibson JM. *Physician to the World: The Life of General William C. Gorgas.* Tuscaloosa, Alabama: University of Alabama Press, 1989.

90. Gillett MC. *The Army Medical Department 1865–1917.* Washington, D.C.: Center for Military History, United States Army, 1995.

91. Goldman EA. *Mammals of Panama.* (Smithsonian Miscellaneous Collections, Vol. 69, No. 5), Washington, D.C.: Smithsonian Institution, 1920.

92. Gorgas MD, Hendrick BJ. *William Crawford Gorgas.* Philadelphia: Lea & Febiger, 1924.

93. Gorgas WC. *A Few General Directions with Regard to Destroying Mosquitoes, Particularly the Yellow Fever Mosquito.* Washington, D.C.: Government Printing Office, 1904.

94. Gorgas WC. *Population and Deaths from Various Diseases in the City of Panama, by Months and Years, from November, 1883, to August, 1906. Number of Employees and Deaths from Various Diseases Among Employees of the French Canal Companies, by Months and Years, from January 1881, to April, 1904.* Washington, D.C.: Government Printing Office, 1906.

95. Gorgas WC. *Annual Report of the Department of Sanitation of the Isthmian Canal Commission for the Year 1907.* Washington, D.C.: U.S. Government Printing Office, 1908.

96. Gorgas WC. *The Expenses Necessary for Sanitation in the Tropics.* (Address of the President of the American Society of Tropical Medicine at the St. Louis Meeting, June 11, 1910.) Chicago: Press of the American Medical Association, 1910.

97. Gorgas WC. *Annual Reports of the Department of Sanitation of the Isthmian Canal Commission for the Years 1906–1913.* Washington, D.C.: U.S. Government Printing Office, 1914.

98. Gorgas WC. *Sanitation in Panama.* New York: D. Appleton and Company, 1915.

99. Harrell W. *Panama's Gorgas Hospital and Staff Doctors.* New York: Carlton Press, Inc, 1976.

100. Harrison G. *Mosquitoes, Malaria & Man: A History of the Hostilities since 1880.* New York: E.P. Dutton, 1978.

101. Haskin FJ. *The Panama Canal.* New York: Doubleday, Page & Company, 1913.

102. Hazlewood, N. *The Queen's Slave Trader. John Hawkyns, Elizabeth I, and the Trafficking in Human Souls.* New York: William Morrow An Imprint of Harper Collins Publishers, 2004.

103. Herbert B. *The Forgotten Heroes. The Heroic Story of the United States*

Merchant Marine. New York: A Forge Book published by Tom Doherty Associates, LLC, 2004.

104. Hibbard E. "The early days in Panama. Isthmus of Panama — A sketch — 1904." (Typed manuscript, 20 pp.) PCC

105. Howard LO. *Mosquitoes. How They Live; How They Carry Disease; How They are Classified; How They May Be Destroyed*. New York: McClure, Phillips & Co, 1901.

106. Huffaker AK. "Laboratory Medicine in the Panama Canal Zone. Past, Present and Future." (Typed manuscript, 13 pp.) PCC

107 Immell MH. *The 1900s*. San Diego: Greenwood Press, 2000.

108. Isthmian Canal Commission. *Annual Reports*. 1904–1914, Ancon, Canal Zone.

109 Isthmian Canal Commission. *Canal Record*. Volumes I–VIII (September 4, 1907 to August 18, 1915), Ancon, Canal Zone.

110. Isthmian Canal Commission. *Manual of Information Concerning Employments for Service on the Isthmus of Panama*. (Revised November 15, 1910), Washington, D.C.: Government Printing Office, 1910.

111. Jackson FE. *The Makers of the Panama Canal*. (No place of publication given): 1911.

112. Jane C. *The Four Voyages of Columbus. A History in Eight Documents, Including Five by Christopher Columbus, in the Original Spanish, with English Translations*. New York: Dover Publications, 1988.

113. Johnson WF. *Four Centuries of the Panama Canal*. New York: Henry Holt and Company, 1906.

114. Kamish RJ. (Untitled manuscript on medical history of the Panama Canal.) Canal Zone: (No date given). PCC

116. Kean BH. *M.D. One Doctor's Adventures Among the Famous and the Infamous from the Jungles of Panama to a Park Avenue Practice*. New York: Ballantine Books, 1990.

116. Kean BH, Mott KE, Russell AJ (eds.). *Tropical Medicine and Parasitology: Classic Investigations* (Vol. 1), Ithaca, New York: Cornell University Press, 1978.

117. Kemble JH. *The Panama Route 1848–1869*. (University of California Publications in History, Vol. 29), Berkeley: University of California Press, 1943.

118. Kitzmiller JB. *Anopheline Names: Their Derivatives and Histories*. (The Thomas Say Foundation, Vol. VIII), Vero Beach, Florida: Florida Medical Entomology Laboratory, 1982.

119. Komp WHW. *The Anopheline Mosquitoes of the Caribbean Region*. (NIH. Bulletin No. 179.) Washington, D.C.: U.S. Government Printing Office, 1942.

120. Laveran A. *Paludism*. (Translated by J.W. Martin), London: The New Sydenham Society, 1893.

121. Le Prince J, Orenstein AJ. *Mosquito Control in Panama. The Eradication of Malaria and Yellow Fever in Cuba and Panama*. New York: G.P. Putnam's Sons, 1916.

122. Ludmerer KM. *Learning to Heal. The Development of American Medical Education*. New York: Basic Books, Inc., Publishers, 1985.

123. Lydston GF. *Panama and the Sierras. A Doctor's Wander Days.* Chicago: The Riverdon Press, 1900.

124. McCarty ML. *Glimpses of Panama and the Canal.* Kansas City, Missouri: Tiernan-Dart Printing Company, 1913.

125. McCullough D. *The Path Between the Seas. The Creation of the Panama Canal 1870–1914.* New York: Simon and Schuster, 1977.

126. Mack G. *The Land Divided. A History of the Panama Canal and Other Isthmian Canal Projects.* New York: Octagon Books, 1974.

127. Marco Polo. *The Travels (Description of the World).* [The translation of William Marsden (1818) in the revised version by Thomas Wright (1854)], Köln: Könemann, 1996.

128. Martin TW. *Doctor William Crawford Gorgas of Alabama and the Panama Canal.* New York: The Newcomen Society of England, 1947.

129. Mears JE. *The Triumph of American Medicine in the Construction of the Panama Canal.* 3rd ed. Philadelphia: Wm. J. Dornan, 1913.

130. Meleney HE. Introduction. In Sweany HC, ed. *Histoplasmosis.* Springfield, Illinois: Charles C. Thomas Publisher, 1960, pp. 3–13.

131. Mellander GA, Maldonado N. *Charles Edward Magoon. The Panama Years.* Rio Piedras, Puerto Rico: Editorial Plaza Mayor, 1999.

132. *Merck's 1899 Manual of Materia Medica.* (Facsimile of 1889 edition), New York: Merck & Co., 1999.

133. Miller HG. *The Isthmian Highway. A Review of the Problems of the Caribbean.* New York: The MacMillan Company, 1929.

134. Minter JE. *The Chagres: River of Westward Passage.* (Allen H, Carmer C, eds. Rivers of America), New York: Rinehart & Company, Inc., 1948.

135. Morison SE. *Admiral of the Ocean Sea. A Life of Christopher Columbus.* Boston: Little, Brown and Company, 1942.

136. Morris E. *Theodore Rex.* New York: The Modern Library, 2002.

137. Murdoch J. "Ancon Hospital in 1904 and 1905." (Typed manuscript, 6 pp.), PCC.

138. *[The] National Formulary of Unofficial Preparations.* 3rd ed. Baltimore: American Pharmaceutical Association, 1906.

139. Nelson W. *Five Years at Panama. The Trans-isthmian Canal.* New York: Belford Company Publishers, 1899.

140. Nida SH. *Panama and its "Bridge of Water."* Chicago: Rand McNally & Company, 1915.

141. Otis FN. *Illustrated History of the Panama Railroad. Together with a Traveler's Guide and Business Man's Handbook for the Panama Railroad and its Connections with Europe, the United States, the North and South Atlantic and Pacific Coasts, China, Australia, and Japan, by Sail and Steam.* 2nd ed. New York: Harper & Brothers, Publishers, 1862.

142. [The] Panama Canal Retirement Association. *The Canal Diggers in Panama 1904 to 1928.* Balboa Heights, Canal Zone, 1928.

143 Paul B. *Health, Culture, and Community: Case Studies of Public Reactions to Health Problems.* New York: Russell Sage Foundation, 1955.

144. Peabody JB. *The Founding Fathers: John Adams. A Biography in his Own Words.* Vol. 1. New York: Newsweek, 1973.

145. Peck AS. *The South American Tour.* New York: George H. Doran Company, 1913.

146. *[The] Pharmacopoeia of the United States.* 7th decennial revision (1890). Philadelphia: J.B. Lippincott Co., 1893.

146. Poser CM, Bruyn GW. *An Illustrated History of Malaria.* New York: Parthenon, 1999.

148. Pringle HF. *Theodore Roosevelt. A Biography.* New York: Harcourt, Brace and Company, 1931.

149. Raine WMM. *The Pirates of Panama.* New York: G.W. Dillinger Company, 1914.

150. Réclus A. *Panama et Darien. Voyages d'Exploration [Panama and Darien. Voyages of Exploration].* Paris: Librairie Hachette et Cie., 1881.

151. Rhoads JB. *Cartographic Records of the Panama Canal.* (Preliminary Inventories No. 91.) Washington, D.C.: The National Archives, National Archives and Records Service, 1956. NAII

152. Robinson T. *Panama: A Personal Record of Forty-six Years 1861–1907.* Panama: The Star & Herald Company, 1907.

153. Rocco F. *Quinine. Malaria and the Quest for a Cure that Changed the World.* London: HarperCollins*Publishers* (Perennial), 2004.

154. Rodrigues JC. *The Panama Canal.* New York: Charles Scribner's Sons, 1885.

155. Roosevelt T. *Message of the President of the United States Communicated to the Two Houses of Congress at the Beginning of the First Session of the Fifty-ninth Congress.* Washington, D.C.: Government Printing Office, 1905.

156. Roosevelt T. "The Panama Canal." In Stephens HM, Bolton HE, eds. *The Pacific Ocean in History.* (Papers and addresses presented at the Panama-Pacific Historical Congress held at San Francisco, Berkeley and Palo Alto, California July 19–23, 1915). New York: The MacMillan Company, 1917, pp. 137–150.

157. Ross WG. *Historical Background of the Panama Canal.* Washington, D.C.: Souvenir Yearbook and Directory, 1947.

158. Rothery A. *Central America and the Spanish Main.* Boston: Houghton Mifflin Company, 1929.

159. Russell PF. *Malaria. Basic Principles Briefly Stated.* Oxford: Blackwell Scientific Publications, 1952.

160. Russell PF. *Man's Mastery of Malaria.* New York: Oxford University Press, 1955.

161. Russell TH. *Glimpses of Panama Canal.* Chicago: Laird & Lee, 1913.

162. *Sanitary Rules and Regulations for the Cities of Panama and Colon.* (Decree No. 14 of 1913), Mount Hope, Canal Zone: Isthmian Canal Commission Press, 1913.

163 Schott JL. *Rails Across Panama. The Story of the Building of the Panama Railroad 1849–1855.* Indianapolis, Indiana: The Bobbs-Merrill Company, Inc., 1967.

164. Scott WR. *The Americans in Panama.* New York: The Statler Publishing Company, 1912.

165. Scruggs WL. *The Colombian and Venezuelan Republics.* Boston: Little, Brown, and Company, 1905.

166. *[The] Sears, Roebuck Catalogue 1902 Edition.* (Facsimile) New York: Bounty Books, Crown Publishers, 1969.

167. Sibert WL, Stevens JF. *The Construction of the Panama Canal.* New York: D. Appleton and Company, 1915.
168. Siegfried A. *Suez and Panama.* New York: Harcourt, Brace and Company, 1940.
169. Simmons JS. *Malaria in Panama.* Baltimore: The Johns Hopkins University Press, 1939.
170. Simons MH. Sanitary conditions on the isthmus of Panama. *Report of the Surgeon-General, U.S. Navy.* Washington, D.C., 1902.
171. Smillie WG. *Studies on Hookworm Infection in Brazil 1919–1920. Second Paper.* (Monographs of the Rockefeller Institute of Medical Research No. 17, May 12, 1922), New York: The Rockefeller Institute for Medical Research, 1922.
172. Smillie WG. *Public Health Administration in the United States.* New York: The MacMillan Company, 1940.
173. Smith DH. *The Panama Canal: Its History, Activities and Organizations.* Baltimore: Johns Hopkins Press, 1927.
174. Society of the Chagres. *Year Book 1914.* Balboa Heights, Canal Zone: John O Collins, Publisher, (no date given).
175. Society of the Chagres. *Year Book 1916–1917.* Girard, Kansas: Girard Shop, (No date given).
176. Sosa JB, Arce EJ. *Compendio de Historia de Panama [Compendium of the History of Panama].* Panama: Casa Editorial del Diario de Panamá, 1911.
177. Speak AS. *The South American Tour.* New York: George H. Doran Company, 1913.
178 Sprague WC. *The President John Adams and President John Quincy Birthplaces, Quincy, Massachusetts.* Quincy, Massachusetts: Quincy Historical Society, 1959 (reprinted 1964).
179. Stapleton DH. *Creating a Tradition of Biomedical Research. Contributions to the History of the Rockefeller University.* New York: The Rockefeller University Press, 2004.
180. Stevens JF. *An Engineer's Recollections.* (Reprinted from Engineering News-Record, 1935), New York: McGraw-Hill Publishing Company, Inc., 1936.
181. Stich V, Minton R. *A Bibliography Covering Medical Activity on the Canal Zone 1904–1954.* (Typed manuscript, 85 pp.), Gorgas Hospital Medical Library, n.d. STDL
182. Stuhl RC, Chevalier GM. *Isthmian Crossings.* (No place of publication given): Xlibris, 2001.
183. Stuhl RC, Chevalier GM. *This Was Panama.* (No place or publisher given), 2002.
184. Sullivan M. *Our Times. The United States 1900 – 1925. I. The Turn of the Century.* New York: Charles Scribner's Sons, 1927.
185. Sweany HC. *Histoplasmosis.* Springfield, Illinois: Charles C. Thomas Publishers, 1960.
186. Taussig RJ. "The American Inter-oceanic Canal, An Historical Sketch of the Canal Idea." In *The Pacific Ocean in History,* Ibid., pp 114–136.
187. Thayer WR. *Theodore Roosevelt. An Intimate Biography.* Boston: Houghton Mifflin Company, 1919.
188. Thayer WS. *Lectures on the Malarial Fevers.* New York: D. Appleton and Company, 1897.

189. Thomas H. *Rivers of Gold. The Rise of the Spanish Empire, from Columbus to Magellan.* New York: Random House, 2003.

190. *Transactions of the Fourth International Sanitary Conference of the American Republics.* Washington, D.C.: Pan American Union, 1910.

191 Trudy AE. *Memoir of Walter Reed. The Yellow Fever Episode.* New York: Paul B. Hoeber, Inc., 1943.

192. Votes P. *Cristobal Colon.* Barcelona: Salvat Editores, 1986.

193. Watson M. *Rural Sanitation in the Tropics: Being Notes and Observations in the Malay Archipelago, Panama and Other Lands.* New York: E.P. Dutton and Company, 1915.

194. Willson FD. The Climatology and Hydrology of the Panama Canal. *Transactions of the International Engineering Congress, 1915.* (San Francisco, California, September 20–25, 1915) Vol. 1, paper No. 9, pp. 223–334.

195. Wilson CM. *Ambassadors in White: The Story of American Tropical Medicine.* New York: Henry Holt and Company, 1942.

196. Winsor J. *Christopher Columbus and How He Received and Imparted the Spirit of Discovery.* Boston: Houghton, Mifflin and Company, 1891.

197. Wright WH. *40 Years of Tropical Medicine Research. A History of the Gorgas Memorial Institute of Tropical and Preventive Medicine, Inc. and the Gorgas Memorial Laboratory.* Washington: Reese Press (Baltimore), 1970.

Articles from Medical Journals and Other Periodicals

1. Adams CF. The Panama Canal Zone. An epochal event in sanitation. *Proceedings of the Massachusetts Historical Society* 1911; 44: 610–646.

2. Agramonte A. The inside story of a great medical discovery. *Scientific Monthly* 1915; 1 (December): 209–237.

3. Ammen D. Proceedings in the General Session of the Canal Congress in Paris, May 23, and in the 4th Commission, May 26, 1879. *Bulletin of the American Geographical Society* 1880; Appendix A: 153–160.

4. Balfour AC. Some British and American pioneers in tropical medicine and hygiene. *Transactions of the Royal Society of Tropical Medicine and Hygiene* 1925; 19: 189–231.

5. Bendiner E. Ronald Ross and the mystery of malaria. *Hospital Practice* 1994; 29 (October 15): 95–97.

6. Brown SH. Personal observations of the Panama Canal. *The St. Louis Medical Review* 1912; (May 12): 132–139.

7. Brown SH. Health conditions in the Canal Zone. *New York Medical Journal* 1912; 96: 366–370.

8. Bruce-Chwatt LJ. Ronald Ross, William Gorgas, and malaria eradication. *American Journal of Tropical Medicine and Hygiene* 1977; 26: 1071–1079.

9. Burr WH. The present aspect of the Panama Canal. *The Independent* 1905: (May 18): 1100–1103.

10. Carr JF. The Panama Canal. The work of the sanitary force. *The Outlook* 1906: (May 12): 69–72.

11. Carter HR. A note on the interval between infecting and secondary cases of yellow fever from the records of the yellow fever at Orwood and Taylor,

Mississippi in 1898. *New Orleans Medical and Surgical Journal* 1900; 52: 617–636.

12. Carter HR. Notes on the sanitation of yellow fever and malaria, from isthmian experience. *Medical Record* (N.Y.) 1909; 76: 56–60.

13. Chaves-Carballo E. Samuel T. Darling and human sarcosporidiosis or toxoplasmosis in Panama. *Journal of the American Medical Association* 1970; 59: 609–612.

14. Chaves-Carballo E. Samuel T. Darling: Studies on malaria and the Panama Canal. *Bulletin of the History of Medicine* 1980; 54: 95–100.

15. Chaves-Carballo E. Ancon hospital: An American hospital during the construction of the Panama Canal. *Military Medicine* 1999; 164: 725–730.

16. Chaves-Carballo E. The cost of running American city hospitals. The Gorgas 1910 survey. *Southern Medical Journal* 2000; 93: 191–194.

17. Chaves-Carballo E. Carlos J. Finlay and yellow fever: Triumph over adversity. *Military Medicine* 2005; 170: 881–885.

18. Christie A. Medical conquest of the "Big Ditch." *Southern Medical Journal* 1978; 71: 717–723.

19. Curtin RG. Medical conditions of the isthmus of Panama with other notes. *Medicine* 1905; 11: 343–349.

20. Dehné EJ. Fifty years of malaria control in the Panama area. *American Journal of Tropical Medicine and Hygiene* 1955; 4: 800–811.

21. Ellman MH. William Crawford Gorgas and the American Medical Association. *Journal of the American Medical Association* 1960; 243: 659–660.

22. Gorgas WC. Sanitary conditions as encountered in Cuba and Panama, and what is being done to render the Canal Zone healthy. *Medical Record* (N.Y.) 1905; 67: 161–163.

23. Gorgas WC. Mosquito work in relation to yellow fever on the isthmus of Panama. *Journal of the American Medical Association* 1906; 46: 322–324.

24. Gorgas WC. Malaria in the tropics. *Journal of the American Medical Association* 1906; 46: 1416–1417.

25. Gorgas WC. The sanitary organization of the isthmian canal as it bears upon antimalarial work. *Military Surgeon* 1909; 24: 261–267.

26. Gorgas WC. Recommendations as to sanitation concerning employees of the mines on the Rand made to the Transvaal Chamber of Mines. *Journal of the American Medical Association* 1914; 62: 1855–1865.

27. Hart FR. Struggle for control of America: The great story of the Caribbean sea. *The Journal of American History* 1907; 1 (No. 4 October, November, December): 640–651.

28. Heffenger AC. The sanitary state of Panama and the interoceanic canal medical service. *Boston Medical and Surgical Journal* 1882; 106: 379–381.

29. Hess FH. Ancon Hospital, Ancon, Canal Zone. *Surgery, Gynecology and Obstetrics* 1920; 30: 424–429.

30. Howard LO. Malaria and certain mosquitoes. *The Century Magazine* 1901; 61: 941–949.

31. Jeffery GM. Malaria control in the Twentieth Century (Presidential Address). *American Journal of Tropical Medicine and Hygiene.* 1976; 25: 361–371.

32. Kamish RJ. Doctor William Crawford Gorgas — 1854–1920. *American Journal of Surgery* 1964; 108: 921–928.

33. Kean BH. Causes of death on the isthmus of Panama based on 14,304 autopsies performed at Board of Health Laboratory, Gorgas hospital, Ancon, Canal Zone, during 40 year period 1904–1944. *American Journal of Tropical Medicine* 1946; 26: 733–748.

34. Lacroisade [JP]. The Panama question. (Letter to the Editor) *Lancet* 1902: 1: 707–708.

35. Landor AHS. The Americans and the Panama canal. *Proceedings of the Royal Institution of Great Britain* 1911; 19: 687–709.

36. Leigh JG. Sanitation and the Panama Canal. The solution of certain climatic and hygienic problems. *Lancet* 1905; 1: 1530–1533, 1597–1601, 1726–1730.

37. Lopez JF, Grocott RG. Demonstration of Histoplasma capsulatum in peripheral blood by the use of methamphetamine-silver stain (Grocott's). *American Journal of Clinical Pathology* 1968; 50: 692–694.

38. McCarthy FP. A review of sanitation in Panama. *Boston Medical and Surgical Journal* 1911; 164: 49–53.

39. Mason CF. Sanitation in the Panama Canal Zone. *Transactions of the International Engineering Congress, 1915.* (San Francisco, California, September 20–25, 1915) 1915: 1(Paper No. 4): 85–116.

40. Mears JE. The triumph of American medicine in the construction of the Panama Canal. *Medical Record* (N.Y.) 1911; 80: 409–417.

41. Minton R, Muller S, Cohen O. Fifty years of American medicine on the isthmus of Panama. *American Journal of Tropical Medicine and Hygiene* 1954; 3: 951–963.

42. Montgomery DW. Impressions of the Panama canal. *American Medicine* 1912; 18: 143–152.

43. Nicolas A. L'Hygiéne dans l'isthme de Panama. *Annales d'Hygiene* (Paris) 1886; 16: 52–70.

44. Oran (no initials given). Tropical journeyings — Panama. *Harper's New Monthly Magazine* 1859; 19 (No. 112, September): 433–454.

45. Parson WB. The Panama Canal. *The Century Magazine* 1905; 71 (No. 1, November): 138–156.

46. Patterson R. Dr. William Gorgas and his war with the mosquito. *Canadian Medical Association Journal.* 1989; 141: 596–599.

47. Pierce JR, Writer JV. Solving the mystery of yellow fever. The 1900 U.S. Army Yellow Fever Board. *Military Medicine* 2001; 166 (Suppl. 1): 1–82.

48. Reed, CAL. The Panama Canal mismanagement — How the Commission makes efficient sanitation impossible. *Journal of the American Medical Association* 1905; 44: 812–818.

49. Riley HD Jr. The history of histoplasmosis. *Journal Oklahoma State Medical Association* 1983; 76: 31–40.

50. Root FM. Studies on Brazilian mosquitoes. I. The Anophelines of the Nyssorhyncous group. *American Journal of Hygiene* 1926; 6: 684–717.

51. Schwartz J, Baum GL. The history of histoplasmosis, 1906 to 1956. *New England Journal of Medicine* 1957; 256: 253–258.

52. [The] Secret of the Strait. *Harper's New Monthly Magazine* 1873; 67, 801–820.

53. Suárez OJ. Ecología y mortalidad en Panamá durante la construcción del canal [Ecology and mortality in Panama during the construction of the canal]. *Revista Cultural La Lotería* 1980; (No. 292, July): 67–73.

54. Turney JJR. Panama or isthmus fever. *Boston Medical and Surgical Journal* 1851; 45: 361–364.

55. Watson M. Finlayson Memorial Lecture. Some pages from the history of prevention of malaria. *Glasgow Medical Journal* 1935; 123: 49, 130, 202.

56. William Crawford Gorgas (1854–1920) medical ambassador to Panama. *Journal of the American Medical Association* 1967; 201: 200–201.

57. Williamson CH. Yellow fever at Panama — Its cause and treatment. *Medical Record* (N.Y.), 1884; (November 8): 509–510.

58. Ziperman HH. The Panama Canal: A medical history. *Americas* (Organization of American States) 1971; 23: 8–18.

59. Ziperman HH. A medical history of the Panama Canal. *Surgery Gynecology & Obstetrics.* 1973; 137: 104–114.

60. Ziperman HH, Wong JC. A medical history of the Isthmus of Panama. *Bulletin of the American College of Surgeons* 1971; 56 (No. 6): 14–18.

Texts about Panama during the Construction of the Canal

1. Allen EA. *Our Canal in Panama.* Cincinnati: (no publisher given), 1913.

2. Ammen D. *The American Inter-Oceanic Ship Canal Question.* Philadelphia: L.R. Hamersly and Co., 1880.

3. Arias H. *The Panama Canal. A Study in International Law and Diplomacy.* London: P.S. King and Son, 1911.

4. Avery RE. *Picturesque Panama and the World's Greatest Canal.* New York: Leslie – Judge Company, 1915.

5. Barrett J. *Panama Canal. What It Is. What it Means.* Washington, D.C.: Pan American Union, 1913.

6. Bishop JB. *Notes and Anecdotes of Many Years.* New York: Charles Scribner's Sons, 1925.

7. Boyce WD. *Alaska and the Panama Canal.* Chicago: Rand McNally and Co., 1914.

8. Byford HT. *To Panama and Back.* Chicago: W.B. Conkey Company, 1908.

9. Diez R. *Panama y el Canal [Panama and the Canal].* New York: Newson and Co., 1913.

10. Edwards A [Arthur Bullard]. *Panama. The Canal, The Country, and The People.* New York: The MacMillan Company, 1911.

11. Gilbert JS. *Panama Patchwork.* Panama: The Star & Herald Company, 1905.

12. Grier TG. *On the Canal Zone Panama.* Chicago: Press of The Wagner & Hanson Co., 1908.

13. Heinemann W. *Joseph Pennel's Pictures of the Panama Canal.* London: William Heinemann, 1913.

14. Howarth D: *The Golden Isthmus.* London: Collins, 1966.

15. Howarth D. *Panama. Four Hundred Years of Drama and Cruelty.* New York: McGraw-Hill Book Company, 1966.

16. Keller U. *The Building of the Panama Canal in Historic Photographs*. New York: Dover Publications, Inc., 1983.

17. Knapp H, Knapp M. *Red, White and Blue Paradise. The American Canal Zone in Panama*. San Diego: Harcourt Brace Jovanovich, Publishers, 1984.

18. Lee WS. *The Strength to Move a Mountain*. New York: G.P. Putnam's Sons, 1958.

19 Miller GA. *Prowling About Panama*. New York: The Abingdon Press, 1919.

20. Mills JS. *The Panama Canal. A History and Description of the Enterprise*. London: Thomas Nelson and Sons, 1913.

21. Miner DC. *The Fight for the Panama Route*. New York: Columbia University Press, 1940.

22. Pepperman WL. *Who Built the Panama Canal?* New York: E.P. Dutton & Company, 1915.

23. Russell TH. *The Panama Canal. Glimpses of the World's Greatest Engineering Feat Linking the Atlantic and Pacific Oceans*. Chicago: Laird & Lee, 1913.

24. Snapp JS. *Destiny by Design. The Construction of the Panama Canal*. Lopez Island, Washington: Pacific Heritage Press, 2000.

25. Thomas J. *Con Ardientes Fulgores de Gloria [With Burning Flares of Glory]*. Bogotá, Colombia: Editorial Grijalbo, Ltda, 1999.

26. Verrill AH. *Panama Past and Present*. New York: Dodd, Mead and Company, 1921.

Name Index

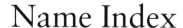

Note: *ff*: and following pages; *passim*: here and there; n (0 n 0): indicates page and note numbers; ref (0 ref 0): indicates Darling's bibliography page and reference numbers.

Subject Index

Ackee poisoning (*see* Jamaica vomiting illness), 138
Aedes (*see* Mosquitoes)
Aedes egypti, 3, 44, 59, 135
Aedes taeniorhyncus, 137
Albany Board of Health, 138
Algicides, 71
Amblyoma cajenens, 78
Alumni Association of the College of Physicians and Surgeons (Baltimore), 23
Amebic dysentery, 74
American Helminthological Society (*see* Helminthological Society), 125, 190, 193
American Medical Association, 78, 173, 190, 193
American Society of Museum Curators, 193
American Society of Tropical Medicine, presidential address, 96, 193
Ancestry, 9*ff*
Ancon Hospital, 50–60 *passim*; admissions, 55; bed space, 52; clinical material sent to Board of Health Laboratories, 64; buildings, 52, 53 illus.; deaths, 57, 59; description, 52, 55–7; entrance, 48, 52, 53 illus., 62; first admissions, 55; living quarters, 55, 56; location, 52; mosquito biting experiments, 69; post-mortem examinations, 62, 65; repairs, 55; staff, 52, 54; yellow fever ward, 49; wards, 55.
Ancylostomiasis (*see* Hookworm, Uncinariasis)
Ancylostoma braziliense, 135, 164, 167
Ancylostoma caninum, 135
Ancylostoma duodenale, 113, 144
Anopheles (*see* Mosquitoes)
Anopheles albimanus, breeding studies, 68; characteristics, 72; habitat, 3, 60; in

Panama, 70, 79, 134; in Puerto Rico, 124; and screening, 71; species-specific control, 3
Anopheles crucians, 139
Anopheles darlingi, 198*ff*, dominant species, 199; and Francis Root, 198, and W. H. W. Komp, 199; habitat, 198; malaria vector, 198; and mosquito repellent, 199
Anopheles punctipennis, 139
Anopheles quadrimaculata, 139
Anthrax, 77
Associacão Christã de Socorros Publicos (Brazil), 110

Bacillus coli, 78
Bacillus dysenteriae, 78
Baltimore City Hospital (*see* Mercy Hospital), 19, 23
Baltimore Orioles (baseball team), 27
Baltimore *Sun*, The (newspaper), 28, 144
Barrasco (fish poison), 133
Bausch & Lomb, 128
Bay View Hospital (Baltimore), 19, 23
Beri-beri, 77
Besnoitia darlingi, 199*ff*, and blind-alley theory, 199; and Émil Brumpt, 200; description by Darling, 199; guinea pig inoculations, 199*ff*; reclassification from Sarcospoidia, 199*ff*
Bibliography, Samuel T. Darling, 225 n 1; abstracts, 165–7; discussions, 160*ff*; journal list, 167*ff*; laboratory notes, 159*ff*; letters, 165; monographs, 165; original articles, 158*ff*; 161–78; pathological reports, 159*ff*; presentations at meetings, 164*ff*
Bilharziasis, 77
Blighia sapida (*see* ackee, Jamaica vomiting illness), 138
Blind alley theory, 76

Subject Index

Parasites (*see* specific nomenclature), 49, 70, 90, 134, 137
Parke-Davis (pharmaceuticals), 10, 16
Pasteur Rabies Institute (Baltimore), 21
Patent medicines, 12, 16
Pathology, 65, 133; faculty in, 18; field selected by Darling, 73; of histoplasmosis, 180–8; laboratories, 19*ff*; lectures in, 21; lure of, 27; of malaria, 3; and Rudolph Virchow, 27; of tropical diseases, 2*ff*; and William Welch, 25, 154*ff*
Pharmacists (in the early Twentieth Century), 16
Phi Beta Zi (Zeta chapter, Baltimore), 23
Philanthropy, and John D. Rockefeller, Sr., 89; and hookworm disease in the South, 90; and International Health Board, 91; and Rockefeller Foundation mandate and mission, 89, 91; and politics in Brazil, 118; and schools of hygiene, 107
Physician salaries in Panama, 41
Pirates of the Spanish Main, 36, 37
Pneumonia, as a leading cause of death in Panama, 68, 81; in South Africa, 81–5 *passim*
Principles and Practice of Medicine (Sir William Osler), 16, 89
Proceedings of the Canal Zone Medical Association, 78, 157, 161; index, 175*ff*
Proceedings of the Medical Association of the Isthmian Canal Zone (*see Proceedings of the Canal Zone Medical Association*)
Public health, 44, 50, 90, 107; careers in, 130; criticism of officers, 103*ff*; propaganda, 115; training in, 112*ff*
Puerta del Cielo Foundation, 199
Pulex irritans, 79
Pure Food and Drug Act, 12

Quinine, doses dispensed, efficacy, synonyms, toxicity, turkey amblyopia, 59

Rabies, 77, 174
Racial discrimination, in Far East, 95–7; in Panama, 177
Rand Mines, 81–5 *passim*; causes of death among workers, 84; and cerebrospinal meningitis, 84; crowded living conditions, 82; death rates, 82, 84; drilling and lashing, 82; and Gorgas commission, 85; medical services, 84; pneumonia among workers, 81; poor diet among workers, 84; recommen-

dations by commission, 84; recruitment of laborers, 82; scurvy, 84; tuberculosis (phthisis), 84
Relapsing fever of Panama, 173*ff*
Reye syndrome (*see* Jamaica vomiting illness), 138
Rockefeller Commission for the Extermination of the Hookworm Disease, 90
Rockefeller Foundation, 89–156 *passim*; creation, 90; and hookworm control, 89–92; mandate, 89; mission, 91; and politics in Brazil, 118; and sanitary inspectors, 90
Rockefeller Institute for Medical Research, 89
Rockefeller Sanitary Commission, 89, 90
Roosevelt, Theodore (President), election, 12, 14; and importance of sanitation in Panama, 50; and "Panama bill", 29; and Panama Canal, 14, 29, 40, 44, 50; personality, 13*ff*; and William Gorgas, 29, 44, 50, 58
Royal palms (*Oredoxa regia*), 47–9
Royal Society of Tropical Medicine and Hygiene, 155

Samuel T. Darling Collection (Johns Hopkins School of Hygiene), 196
Samuel T. Darling Memorial Library (Panama), 196*ff*; bronze plaque inscription, 197; dedication ceremony, 196*ff*; exhibits, 197; transfer to Stimson Library, Fort Sam Houston, Texas, 197; and Virginia Ewing Stich, 197
Samuel T. Darling, S.S., 197*ff*
Sanitation of Panama, 29, 70
Santa Casa (Hospital, São Paulo), 110
São Paulo Polytechnic Institute, 108
Sarcocystis, 76
Sarcocystis muris, 199
Sarcosporidia darlingi (*see* Besnoitia), 200
Sarcosporidiosis, 76, 174
School of Hygiene (São Paulo), 108, 111
Sears, Roebuck Catalogue [*The*], 11*ff*
Silver force, 177
Sisters of Charity of St. Vincent de Paul, 52, 54*ff*
Southeastern Shipbuilding Company (Savannah, Georgia), 198
Splenomegaly (spleen enlargement), 139, 180
Station for Field Studies in Malaria (Leesburg, Georgia), 127–43; books requested, 132; complaints about food and hotel, 130; and Francis O'Connor, 128; location selection,

.